Health Informatics

(formerly Computers in Health Care)

Kathryn J. Hannah   Marion J. Ball
Series Editors

Harold P. Lehmann   Patricia A. Abbott
Nancy K. Roderer   Adam Rothschild
Steven F. Mandell   Jorge A. Ferrer
Robert E. Miller   Marion J. Ball
Editors

Aspects of Electronic Health Record Systems

Second Edition

With a Foreword by Herbert Pardes

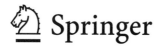 Springer

Harold P. Lehmann, MD, PhD
Associate Professor
Health Sciences Informatics
Joint Appointments Pediatrics
Health Policy and Management
Johns Hopkins University
Baltimore, MD 21205
USA

Patricia A. Abbott, PhD, RN, BC,
    FAAN
Assistant Professor
School of Nursing
Joint Appointment
Health Sciences Informatics
School of Medicine
Johns Hopkins University
Baltimore, MD 21205
USA

Nancy K. Roderer, MLS
Assistant Professor and
    Interim Director
Health Sciences Informatics
School of Medicine
and
Director
Welch Medical Library
Johns Hopkins University
Baltimore, MD 21205
USA

Adam Rothschild, MD
Fellow, Post-doctoral Fellowship
    Program
Department of Biomedical
    Informatics
Columbia University
New York, NY 10032
USA

Steven F. Mandell, MS, MLA
Senior Director for Information
    Services
Center for Information Services
Johns Hopkins University
Baltimore, MD 21205
USA

Jorge A. Ferrer, MD, MBA
Health Informatics Specialist
Veterans Health Administration
Office of Health
    Data and Informatics
Bay Pines, FL 33708
USA

Robert E. Miller, MD
Associate Professor
Department of Pathology
Biomedical Engineering and
    Health Sciences Informatics
The Johns Hopkins University
    School of Medicine
Baltimore, MD 21205
USA

Marion J. Ball, EdD
Professor, Johns Hopkins
    School of Nursing
Joint Appointment
Health Sciences Informatics
Johns Hopkins University
    School of Nursing
and
Affiliate Professor
Information Systems
University of Maryland
Baltimore
and
Fellow
Global Leadership Initiative
Center for Healthcare Management
Baltimore, MD 21210
USA

Series Editors:
Kathryn J. Hannah, PhD, RN
Adjunct Professor
Department of Community
    Health Science
Faculty of Medicine
The University of Calgary
Calgary, Alberta T2N 4N1
Canada

Marion J. Ball, EdD
(see above)

Library of Congress Control Number: 2006921546

ISBN: 0-387-29154-7
ISBN: 978-0387-29154-3

Printed on acid-free paper.

© 2006 Springer Science+Business Media, Inc.

Printed in the United States of America.   (BS/EB)

9 8 7 6 5 4 3 2 1

springer.com

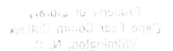

To Nina Matheson, who has provided us a vision of informatics encompassing all the many needs embraced by this book, and so much more,

and

To Morrie Collen, coeditor of the first edition, chair of the IT Section for the IOM Committee in 1991, and visionary in our field

and

To Sharon Coleman (1964–2005), one of the most empowering informaticists many of us have ever had the opportunity to work with. Sharon's combination of intelligence, confidence, and a true flair for living empowered her colleagues at the Veterans Health Administration, the US Army, and her nursing students to be better informaticists than they ever knew they could be.

Foreword

When a doctor sees a patient for the first time, there are a few things he will know and a million things he will not. As a doctor, educator, and administrator, I have become more and more frustrated by those million things.

These are the bits of data and history that are knowable, but hidden. Something registered about a patient in one office or another that has stayed in that office and could be useful now to the treating physician as they begin to consider treatment options.

Consider a patient who presents unconscious after complaining of chest pain. What prescriptions and over-the-counter medications does he take? Has he had surgery. If so, for what? Does he have allergies? Does he have a history of heart trouble or stomach disorders? This patient is in an emergency situation, vital questions remain unknowable, and something must be done.

Herein lies a medical knowledge gap: The distance between what we know about a patient and what we should know to make a correct diagnosis and provide the correct treatment. And this is why medical information, the basis of knowledge, is so important. Without it, mistakes and errors may occur; treatment may be unnecessarily delayed, so health care suffers.

Information technology is the most efficient way to share large amounts of data quickly. It has the potential to bring information together for better understanding and better outcomes. It offers knowledge and with it the promise of better health care. Interoperability, a word once unknown, has become the new goal in health care because it is so important. This concept is linked to what we call the electronic patient record—something most people consider to be a terrific idea but a concept that has been difficult to make a reality.

Look at a first-hand experience in record keeping. New York-Presbyterian has seen the need for an electronic patient record for some time. In 1987, before installation began, a nursing station typically had four incompatible computers: One for patient registry, another for laboratory results, another for narrative reports, and the last for OB/GYN reports. The incompatible systems were light years ahead of the paper record—more up to date and easy to share between medical teams, but much more difficult to cross-check than the paper records.

So, teams of people began to explore the issue. More than a dozen years and hundreds of millions of dollars later, banks of computers have been replaced. Our hospital has a patient database with 2.5 million records that can be read by any authorized clinician through a secured link from anywhere over the Internet. This is a true, fully functional electronic medical record. So we know it works, but there is more to do and improve. Despite all our work, we are still developing our capacity and making considerable progress.

What began as a good idea was realized only through an incredible effort of will by the institution and its people. Not only did technology need to be developed, but attitudes within the institution needed to change. People needed to think about their information as something to be shared with others, rather than something that was unique to their group.

These are just a few of the issues, both anticipated and unanticipated, as one hospital tried to make the change. Imagine the struggles of hundreds of hospitals or the entire hospital system, not to mention individual medical offices, as they attempt the same effort. Without funding. Without standards. Without security. Without a clear sense of how to accomplish the goal.

Fortunately, a few people have imagined it. In this book, some of the finest minds and innovators in information technology have set forth their findings about the obstacles to true interoperability. It will help us all as a map to the issues we must answer as we move forward.

The largest hurdle could be convincing the vast medical community to use such a system. Despite a national emphasis on using information technology to improve patient care, the vast majority of America's physicians do not possess the technology to perform basic functions such as writing electronic prescriptions, the Center for Studying Health System Change, has said. According to a survey by the nonpartisan research group, less than 25% of U.S. physicians were able to generate treatment reminders for use during patient visits in 2001, and only about 10% could write electronic prescriptions.

Clearly, there are more dynamics at stake. Although the technology is available, there are other barriers, some may be financial, some legislative, and some based on confidence in the product. There could be a million things. But rather than be frustrated, we must seek the answers and begin to address them—one at a time.

Herbert Pardes, MD
President and Chief Executive Officer
New York-Presbyterian Hospital

Series Preface

This series is directed to healthcare professionals who are leading the transformation of health care by using information and knowledge. Launched in 1988 as *Computers in Health Care*, the series offers a broad range of titles: some addressed to specific professions such as nursing, medicine, and health administration; others to special areas of practice such as trauma and radiology. Still other books in the series focus on interdisciplinary issues, such as the computer-based patient record, electronic health records, and networked healthcare systems.

Renamed *Health Informatics* in 1998 to reflect the rapid evolution in the discipline now known as health informatics, the series will continue to add titles that contribute to the evolution of the field. In the series, eminent experts, serving as editors or authors, offer their accounts of innovations in health informatics. Increasingly, these accounts go beyond hardware and software to address the role of information in influencing the transformation of healthcare delivery systems around the world. The series also will increasingly focus on "peopleware" and organizational, behavioral, and societal changes that accompany the diffusion of information technology in health services environments.

These changes will shape health services in the new millennium. By making full and creative use of the technology to tame data and to transform information, health informatics will foster the development of the knowledge age in health care. As coeditors, we pledge to support our professional colleagues and the series readers as they share advances in the emerging and exciting field of health informatics.

Kathryn J. Hannah, PhD, RN
Marion J. Ball, EdD

Contents

Section 3   Technology Infrastructure

Section 4   Going Forward

Contributors

Patricia A. Abbott, PhD, RN, BC, FAAN
Assistant Professor, School of Nursing, Joint Appointment, Health Sciences Informatics, School of Medicine, Johns Hopkins University, Baltimore, MD 21205, USA

Marion J. Ball, EdD
Professor, Johns Hopkins School of Nursing, Joint Appointment, Health Sciences Informatics, Johns Hopkins University School of Nursing; Affiliate Professor, Information Systems, University of Maryland, Baltimore County; Fellow, Global Leadership Initiative, Center for Healthcare Management, Baltimore, MD 21210, USA

Zakir Bickhan, MSc, BSc (Hons), RGN
Health Informatics Design Consultant, National Health Service (NHS) Connecting for Health, Department of Health, London, UK

Jeffrey S. Blair, MBA
Vice President, Medical Records Institute, Albuquerque, NM

George H. Bowers, FHIMSS
Principal, Health Care Information Consultants, LLC, Baltimore, MD 21202, USA

Alan Coltri
Chief Systems Architect; Assistant Professor, Health Science Informatics, Johns Hopkins Medicine Center for Information Services and Johns Hopkins University, Baltimore, MD 21205, USA

Don E. Detmer, MD, MA, FACMI
President and Chief Executive Officer, American Medical Informatics Association; Professor of Medical Education, University of Virginia, Charlottesville, VA 22908, USA

Joan R. Duke, FHIMSS
Managing Principal, Health Care Information Consultants, LLC, Baltimore, MD 21231, USA

Peter L. Elkin, MD
Professor of Medicine, Mayo Clinic College of Medicine, Rochester, MN 55905, USA

Jorge A. Ferrer, MD, MBA
Health Informatics Specialist, Veterans Health Administration, Office of Health, Data and Informatics, Bay Pines, FL 33708, USA

Linda F. Fischetti, RN, MS
Health Informatics Architect, Veterans Health Administration Office of Information, Silver Spring, MD 20910, USA

Paul Fitzgerald, BA (Hons), BS, Dip, Ed
Former Assistant Secretary, National Health*Connect* Program Office, Federal Government Department of Health and Ageing, Canberra, Australia

Dennis Giokas, MS, MM
Chief Technology Officer, Canada Health Infoway, Inc., Montreal, Canada

Connie A. Gladding, MA, MS, CPHIMS
Chief Enterprise Architect, Director Enterprise Architecture, Integration and Communications, Office of the Assistant Secretary of Defense, Health Affairs, Washington, DC 20301, USA

Paul N. Gorman, MD
Associate Professor, Department of Medical Informatics and Clinical Epidemiology, Joint Appointment, Department of Medicine, Oregon Health and Science University, Portland, OR 97239, USA

Michael L. Henderson
President and Principal Consultant, Eastern Informatics, Inc., Silver Spring, MD 20910, USA

Kevin B. Johnson, MD, MS
Associate Professor, Biomedical Informatics and Pediatrics, Vanderbilt University, Nashville, TN 37232, USA

Rita Kukafka, DrPH
Assistant Professor, Biomedical Informatics and Public Health, Columbia University, New York, NY 10032, USA

Gilad J. Kuperman, MD, PhD
Director, Quality Informatics, New York Presbyterian Hospital; Assistant
Professor, Public Health, Weill-Cornell Medical College; Associate Pro-
fessor, Biomedical Informatics, Columbia University, New York, NY 10032,
USA

Darren Lacey, JD
Chief Information Security Office, The Johns Hopkins School of Medicine,
Baltimore, MD 21205, USA

Harold P. Lehmann, MD, PhD
Associate Professor, Health Sciences Informatics, Joint Appointments
Pediatrics, Health Policy and Management, Johns Hopkins University,
Baltimore, MD 21205, USA

Nancy M. Lorenzi, PhD
Professor of Biomedical Informatics and Assistant Vice Chancellor for
Health Affairs, Clinical Professor of Nursing, Vanderbilt University Medical
Center Informatics Center, Eskind Biomedical Laboratory, Nashville, TN
37232, USA

Yves A. Lussier, MD
Director, Biomedical Informatics Core, Northeast Research Center in
Biodefense and Emerging Infectious Diseases; Assistant Professor, Depart-
ment of Biomedical Informatics and Department of Medicine, Columbia
University, New York, NY 10032, USA

Steven F. Mandell, MS, MLA
Senior Director for Information Services, Center for Information Services,
Johns Hopkins University, Baltimore, MD 21205, USA

Stacy Melvin, MBA
Senior Manager, Healthcare Consulting Division, Kurt Salmon Associates,
New York, NY 10019, USA

Robert E. Miller, MD
Associate Professor, Department of Pathology, Biomedical Engineering
and Health Sciences Informatics, The Johns Hopkins University School of
Medicine, Baltimore, MD 21205, USA

Frances Morrison, MD, MPH
Postdoctoral Fellow, Department of Biomedical Informatics, Columbia
University, New York, NY 10032, USA

Rosemary Nelson, MSN, MA, CPHIMS
President and CEO, MDM Strategies, Inc., Merritt Island, FL 32953, USA

Joyce C. Niland, PhD
Chair and Professor, Information Sciences, City of Hope National Medical Center, Duarte, CA 91010, USA

Gerard M. Nussbaum, MS, CPA, CMA
Senior Manager, Healthcare Consulting Division, Kurt Salmon Associates, New York, NY 10019, USA

Jason Oliveira, MBA
Senior Manager, Healthcare Consulting Division, Kurt Salmon Associates, New York, NY 10019, USA

Aysha Osborne, BA (Hons)
Former Program Officer, National Health*Connect* Program Office, Federal Government, Department of Health and Ageing, Canberra, Australia

Stephanie L. Reel, MBA
Chief Information Officer and Vice Provost for Information Technology, Johns Hopkins University; Vice President for Information Services, The Johns Hopkins School of Medicine, Baltimore, MD 21205, USA

Elaine Remmlinger, EdM, MPA
National Practice Leader, Healthcare Consulting Division, Kurt Salmon Associates, New York, NY 10019, USA

Helga E. Rippen, MD, PhD, MPH
Senior Advisor, Health Informatics, Assistant Secretary of Health and Human Services, Department of Health and Human Services, Washington, DC 20201; Rand Corporation, Arlington, VA 22202, USA

Nancy K. Roderer, MLS
Assistant Professor and Interim Director, Health Sciences Informatics, School of Medicine; Director, Welch Medical Library, Johns Hopkins University, Baltimore, MD 21205, USA

S. Trent Rosenbloom, MD, MPH
Assistant Professor, Biomedical Informatics, Vanderbilt University, Nashville, TN 37232, USA

Adam Rothschild, MD
Fellow, Post-doctoral Fellowship Program, Department of Biomedical Informatics, Columbia University, New York, NY 10032, USA

Layla Rouse, MS
Project Administrator, Information Sciences, City of Hope National Medical Center, Duarte, CA 91010, USA

Peter Schloeffel, MB, BS, BSc(Hons), FACHI
Director, Ocean Informatics Pty. Ltd.; Adjunct Professor, Health Informatics, Central Queensland University, Queensland, Australia

Edward H. Shortliffe, MD, PhD
Rolf H. Scholdager Professor and Chair, Department of Biomedical Informatics, Deputy Vice President for Strategic Information Resources, Columbia University Biomedical and Health Information Services, Columbia University Medical Center, New York, NY 10032, USA

Khan M. Siddiqui, MD
Chief, Imaging Informatics and Body MR Imaging, Veterans Affairs Maryland Health Care System; Assistant Professor, Department of Radiology, University of Maryland School of Medicine, Baltimore, MD 21201, USA

Eliot L. Siegel, MD
Professor of Radiology, University of Maryland School of Medicine; Chief, Imaging Services, Veterans Affairs Maryland Health Care System, Baltimore, MD 21201, USA

Walter W. Wieners, MA
National Advisory Council, School of Nursing, Johns Hopkins University; Director, Europe, Middle East and Africa, Oracle Nederlands BV, Amsterdam, The Netherlands

David Williams, Colonel, AN
Deputy Director, Information Management, Chief, E-Health Requirements and Operational Architecture, Office of the Assistant Secretary of Defense, Health Affairs, Washington, DC 20301, USA

William A. Yasnoff, MD, PhD
Managing Partner, NHII Advisors, Arlington, VA 22201, USA

1
Introduction

HAROLD P. LEHMANN, JOAN R. DUKE, and GEORGE H. BOWERS

Purpose

The nation's attention to health information technology has never been more focused than it is today. The new attention derives from the efforts of the federal government and the Office of the National Coordinator for Health Information Technology to achieve the vision of broad and deep use of information technologies, especially the electronic patient record.

This second edition also reflects the great changes made since, and because of, the Institute of Medicine's (IOM) report on computer-based patient records (CPRs), 15 years ago.[1] In particular, with the subsequent IOM report on patient safety,[2] the general-medical and political communities have adopted the perspective that the CPR plays a vital role in improving the quality of American medical care at systemic and strategic levels. In addition, the perennial concern with increasing healthcare costs has led to the consensus that computerizing information flow in clinical care should lead to increased systemic efficiencies and reduced costs. There has been a broadening in ethical perspective, from the focus of the health professional's work to the broader imperative to support individual patients' decision making as well as the public's health. Finally, the notion of going "national" probably could not have been conceived without the Internet and the World Wide Web, the latter having been only a research protocol at the time of the first edition.

The CPR has been the focal point for researchers, developers, and vendors for more than 40 years, but never like today. The last crest of attention came 15 years ago with the IOM's report on the CPR.[1] A series of white papers was developed by IOM committee members to support that report; those white papers were assembled into the first edition of *Aspects of the Computer-based Patient Record*.[3] The current edition updates those articles and extends them.

There is some confusion about the terms used for the electronic patient record. The following discussion describes the derivation and use of the various terms. The 1991 IOM report[1] defined the CPR as an electronic

1

patient record that resides in a system specifically designed to support users through availability of complete and accurate data, practitioner reminders and alerts, clinical decision support systems, links to bodies of medical knowledge, and other aids. The CPR, residing in a particular system, should have the ability to capture discreet, analyzable data that can be used to provide clinical decision support and to extend medical knowledge.

The vendor community and trade magazines use the terms CPR and electronic medical record (EMR) for any system that collects patient record data in any electronic form including scanned images of documents. The classification of a product as an EMR, CPR, or sometimes EPR (electronic patient record) can mean a system that captures any patient data, from any aspect of the healthcare organization. Even though a system might encompass only one area of the organization, such as the emergency room, collect clinical data from one healthcare setting such as home health, or simply capture scanned images from the paper medical record, the system may be categorized with any of these acronyms. This has led to some market confusion, but even more harmful, the systems so classified did not always address building some type of repository to capture and integrate patient information; nor do they encourage the collection of discrete data about patient care that can be shared by various providers and various settings of care.

The definition of CPR today has expanded to encompass a broader view of the patient record than in 1991. The CPR is moving from the notion of one location, one patient care event, one device to a much enhanced information utility for the care of patients including the ability to provide a longitudinal account of care and an extension of medical knowledge. The term "electronic health record (EHR)," first coined by the American Society for Testing and Materials, is now used by the National Committee on Vital and Health Statistics (NCVHS) to describe the patient record that is the centerpiece of the National Health Information Network (NHIN).[4] EHR is now the more expansive term referring to an interoperable electronic patient record that collects information about a person from CPR (EMR and EPR) systems that reside in various provider settings. Electronic health record systems (EHR-Ss) is the broadest term.

To document the increase in attention to EHR-Ss over the past decade, we used these terms to search PubMed and the business literature. Figure 1-1 shows the results. First, the number of mentions in PubMed has increased steady to about 3000 annually, today, for a total of more than 36,000 mentions over 10 years. The *proportion* of those articles representing scientific research has remained low, suggesting that the focus since 1995 has been on implementation and practice. A search of the business literature (not shown) provided a total of only 951 mentions over 10 years; however, the number of mentions doubled from 100 to 200+ in 2003. This figure and these numbers attest to growing interest in electronic records.

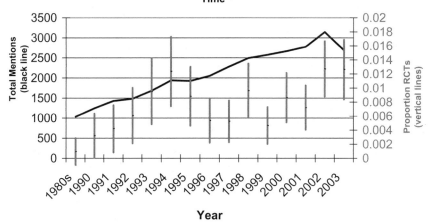

FIGURE 1-1. EHR-S in the literature. The gray line shows total mentions in PubMed title/abstracts of terms related to EHR-S (CPR, PHR, etc.). The vertical bars show what proportion of those articles in any year represent research (randomized trials); the bars show the confidence intervals for those proportions.

The 2003 IOM Letter Report, Key Capabilities of an Electronic Health Record System[5] defined the EHR-S as follows. An EHR-S includes:

1. Longitudinal collection of electronic health information for and about persons, where health information is defined as information pertaining to the health of an individual or health care provided to an individual.
2. Immediate electronic access to person- and population-level information by authorized, and only authorized, users.
3. Provision of knowledge and decision support that enhance the quality, safety, and efficiency of patient care.
4. Support of efficient processes for healthcare delivery.[5]

Critical building blocks of an EHR-S are the EHRs maintained by individual providers (e.g., hospitals, nursing homes, ambulatory settings) and by individuals (also called personal health records).

The functional model for the EHR-S has been developed under the auspice of Health Level-7 (HL7). HL7 is an accredited standards organization which initially focused on interchange of healthcare information, but has expanded its scope to include the sharing of the health record. The functional model was balloted by HL7 and approved for Draft Standard for Trial Use (DSTU) (Figure 12-1) in July 2004. The EHR-S standard distilled the contents of a patient record into direct care, supportive functions, and Information Infrastructure as follows:

- *Direct care* includes care management, decision support, and operations management and communications.
- Supportive functions include clinical support; measurement, analysis, research and reports; and administrative and financial support.
- The information infrastructure addresses such functions as identification, authentication, security, confidentiality, and terminology.

The functional model offers a first-time opportunity for an organization to identify whether a vendor of a system for any aspect of an EHR meets or exceeds this set of functions using a consistent industry definition. The functions identified can be used within a request for a system proposal or during a vendor demonstration to see if all of the key aspects of an EHR are available.

The goal of this book is to tell the story of where we are today in the con-tinuing evolution of EHR-S concepts. With the help of experts in the field, including researchers, developers, and vendors, we hope to provide healthcare decision makers the information and referral to the tools they will need to decide whether to implement EHRs and how to implement them, as well as to provide the background needed to follow these topics over the coming decade.

Outline

The book is divided into four sections; an asterisk (*) denotes topics newly added to this edition. The sequence of chapters follows the prescription for appropriate system design and implementation: Needs assessment and requirements specification, followed by system design and implementation, and then system evaluation and critique. The first section focuses on *Needs*, which provides a more detailed *History* (Chapter 2) of EHR-S and the needs of stakeholders beyond clinicians: *Researchers* (Chapter 3), *Patients* (Chapter 4), and *Population Health* (Chapter 5). These groups were not fully addressed in the first edition, and the realization of the importance of EHR to these needs has blossomed over the past decade. *Clinicians'* needs are reflected in the Standards chapter (Chapter 12), where the HL7 Draft Standard for Trial Use for the EHR System Functional Model is described.

Section 2 continues concerns of needs and requirements, but in terms of the decision maker's perspective and specific functionalities. *Current State* provides the current context. *Scoping an EHR* (Chapter 6) addresses con-crete sites of the functionalities needed in specific clinical venues, as well as the issues in implementing and operating an EHR-S. *Provider Order Entry* (Chapter 7) discusses the functionality that most represents the hope for EHR-S to impact on patient safety and the quality of clinical care. *Public

Policy Issues (Chapter 8) provides the larger contemporary context for EHR-S. **DOD System* (Chapter 9) provides details about a successful, yet evolving exemplar system. **The Global Perspective* (Chapter 10) presents an even wider context, as countries around the world address the same EHR-S questions we are facing in the United States.

Section 3, *Technology,* provides more details about the technical state of EHR-S and allied efforts. The first three chapters discuss general design issues. *Databases in Health Care* (Chapter 11) goes into theoretical and pragmatic details about the core technology underlying EHR-S. The title of *Standards, Standards, Standards* (Chapter 12) takes cognizance of the central role that standards play in EHR-S and will play in the NHIN, and has been the area that perhaps has seen the most activity in the past decade. *Privacy and Security* (Chapter 13) addresses the concerns about which the last 8 years' experience with HIPAA (Health Insurance Portability and Accountability Act) has sensitized the medical community, from the perspective of a chief information security officer. The next three chapters deal with issues specific to EHR-S. *Clinical Documentation* (Chapter 14) discusses the thorny issue of getting clinical data entered into the system: The entire promise of EHR-S depends on getting that data, yet it may be the most brittle step in the process. *Health Text Analysis* (Chapter 15) addresses the text component of EHR-S, including the emerging capabilities for systems to encode free text automatically into controlled vocabularies, thereby decoupling the user's desire for flexible data entry from the administrator's need for systematic representations of clinical findings, diagnoses, and treatments. *Digital Imaging* (Chapter 16) updates the book regarding these large datasets, which are now available to clinicians at the point of care, a development already radically changing workflow and the impact of radiology on clinical care. Finally, **Clinical Adoption* (Chapter 17) addresses the human and organizational realities of implementing and deploying the large and complex systems.

The last section, Section 4, is entitled, *Going Forward*. **Evaluation* (Chapter 18) is an important aspect of all implemented systems, and completes the cycle by telling us whether our needs have been met and what future innovations are needed to close the gap between what we have and what we need. The two Grand Challenges chapters take two perspectives. **Grand Challenges of Information Technology in Medicine* (Chapter 19) addresses how medicine may have to change to accommodate the technologies that are increasingly available. **Grand Challenges of Medicine and Health for Information Technology* (Chapter 20) ends the book with a description of needs that developments in medicine will elicit in the near future, preparing the groundwork for the next generation of EHR-Ss.

A major strength of this book is the range of backgrounds that the authors represent. In keeping with the themes of decision making and perspectives, we have academics, chief information officers (CIOs), consultants, vendors, end users, clinicians, radiologists, technologists, applied informatics researchers, and basic scientists as contributors. We hope that these different perspectives will enable a wide range of readers to find what they need within these pages to make the decisions they need to implement the vision of the EHR-S.

Acknowledgments

We would like to thank a number of people who helped in the creation of this book: Hansie Methelier for helping with evidence collection for the Introduction; Scott Wallace from the National Alliance for Health Information Technology provided initial thoughts; and David Liss at New York-Presbyterian-Cornell. The Division of Health Sciences Informatics of the Johns Hopkins School of Medicine for supporting this effort. Michelle Schmitt-DeBonis and Springer guided us through the publications process. Finally, our thanks to Marion Ball for her constant support, anticipatory guidance, and encouragement.

References

1. Institute of Medicine. Committee on Improving the Patient Record. The Computer Based Patient Record: An Essential Technology for Healthcare. Washington, DC: National Academy Press; 1991.
2. Aspden P, Corrigan JM, Wolcott J, Erickson SM, eds., Committee on Data Standards for Patient Safety. Patient Safety: Achieving a New Standard for Care. Washington, DC: National Academy of Sciences; 2003.
3. Ball MJ, Collen M, eds. Aspects of the Computer-based Patient Record. 1st ed. New York: Springer-Verlag; 1992.
4. HIMSS standard insight—an analysis of health information standards development initiatives. April 2003. Available at: http://www.himss.org/content/files/StandardsInsight/2003/04-2003.pdf. Accessed November, 2005.
5. Institute of Medicine, Committee on Data Standards for Patient Safety, Key Capabilities of an Electronic Health Record—Letter Report, July 31, 2003.

Section 1
Needs

2
History

Stephanie L. Reel and Steven F. Mandell

Overview

In order to discuss and analyze aspects of the computer-based patient record (CPR), it is important to note that many definitions of the CPR have been posited over the past few decades. These range from focused descriptions of functions and features of the CPR in the 1970s and 1980s, to global views of a portable continuity of care record in most recent years.[1-4] The original goal was to move as much of the inpatient paper chart into an electronic format. This included capturing patient data, retrieving patient data, and supporting business and administrative functions. Because healthcare providers, and only healthcare providers, created and maintained a record of their encounters with their patients on paper, it seemed reasonable that moving portions to an electronic format would improve care, reduce redundancy, and facilitate administrative and fiscal improvements.[5] As time passed, the American healthcare model changed from inpatient to an inpatient/outpatient paradigm, our society became more mobile, and technology improved at a phenomenal rate. Thus, the modern CPR evolved to capture more data types from more sources and with richer technology platforms. It is now generally agreed that a CPR is a longitudinal collection of personal health information concerning a single individual, entered or accepted by healthcare providers, and stored electronically. The information is organized and securely stored primarily to support safe, efficient, and quality health care.[6] However, the modern healthcare record has ended up being equally fragmented as in the early days, because many of the record components remain paper based, and many provider groups have created their own electronic silos.

The most recent "official" definition of a CPR has been provided by the Institute of Medicine (IOM).[7] The system should include:

1. Longitudinal collection of electronic heath information for and about persons, where health information is defined as information pertaining to the health of an individual or health care provided to an individual

2. Immediate electronic access to person and population-level information by authorized, and only authorized, users
3. Provision of knowledge and decision support that enhances the quality, safety, and efficiency of patient care
4. Support of efficient processes for healthcare delivery

The IOM posited five criteria to provide guidance in determining CPR functionality. These included improving patient safety, supporting the delivery of effective patient care, facilitating management of chronic conditions, improving efficiency, and determining the feasibility of implementation. The IOM further identified core CPR functionalities as:

- Health information and data
- Order entry/management
- Decision support
- Results management
- Electronic communications and connectivity
- Patient support
- Administrative processing
- Reporting and population health management

The IOM Committee recognized that the CPR will be built incrementally utilizing clinical information systems and decision support tools as building blocks. In addition, the four settings where a CPR should be sited are the hospital, ambulatory care, nursing home, and care in the community. Further effort in home health agencies, pharmacies, and dental practices will follow. Thus, the IOM has provided a broad framework through which data structures and systems could be developed to meet the challenges of a lifetime CPR that spans providers and care settings.[7]

History

The use of a computer to record a medical history was first described in 1966 at the University of Wisconsin. This early attempt was foiled by the massive machinery required and the limited capacity of the software. However, the university's medical leaders optimistically predicted that computers would someday be used to capture the patient's entire medical history.[8] About the same time, Morris Collen led the effort at Kaiser Permanente to collect, format, and electronically store patients' health screening examinations. The system had the ability to input data from encounter forms, optical scanning forms, and machine readable cards. By 1971, it was reported that more than one million patient records were maintained in its database.[9] It was at this time that an array of new systems came into being, ranging from full fledged hospital systems to medical decision support tools. Although most were developed under the auspices of acade-

TABLE 2-1. Early CPR systems

Year	System	Facility	Pioneer
1968	COSTAR	Harvard Community Health Plan	Octo Barnett
1969	Computerized Medical Records	Kaiser Permanente	Morris Collen
1970	TMR—The Medical Record	Duke University Medical Center	William Stead
1971	Computer-aided diagnosis		Howard Bleich
1971	PROMIS—Problem Oriented Medical Record	Medical Center of Vermont	Lawrence Weed
1971	Computer-based medical interviews		Warner Slack
1972	Technicon Medical Information System	El Camino Hospital	
1972	Regenstrief Medical Record System	Regenstrief Institute, Indiana University	Clement McDonald, William Tierney
1973	HELP	LDS Hospital	Homer Warner
1978	STOR—Summary Time Oriented Record	University of California, San Francisco Medical Center	
1978	Automated adverse drug reactions	Stanford University Medical Center	Stanley Cohen

mic medical systems and universities, some came from the burgeoning commercial hospital information system vendor marketplace. Prime examples of these pioneering efforts are listed in Table 2-1 and described in more detail in the following six sections.

COSTAR: Computer Stored Ambulatory Record System—The Harvard Community Health Plan, Boston, MA (1968)

The Harvard Community Health Plan (HCHP) was conceived as a prepaid ambulatory group practice to service the patients in the Boston area. It provided its members comprehensive care including medical, surgical, nursing, laboratory, radiology, and emergency care. Octo Barnett led an HCHP collaboration with the Laboratory of Computer Sciences (LCS) at the Massachusetts General Hospital to develop and implement a CPR system to facilitate quality patient care. Using specialty-based encounter forms onto which patient information was captured, medical records clerical staff used video terminals to enter data into MGH utility multi-programming system (MUMPS)-based programs. Other data were keyed into terminals in the laboratory, radiology, etc. As such, COSTAR was able to store, retrieve, and print patient information is an electronic format. Tied into a patient appointment list, COSTAR was able to automatically print out a patient status report for the physician that included basic demographics, a problem list, current and past medications, laboratory and radiology results, etc. COSTAR also supported quality assurance programs and administrative and reporting functions. It was eventually installed at hundreds of sites.[10,11]

PROMIS: Problem Oriented Medical Information System—Medical Center Hospital, University of Vermont, Burlington, Vermont (1971)

PROMIS was a unique system in that it was structured around the patient's problems, as pioneered by Lawrence Weed. The patient record was structured around four phases of medical action: A patient record including medical history and physical examination, a list of the patient's problems, diagnostic and treatment plans for each problem, and progress notes on each of the patient's problems. Except for the initial basic data, all entries in the system relate to the problem, and thus the presentation of the data is organized for review by the physician in a unique way. PROMIS guided the medical care provider using structured vocabulary, content, and organization for the computerized patient record. As the provider entered data, the program would branch based on the input, and at times provide medical knowledge. Weed and the PROMIS developers sought out experts in relevant fields to provide decision support in a variety of settings. The system used touch screens as an input device, was written in Assembly and SETRAN, and was built in conjunction with the Control Data Corporation and by grant funding from a variety of federal and private granting agencies.[10,12]

TMR: The Medical Record—Duke University Medical Center, Raleigh, North Carolina (1970)

TMR derived at Duke University Medical Center was designed to permit a variety of healthcare personnel to obtain data about a patient and to enter the data directly into a database during the encounter. It evolved to manage all aspects of the encounter including registration, scheduling, ordering a diagnostic test, result reporting, and check out. The system satisfied the core needs for clinical care, patient management and billing, as well as research. The overall strategy was to create an electronic record that would provide legible views of the clinical encounter, make the record accessible in multiple locations simultaneously, provide basic decision support, and create a rich store of data for the medical and scientific communities. The developers created their own proprietary database management language, GEMISCH, which allowed for them to expand and port the system to newer and more complex platforms as they became available. In addition, it provided a mechanism for TMR to be coupled with the Duke Hospital Information System as it grew in importance. Over its 25-year life, the TMR provided the solid foundation for the growth of a robust computer-based electronic record and Duke University Medical Center, and provided guidance and leadership for design and creativity to the informatics community.[13]

TMIC: Technicon Medical Information System (Lockheed Corporation)—El Camino Hospital, Mountain View, California (1972)

In the 1970s, the deployment of the TMIC at El Camino Hospital was one of the first commercial electronic patient record (EPR) systems. Developed by Technicon at a cost of about $25 million, the 450-bed community general hospital was chosen as a demonstration site. The system was a hospital-wide product that was designed to store patient data and to display the data to healthcare providers throughout the hospital. It was the first system that included direct physician order entry. Data were entered through video terminals using light pens and were broadly used by the physicians. Orders, laboratory results, radiology reports, patient care plans, and medications were all available. The result was a patient record composed of both electronic and paper sections. Printouts of all records were assembled after patient discharge and were only available electronically for 48 hours from that time. Electronic data were then transferred to magnetic tape for permanent storage. The system was hosted on IBM Mainframe computers at Technicon's regional data processing center.[14] An outcomes study demonstrated a 5% reduction in nursing costs, a 4.7% shorter length of stay, and an overall decrease in hospital costs.[15] A similar system was eventually deployed by Techicon at the National Institutes of Health, and a framework was developed for nursing documentation as well.[16]

RMS: Regenstrief Medical Record System, Indiana University, Indianapolis, Indiana (1972)

Under the leadership of Clement McDonald and William Tierney, the RMS has evolved over 30 years from a summary medical record in a diabetes clinic to a complex EPR. The system was originally designed to reduce the size of the paper record and provide a more organized and systematic method of storing patient data. An important component of the system provided physicians with alerts about problems in the record, which led to a number of important studies about the usefulness of decision support.[10] By 1990 it had the capacity to store patient observations, laboratory test results, and imaging studies as well as generate flow sheets and capture orders directly from physicians.[17] The system had interfaces to an array of ancillary and boutique systems which sent data of all types to the host for storage and display. All inpatient and outpatient services at the Indiana University Medical Center, its clinics, and ancillary facilities throughout Indianapolis were eventually included.

HELP: Health Evaluation Through Logical Processing— LDS Hospital, Salt Lake City, Utah (1973)

In the early 1960s, Homer Warner worked with computers to provide decision support in cardiology and set the stage for the development of medical informatics. Through his work and his colleagues at the LDS Hospital and University of Utah, the HELP system was developed. The HELP system was developed over the next 30 years and now serves more than 22 hospitals and 150 clinics and physician offices in Utah and Idaho. HELP is a complete knowledge-based hospital information system. It supports not only the routine applications of a hospital information system including ADT, order entry/charge capture, pharmacy, radiology, nursing documentation, ICU monitoring, but also supports a robust decision support function. The HELP system was one of the first information systems in a hospital to combine the use of computers for storing and transferring information with using them for giving advice to solve clinical problems. The decision support system has been actively incorporated into the functions of the routine hospital applications.[18] Decision support has been used to provide alerts/reminders, assist in data interpretation and patient diagnosis, as well as providing patient management suggestions. Activation of the decision support is provided both synchronously and asynchronously through data and time drive mechanisms. The data-driven activation is instantiated as clinical data is stored in the patient's computerized medical record. Time-driven activation of medical logic is triggered at defined time periods. In recent studies, use of the HELP integrated system showed that the risk of wound infection decreased significantly when antibiotics were given in the 2 hours before surgery at LDS Hospital in Salt Lake City. This was the first study of how timing of prophylaxis affects surgical wound infections in actual clinical practice. The HELP system detected 60 times as many adverse drug reactions in patients as the traditional method at LDS Hospital. The computer-detected reactions—95% of which were moderate to severe—occurred in 648 patients over 18 months.[19]

Case Study: Johns Hopkins—The Johns Hopkins EPR, Baltimore, Maryland (1984)

There are many opinions about which parts of the medical record must be included in an EPR, and nearly all of them must at least be considered when defining, designing, constructing, or deploying systems. As noted above, the computerized patient record must allow for the inclusion of relevant factors and the exclusion of those not pertinent for patient care. It must know if a pertinent relative factor is missing or is likely to be missing. It must know when data are expected to be present or when data are likely to arrive. It must be linked to external reference material that is either locally stored or connected via the Web. It must be able to be easily modified or adjusted to react to the subtle differences within and among various patient populations. It must be able to assist the provider, as she/he attempts to assist referring or consulting physicians. It must provide the vehicle for informing all members of the care team when orders, results, or clinical commentary have been posited. It must be a longitudinal collection of electronic health information for and about patients. This record must present a longitudinal view of the patient for all the practitioners. It must become the standard that is used by all members of the care delivery team. It must be the primary source of knowledge about a patient, and there must be a well-understood, very good reason for using it. What must it contribute to the process of delivering care for it to be worth the investment? The incentives must be apparent and realized within a reasonable time frame. For the EPR to effectively evolve, it must be responsive to the "law of unpredictable outcomes," remaining flexible in its architecture and presentation format. Although it must be shareable, it must be capable of being customized and personalized to the needs, location, and status of the provider of care. Above all, its designers and the system must be able to "learn" from all of its past experiences.

As with most large academic medical institutions, the history of the development of the EPR at The Johns Hopkins Hospital has been one of evolution rather than revolution. In the mid-1980s, it became apparent to a number of clinical and technical leaders that automated medical information systems would have to play a major role in improving the continuity of care issues demanded by the new diagnostic related groups (DRG) system, which emphasized shorter hospital stays and maximized the use of outpatient and home care. One such initiative at Johns Hopkins was the development of AUTRES, the automated discharge resume.[20] Designed as the first major computer-generated report to provide complete discharge information for a referring physician or other healthcare provider, it was piloted in 1984 and went into full production serving the Department of Medicine in 1988. It was seen as the first part of an automated record that would provide data for future treatment and research.[21] An important component of the AUTRES project was the development of a technical infrastructure that included connectivity among diverse platforms including an IBM mainframe, Digital Equipment Company (DEC) mini computers, and personal computers. In addition, it relied on heterogeneous data sources accessed in part through a middle tier of Remote Procedure Calls (RPC), software designed to transparently deliver data to the user regardless of where it is stored. The goal was to build a library of such software so that any number of systems could retrieve the data without rewriting the code.

The development of the earliest version of the Johns Hopkins EPR, conceived in 1989 to provide a patient-centered view of the patient's healthcare experience in the inpatient wards, was layered on the AUTRES technical foundation. Using the hospital's mainframe computer as the main repository, the application provided the physician with the ability to select and view all of the patient's laboratory values, radiology reports, discharge summaries, and operative notes. Written in a computer language known as CSP, and displayed on dumb terminals or personal computers in terminal emulation mode, the application also allowed for online editing and signature of summaries and notes using specially written scripts. Laboratory results and radiology reports were also available for outpatient episodes of care. Even though it was a text-based non-Windows system, the EPR provided physicians at Johns Hopkins a significant set of data in an electronic format. Although it became the standard for electronic information and initiated considerable interest among the faculty for use in patient care, teaching, and research, it was clear that a more robust version needed to be developed that would provide fast and efficient access to every patient's record across the entire continuum of care at Johns Hopkins.

The second version of this electronic record named "EPR 95," developed in 1995, was created by a select group of Johns Hopkins' clinical faculty and the Johns Hopkins Medicine Center for Information Systems programming staff.[21] In order to take advantage of the technology of the day, the clinicians and technical staff designed the new system to use a client-server architecture. In this way they were able to craft a physician workstation with a graphical user interface that provided an elegant interaction to an array of functions, seamlessly tied to servers across the enterprise from personal computers to an Amdahl mainframe. The data were "served" via the Remote Procedure Calls from the mainframe's DB2 database and VSAM files, and from databases of other, smaller computer servers.

The Johns Hopkins Health System is a large complex academic medical institution with more than a hundred thousand inpatient visits and more than a million outpatient visits per year. Its physical plant is dispersed throughout the state of Maryland. There is no single place where a patient's medical record is stored on paper. Even within the main East Baltimore campus, there is no single unified patient record. Therefore, EPR has become the primary source for fast, reliable access to the patient's clinical information. At present, there are about 3500 client workstations connected to the EPR. The latest version of the product is being used by more than 5000 clinicians in clinics, nursing units, physicians' offices, and in the medical records department. The system records more than 3.5 million transactions every week. The EPR is available at the Johns Hopkins Hospital, the Johns Hopkins Bayview Medical Center, the Johns Hopkins Howard County General Hospital, and at dozens of ambulatory sites throughout the state of Maryland. The global access allows caregivers in both inpatient and out-patient settings to see visit histories, laboratory results, documents, radiology images, etc. wherever they are providing care. Although there are some data not available at this time, more notes, reports, and data sources are being regularly coupled or stored in EPR.

Any healthcare provider (with appropriate security rights) using EPR can make use of the following features:

- Selection from more than 4 million patient records by patient's identification number, patient's name, provider, inpatient census by nursing unit, or outpatient census by clinic, and by date of service.
- View of the patient's problems, medications, and allergies, with online capability to add, modify, and change.
- View of all inpatient and outpatient visits, with "drill-down" to associated information.
- View of more than 110 million laboratory results, with stop-light highlighting of normal, out-of-range, and panic values, and all associated pathology comments, searchable by department (pathology, hematology, microbiology, etc.) and date range.
- View of 5 million radiology reports posted over the past decade, searchable by patient, department, and date range. View radiologic images from all modalities through a Web viewer with zoom, rotation, and annotation capabilities.
- Ability to view nearly 10 million documents including clinic notes, operative notes, and discharge summaries.
- Ability to create, modify, print, and electronically sign and/or view documents via word processing and specialized templates.
- Ability to dictate into a central dictating service, have those notes electronically posted to the EPR, and then view, edit, print, and electronically sign them.
- Ability to create, modify, and print a pediatric health maintenance record including immunizations.
- View of an array of other patient documentation including echocardiograms, electroencephalograms, progress notes, sonograms, and so on.
- Ability to access the Central Physician Directory of 80,000 referring physicians and to cut and paste relevant data into notes and other documents.
- Ability to create and store template-driven Cancer Staging Notes that meet ACOS guidelines.
- Ability to provide Decision Support via Web access to an array of knowledge bases, including Micromedex drug database, MEDLINE, consultants pager information, and so on.

A Web-enabled read-only version of EPR has also been developed using Java Script and Cold Fusion™ which is being widely used across the Johns Hopkins' continuum of care for remote access. This version is expected to grow in functionality as the security and patient confidentiality issues associated with Web-based electronic records are resolved.[22]

The EPR at Johns Hopkins is an evolving product with many attributes that support patient safety and evidence-based medicine. However, like all systems there are always new features and functions that will make the product richer in usability and functionality.[23] It is expected that the clinical leadership will focus their efforts to continually improve the EPR and to use the newest technologies available. It is clear that sophisticated decision support services, scanned document management, telemedicine, telesurgery, and full-motion video technologies must be fully incorporated into the EPR of the future to ensure that its full potential can be realized.

Decision Support Capabilities

A key component in many of the CPRs cited has been their ability to provide some measure of decision support during the care process. Physicians have sought to use computers to aid them in clinical care since the earliest days that processors became available in healthcare settings. Early decision support systems such as Mycin and Internist were designed at academic medical institutions to assist physicians in the diagnosis and treatment of complex problems. However, these early systems were limited in scope and capabilities. As the clinical community learned more about how computers could play a role in communications and decision making, as programming tools became more robust, and as the prices of hardware systems decreased, more broad-based applications were developed. Some of the most significant products were developed at Latter Day Saints Hospital (LDS), Regenstrief Institute, Brigham and Women's Hospital, Duke University Medical Center, and at Vanderbilt University Medical Center. In general, these products were developed to integrate the computer and its power to instantaneously execute millions of complex algorithms directly into the healthcare process. The goal was to move the computer from its traditional role as a reporter of facts to a role as an active partner in improving the quality of care for the patient. The general constructs of a decision support system include: 1) alerting the care provider to situations of concern, 2) critiquing previous decisions, 3) suggesting interventions to the care provider, and 4) providing a retrospective quality assurance analysis. Major features of the leading systems included antibiotic consulting, adverse drug reaction warnings, duplicate order checking, and protocol-based reminders.[24] To integrate the decision support capabilities into a CPR, the following system attributes should be included:

• Data warehousing with rapid access to as much relevant clinical information as possible

- Focus on the use of encoded data so that relationships between data elements can be linked, clinical rules related to these data can be established, and messages or actions are triggered when rules are met or broken
- Logical display of all the relevant available information that the caregiver requires
- Simple computerized navigational processes to access auxiliary data
- Screen design and information flow that closely match clinical practice
- Support of clinical pathways and identification of variance from pathways
- Guidance and alerts to physicians regarding duplicate order checking for medications and laboratories, drug–drug interactions, allergy checking, checking of dose range limits, and so on

CPR Systems Design

Underlying Architecture

The development of a CPR requires an underlying design that reflects the use of clinical data in practice settings. As such, medical information systems have evolved into three major categories: transactional systems, data repositories, and data warehouses. Transactional systems capture real-time activity and satisfy the specific needs of a defined area of practice. Most of these transactions can be initiated directly by a clinician, through an electronic interface with instruments, analyzers, or physiologic monitors. Transactional data are stored in database management systems that can be queried as needed by an array of reporting tools. These niche systems are the foundation for the construction of a comprehensive database of clinical information. Standardized data collection methods among these systems are important, but the general recognition that each of these systems is designed to satisfy a particular need often overshadows cross-platform data integrity. Interfaces and integration tools are often used to mitigate the differences between and among these systems. These are, by their nature, complex processors that require enormous engineering and design. Data repositories are often created as a result of several transactional systems interacting together to complete a patient-centered view for a provider. Each transactional system must transmit data in a standard format to a repository where the data can be aggregated and used for display and decision support. Repositories typically allow for real-time online access to this information, often allowing for complex queries to be generated through analytic software programs. These systems can provide views of the data that cut across the transactional systems and can be displayed as text, graphics, or tables.

Warehouses and "data marts" are more often large, complex repositories used for retrospective analyses. These warehouses are designed to ensure accurate and complete data collection and contain vast amounts of information that is refreshed at regular intervals (e.g., weekly, monthly, etc.). These systems often consist of archived data that may not be available online and that lend themselves to complex longitudinal queries. This form of repository is often most valuable when large populations of patients are aggregated to perform comparative studies or to determine the presence or absence of trends. Warehouses also provide a mechanism for queries that might otherwise adversely affect the performance of transactional systems used for direct patient care. Despite the obvious value of data warehouses, there are risks associated with their construction. Because of the absence of data standards, including standard data definitions, these warehouses often fall victim to the problems inherent in all poorly managed data. The data lack integrity, their value and range vary, duplication is widespread, and many data elements lack the power to be stored in a formal hierarchy. To minimize the impact of this weakness, "data-scrubbing" techniques such as editing algorithms are used to reduce redundant records and correct obvious errors. This effort is often the most complex and time-consuming aspect of creating a comprehensive clinical repository. The ultimate CPR is typically a combination of the three architectural solutions described above, with a focus on data accuracy and reliability. Designed properly, the CPR will provide the clinician with access to current medical literature as well as all related medical knowledge derived from patient experiences. Last, the CPR must provide the needed information in a format that can be easily and readily appreciated and understood. It must capture relevant data from other electronic sources with minimal human intervention, performing required data validation to ensure accuracy and reliability. As indicated by Figure 2-1, these data must then be aggregated and assimilated so that they have meaning between and among the various components of the CPR.

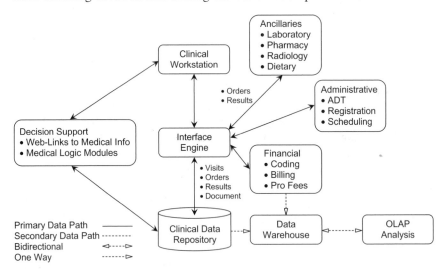

FIGURE 2-1. Sample architecture of a CPR.

Clinical Decision Support Design

Computer-assisted rules-based medicine is intended to guide the behavior of clinicians and other members of the healthcare team. In general, clinicians know the "rules" but are often deprived of the knowledge of the occurrence of a clinical event that might necessitate the application of a rule. A caregiver can react only to facts that are known and can base decisions only on requirements that are understood. Therefore, the first rules to be defined and implemented must focus on the need to notify appropriate staff of the occurrence of an event, or the failure of an event to occur. Only when the data are available can interventions be planned. The challenges associated with providing clinical alerts are not trivial, however, because the magnitude of data input is staggering. There is recognition that computers can enhance the ability of a caregiver to manage information, assess inputs, and make informed decisions. This is often different, however, from compliance with automated guidelines. Adherence to computerized pathways or practice guidelines, at least in some disciplines, has been embraced slowly because of the failure of these guidelines to incorporate the inherent decision making that many physicians perform as part of care delivery. There are thought processes that emerge from past experiences or "lessons learned" and from the "art" of medicine. It is often difficult for systems to emulate these processes, or to allow for deviations or variations in practice that might result from them. Within each electronic record available today there are some expected sets of functionality that will support the physician in all aspects of patient care. Although not every software product provides every component, most are clearly migrating toward a full-service system that can support a patient across the continuum of care. Examples of this functionality include problem lists that can be linked to encounters, providers, diagnoses, orders, and results; health status metrics; input data that led to an intervention; access to knowledge bases; cost metrics and compliance data elements; controlled vocabulary and coding mechanisms; and a data dictionary that allows for varying degrees of granularity. It must be patient centered when needed, provider-specific in its presentation format, and disease-aware when guiding decisions. To build all of this in an easy-to-use format is a challenge for even the most gifted software developers.

Computerized decision support and pathway development have also evolved over the past 15 years. The delineation of a medical taxonomy has hastened the growth of pathway development. Now widely acknowledged as a standard, the Arden Syntax is an accepted language for the definition of clinical rules that drive alerts, reminders, clinical guidelines, and data interpretations. The standard was defined in 1989, at the Arden Homestead Conference in Harriman, New York. It has become the standard language for the definition of rules-based computer electronic records, particularly when integrated with order management systems. It is within these rule sets that standard pathways and guidelines can be defined. The Arden Syntax is one important step in a long process of defining and deploying standards to support computer-assisted care delivery.[25]

Clinical Information and Decision Support Resources

In his seminal work, *The Science of Decision Making*, Nobel laureate Herbert Simon posits the proposition that decision making is composed of three parts: Collecting the data, considering all the options, and then selecting the best option.[26] The first task, collecting the data, is remarkably complex when one considers the amount of data published in any one given field in today's global medical marketplace. Medical professionals are facing an information explosion, and medical knowledge is expanding at an unprecedented rate. More than 400,000 articles are published in medical journals each year. The diffusion of knowledge to practitioners is so slow that one study found that 2 years after wide publication, fewer than 50% of general practitioners knew that laser surgery could save the sight of some of their diabetic patients.[27] Each day, more and more of the data are available almost as soon as the results are known via publishing on the Internet and the World Wide Web (www). Internet World Statistics indicate that the number of users of the internet has reached nearly one billion, with nearly 470 million persons using the English, Chinese, or Japanese languages. In early 2004, Google reported that it covered 6 billion items, 4.28 billion Web pages, 880 million images, and 845 usenet messages. These connections are made possible via the linking of over nearly 250 million host computers.[28] A recent keyword search of the Web revealed that more than 83.4 million documents contained the word "cancer," 8.77 million contained the term "skin cancer," and more than 3 million contained the word "melanoma." These numbers grow at a phenomenal rate each year, which is remarkable considering that Tim Berners-Lee "invented" the World Wide Web protocols in 1989 and that the first multi-computer browser, Mosaic, only became available in late 1993.[29]

There is general agreement that the problems clinicians face are lack of robust tools to access data quickly, effectively, and in context for the answer they are seeking to find. They generally complain that they lack the time to launch an inquiry, decry the poor organization of the available material, and the poor performance of "content-aware" search engines. It is believed that the Web is a powerful tool for delivering online clinical information. However, many have pointed out that its value to healthcare professionals is limited because its information is highly distributed and difficult to locate, its retrieval tools are modest, and its indexing methodologies are suspect. The result is the development of suboptimal and "fuzzy" searches that interweave clinical content, consumer-oriented clinical information, and nonrelevant information. Even the most mainstream sources such as the National Library of Medicine has so much data that targeted searches are complex. The PubMed service MEDLINE has more than 12 million journal article references and abstracts dating to the mid-1960s with another 1.5 million references back to the 1950s. The available guide to nearly 4000 journals garners more than 500 million searches per year.[30] Although queries may yield exquisite results, the search may require considerable refinement through multiple filters and granular probing.

Medical informaticians have been developing tools and methods to resolve this conundrum and enhance the CPR. One application, CliniWeb, was an index to clinical information on the Web, providing a browsing and searching interface to clinical content at the level of the healthcare provider or student. Its database contained a list of clinical information resources on the Web that were indexed in terms from the Medical Subject Headings (MeSH) disease tree and is assisted by the concept-mapping engine of the SAPHIRE system. The CliniWeb database included links to more than 50,000 fully indexed Uniform Resource Locators (URLs), but admittedly suffered from its inability to maintain the database in the dynamic Web environment and provide more sophisticated indexing and retrieval capabilities. It stopped its service in 2003.[31]

WebMedline, developed in 1994 by Bill Detmer at Stanford University, facilitated searching of the medical literature using a standard Web browser. The application authenticated the user, allowed input of search criteria, and then composed a legal MEDLINE search statement by removing stopwords from the input, qualifying input terms with appropriate field descriptors, and then joining these qualified input terms with Boolean operators. In addition, it attempts to map keywords to controlled indexing terms and returned MeSH terms to assist in choosing more precise query variables. The results were then output in MEDLINE format, creating links to full-text documents when it found a corresponding full-text URL. In 1995, WebMedline was licensed to Ovid Technologies and was used as the foundation for the Ovid Web Gateway.[32] WebMedline is no longer operational because of a change in the way the National Library of Medicine processes requests. Users have been pointed to Unbound Medline, which is a supported interface based on WebMedline.

DXplain is a Web-based diagnostic decision support program, designed as an educational tool to assist physicians and medical students in formulating a differential diagnosis based on one or more clinical findings. It was developed at the Massachusetts General Hospital with grant support for the Web version from the National Library of Medicine (producer of the MEDLINE database) and Hewlett-Packard.[33] In practical use, DXplain has the capabilities of an electronic medical textbook, a decision support tool, and a medical reference application. DXplain covers more than 2000 diseases, more than 5000 clinical manifestations, and 65,000 interrelationships including laboratory, X-ray, and electrocardiogram abnormalities. In addition to suggesting possible diagnoses, DXplain can provide brief descriptions of every disease in the database. This program generates a list of possible diagnoses, using a probabilistic algorithm. It first evaluates the term importance and term-evoking strength of each finding diagnosis pair and then calculates a summary score for each disease. A disease score is most influenced by positive findings that have high term evoking strength. After DXplain evaluates each clinical finding, it displays the highest ranked diagnoses divided into "common diseases" and "rare or very rare diseases." Entries are continually updated and revised, with input from users strongly encouraged.

Using Dxplain as a service, other medical informatics groups are connecting DXplain to their own services. In one case, the Columbia University Department of Medical Informatics developed an experimental link between Dxplain and their laboratory reporting system to transform its unstructured results terminology into an acceptable Dxplain term.[34] By providing newer and more efficient ways of classifying data, developing more sophisticated matching tools based on "universal" medical syntax, and designing "expert" rules and algorithms, informaticians have made the modern clinical decision support tools more powerful than ever. Yet, these systems still require a large amount of effort to maintain, generally require clinicians to distill what they need from a plethora of relevant and irrelevant information, and require active involvement by clinicians to launch and refine searches.

The Brigham Integrated Computing System (BICS), introduced by Brigham and Women's Hospital in 1989, includes a full ambulatory medical record, an inpatient order entry system, an event engine, and a lifetime record of a wide variety of tests, clinical summaries, and procedures.[35] It was developed with the principles of including broad content, workflow support, clinical decision support, efficient communications of data, and providing advanced services. It is used 24 hours a day throughout the facility and has had a substantial positive impact on the way medicine is practiced. Orders can be placed for any patient from any workstation, including remote workstations from offices and homes, greatly improving order accuracy, legibility, and timeliness while reducing the number of verbal orders. By inserting practice guidelines, rules, and reminders at the point where the physician places the order, the BICS is able to intervene and reduce 20% or more of adverse in-hospital events.[36] It is currently estimated that the system provides alerts for about 30 potential adverse reactions from 4000 daily medication orders, with almost 50% of those warnings resulting in changes to the order. Significant numbers of redundant laboratory and medication orders are similarly flagged, with nearly 35% of those orders being canceled. Thus, not only is patient care enhanced, but it is estimated that the clinical decision support system saves Brigham and Women's Hospital nearly $5 million per year.

The development of WizOrder at Vanderbilt University Medical Center (VUMC), begun in 1994, was an effort to implement a medical decision support system by understanding that such a system could gain widespread acceptance when a "critical mass" of functionality was delivered to the clinical community through an easy-to-use interface on a readily available platform. The core of the WizOrder application is the assumption that the system enables clinicians to convert their decisions into actions at the time of order writing so that patient-specific decision support is implemented optimally through the order entry process. The design specifications include:

- A single-screen layout that remains stable during the session and has as few dialog boxes as possible
- A list of current active orders visible at all times and displayed in a clinically relevant sequence
- A mechanism to enter orders in a manner similar to handwritten orders
- Problem-driven sets of orders that resemble familiar preprinted order sheets
- Seamless access to decision support tools

Decision support tools include: Drug monographs; drug–drug and drug–laboratory interaction warnings; allergy warnings; patient-specific dose-range checking; decision trees for selecting empirical anti-biotherapies; diagnosis- and procedure-based order sets; an automated link to relevant biomedical literature citations; and various tightly integrated Web-based resources such as extensive drug references, patient education sheets, radiology reference manuals, and so forth.[37] This is supported by importing data and knowledge from other systems known to WizOrder from Ovid, PubMed, etc. The ability to notify users and applications of new events is an essential part of the decision support function within the CPR at VUMC.

Technologic Barriers in Decision Support

Most traditional systems rely on the request-reply model to query databases for new data. The systems noted above, for the most part, are synchronous, event-based, clinical systems developed to notify physicians and nurses of critical interactions and results at the time of order entry. Thus, the machine and the clinician must be coupled and in direct communication to complete the transaction. However, the ubiquitous presence of asynchronous events in clinical experience argues for the delineation of a general notification engine as a new component of an extended decision-making tool.[38] In this manner, the machine and the clinician are decoupled, but the asynchronous event launches processes that facilitate communication in a way that permits the clinician to respond appropriately. For example, if a laboratory value is posted to the patient's record and the system recognizes that there are negative implications for a drug the patient is on, a notice to the clinician in the form of a page, e-mail, or some other alert can be facilitated. Clinical outcomes may thus be improved by proactive patient management or by averting adverse reactions.

The medical information systems architecture of transactional systems, data repositories, and data warehouses are coming to fruition because of technologic developments that enable massive data warehousing and analytic query capabilities. Sophisticated and powerful database systems, huge and efficient storage area networks, and increasingly powerful symmetric parallel processing capabilities are all available today at ever-decreasing costs. However, there is a paucity of rigorous standards that would facilitate the exchange of healthcare data across disparate systems, and the development of a naturally intuitive human–machine interface remains a major challenge despite such advances as template-driven formats and voice input. The medical informatics literature is rich with details of projects that try to solve this dilemma with techniques such as speech recognition, digital dictation, structured data entry, content-to-speech generation, and new graphical interaction models.[39,40] Data entry is not typically a strength of the physician, and all of these systems require some form of data entry. Given the frenetic pace of academic medicine and the demand for more and more documentation, there is even greater pressure to create an input methodology that closely emulates the time frame of documenting with pen and paper. Most activity in this area attempts to do two things: Reduce the time for data input to "near-paper-and-pen time" and provide value to the healthcare provider in exchange for the extra time required for electronic input. Until the time difference between paper-and-pen entry and electronic data entry nears zero, and/or continuous speech voice recognition is error-free and speaker-independent, interface issues will remain a significant impediment to making the CPR ubiquitous.

Another barrier that continues to hamper the development of the computer based medical record is the lack of standards that would facilitate the collection and exchange of healthcare data so that they may be aggregated and analyzed to support clinical decision making. With the current efforts by the federal government to support pooled data in regional databases (regional health information organizations), and to make them available through reliable, secure networks, EPRs will be more easily adopted. As previously noted, clinical data are stored in an array of systems across the healthcare continuum. International protocols established by the Institute of Electrical and Electronic Engineers (IEEE), the American National Standards Institute (ANSI), and so forth, set message standards for computer-to-computer communications and define the structure and content that can be exchanged between systems. Given the variety of clinical data formats (e.g., text, image, voice), the numbers and maturity of standards make messaging and connectivity a complex problem. The development of interfaces between disparate systems has been a medical informatics topic for nearly 20 years, leading to the creation of a number of groups within international standards organizations.[41] The American College of Radiology (ACR) and the National Electrical Manufacturers Association (NEMA) developed the first Digital Imaging and Communications in Medicine

(DICOM) standard in 1983 whereas the ANSI accredited the Health Level-7 (HL7) standard for patient admissions, clinical observations, pharmaceutical and dietary issues, appointment scheduling, and so on, in 1994.[42,43]

Importantly, the United States Health Insurance Portability and Accountability Act of 1996 (HIPAA) requires that standards for electronic exchange of administrative, financial, and clinical data be established. Work is in progress on all fronts in this area, but it will take time for standards to be selected, adopted, and proliferated. In addition to clinicians seeking more robust data, major beneficiaries will be healthcare policy makers, clinical researchers focusing on the effectiveness and appropriateness of care, regulatory agencies, and third-party payers.

Clearly, the goals posited by the IOM for a robust CPR are coming to fruition. With new technology, powerful computers, programming tool sets, and medical informatics skills, the deployment of fully functioning CPRs is moving forward in many medical centers. Although there are many difficulties in deploying a system of such breadth and depth, the rewards for patient care, education, and research appear to be rich. However, it should be noted that these systems only scratch the surface in terms of providing the decision support that will be commonplace in the next decade. Although there is great complexity in the system design, these are relatively simple processes that take known data, compare it with certain sets of rules coded in the application, and then trigger events based on the testing of those rules. The continuing pressure to collect more information, make it available to all healthcare providers whenever it is needed, to do so in a more timely and efficient manner, and to ensure that patient safety is the driving force in each of the transactions, will finally lead to a ubiquitous CPR. The goal is not to have these systems available only in the Hopkins, Harvards, and Dukes in the nation, but in every community hospital and physician's office as well.

Conclusion

In his 2004 State of the Union Address, President George W. Bush noted: "By computerizing health records, we can avoid dangerous medical mistakes, reduce costs, and improve healthcare." This bold statement by the President has provided a call to action for all sectors of the healthcare industry to examine its focus and become more aggressive in moving toward an electronic patient-based medical record. This is a culmination of a series of events over the last 5 years that have pointed in this direction. The IOM has provided two reports that have challenged many long held beliefs. The first, *To Err is Human*, was published in 1999 and described the reasons why we should be using information systems and communication technologies in health care to reduce errors, improve outcomes, and reduce costs. *Crossing the Quality Chasm*, published in 2001, discussed the importance of the entire healthcare system including the cultural, organization, and technical aspects in creating a safe and efficient healthcare environment.[44,45]

References

1. Barnett GO. The application of computer-based medical records systems in ambulatory practice. N Engl J Med 1984;310:1643–1650.
2. Weed LL. Medical records that guide and teach. N Engl J Med 1968;278: 593–600.
3. Stead WW, Hammond WE. Computer based medical records: The centerpiece of TMR. MD Comput 1988;5:48–62.
4. McDonald CJ, Blevins L, Tierney WM, Martin DK. The Regenstrief medical records. MD Comput 1988;5:34–47.
5. Dick RS, Steen EB. The Computer-based Patient Record: An Essential Technology for Health Care. Washington, DC: National Academy Press; 1991.
6. Standards Insight: An Analysis of Health Information—Standards Development Initiatives, April 2003, HIMSS: 9.
7. Key Capabilities of an Electronic Health Record System—Letter Report, Committee on Data Standards for Patient Safety, Board on Health Care Services, Institute of Medicine of the National Academies. Washington, DC: The National Academies Press; 2003:1–5.
8. Slack WV, Hicks GP, Reed CE, Van Cura LJ. A computer based medical history. N Engl J Med 1966;274:194–198.
9. Policy implications of medical information systems. Available at: www.wws. princeton.edu: 28.
10. Fitzmaurice JM, Adams K, Eisenberg J. Three decades of research on computer applications in health care. J Am Med Inform Assoc 2002;9:144–160.
11. Policy implications of medical information systems. Available at: www.wws. princeton.edu: 30–36.
12. Ball MJ, Collen M, eds. Aspects of the Computer-based Patient Record. New York: Springer-Verlag, 1992.
13. Policy implications of medical information systems. Available at: www.wws. princeton.edu: 21–26.
14. Coffey R. How Medical Information Systems Affect Costs: The El Camino Experience. Washington, DC: Public Health Service, 1979.
15. Staggers N, Thompson CB, Snyder-Halpern R. History and trends in clinical information systems in the United States. J Nurs Scholarsh 2001;33(1):75–81.
16. McDonald C. Protocol based computer reminders, the quality of care, and the non-perfectability of man. N Engl J Med 1976;295:1351–1355.
17. Kuperman GJ, Gardner RM, Pryor TA. HELP: A Dynamo Hospital Information System. Computers and Medicine. New York: Springer-Verlag, 1991.
18. www.AHRQ.gov/Research?computer.htm, 2004.
19. Menlove RL, Burke JP. The timing of prophylactic administration of antibiotics and the risk of surgical-wound infection. N Engl J Med 1992;30:326(5):281–286.
20. Lenhard RE, Buchman JP, Achuff SC, et al. The Johns Hopkins Hospital automated resume. J Med Syst 1991;15(3):237–247.

21. Mandell SF, Szekalski S. The use of an enterprise wide electronic patient record. Proc AMIA Symp 1997:1029.
22. Wang DJ, Harkness KB, Allshouse C, et al. Development of a Web based electronic patient record extending accessibility to clinical information and integrating ancillary applications. Proc AMIA Symp 1998:131–134.
23. Staggers N, Thompson CB, Snyder-Halpern R. History and trends in clinical information systems in the United States. J Nurs Scholarsh 2001;33(1):77.
24. Teich JM. Clinical systems for integrated healthcare networks. J Am Med Inform Assoc 1998;4(1):19–28.
25. Arden Syntax, Mission and Charter. Available at: www.HL7.org. 2004.
26. Simon H. The New Science of Decision Making. New York: Prentice Hall; 1977:14.
27. Detmer WM, Shortliffe EH. Using the Internet to improve knowledge diffusion in medicine. Commun ACM 1997:101–108.
28. Caslon Analytics: net metrics and statistics guides. Available at: www.caslon.com.au. 2005.
29. Berners-Lee T. A little history of the World Wide Web. Available at: www.org/history.html. Nov 1998.
30. National Library of Medicine: fact sheet. Available at: www.nlm.nih.gov. 2005.
31. Hersh WR, Brown KE. CliniWeb: managing clinical information on the World Wide Web. J Am Med Inform Assoc 1994;3(4):273–280.
32. Detmer WM, Shortliffe EH. A model of clinical query management that supports integration of biomedical information over the World Wide Web. Proc Annu Symp Comput Appl Med Care 1995:898–902.
33. Barnett GO, Cimino JJ, Hupp JA, Hoffer EP. DXplain: an evolving diagnostic decision support system. JAMA 1987;258(1):67–74.
34. Barnett GO, Fanighetti KT, Kim RJ, Hoffer EP, Feldman MJ. DXplain on the Internet, AMIA.org.pubs/symposia, 2002.
35. Teich JM, Glaser JP, Beckley RF, Aranow M. Brigham and Women's Hospital information system. Davies recognition submission. Computer Based Patient Record Institute. 1996.
36. Teich JM, Glaser JP, Beckley RF, et al. The Brigham integrated computing systems (BICS): advanced clinical systems in an academic hospital environment. Int J Med Inform 1999;54:197–208.
37. Guissbuhler A. WizOrder: a physician order management system developed by Vanderbilt University Medical Center. Available at: www.mc.Vanderbilt.Edu/dbmi/antoine/wizdemo. Dec 1998.
38. Sullivan SJ. White paper: clinical decision support—why does it matter? Eclipsys Corporation; 1997.
39. Simborg DW. Networking and medical information systems. J Med Sys 1984; 8:43–47.
40. Bierner G. TraumaTalk: content to speech generation for decision support at point of care. J Am Med Inform Assoc 1998;4(2):698–702.
41. Sittig DF, Yungton JA, Kuperman GJ, Teich JM. A graphical user interaction model for integrating complex clinical applications: a pilot study. J Am Med Inform Assoc 1998;4(2):708–712.
42. Huff SM. Clinical data exchange standards and vocabularies for messages. J Am Med Inform Assoc 1998:62–67.

43. McDonald CJ. Need for standards in health information health affairs. 1998; 6(17):44–46.
44. Kohn L, Corrigan J, et al. Committee on Quality in Health Care in America. To Err is Human: Building a Safer Health System, Institute of Medicine. Washington, DC: National Academy Press; 2000.
45. Committee on Quality of Health Care in America. Crossing the Quality Chasm: A New Health System for the 21st Century. Institute of Medicine. Washington, DC: National Academy Press; 2001.

3
Clinical Research Needs

Joyce C. Niland and Layla Rouse

Advances in biomedical research and the development of new therapeutic interventions follow a natural clinical research life cycle, as depicted in Figure 3-1. Observational studies and case series may point toward a possible association between certain treatments and patient response. Basic science and animal studies are conducted to elucidate the proposed mechanism and to confirm or refute the potential for improved efficacy and acceptable side effects.

Clinical trials are then performed to test the new interventions in humans for the first time, to determine the optimal dose (Phase I trials), establish whether there is a reasonable response rate (Phase II trials), and then test the new intervention against the standard or a placebo via randomized assignment (Phase III). Once true benefit of the new treatment has been statistically proven in a Phase III trial, clinical research moves to the arena of outcomes research, i.e., collecting treatment and outcomes data on all patients treated under the new standard of care established via clinical trials evidence to determine generalizability to the global patient population.

All phases of the clinical research life cycle could be greatly enhanced and facilitated by means of electronic data made available via an electronic health record system (EHR-S). There is no doubt that the EHR-S holds great promise for improving the efficiency, quality, and cost of patient health care. Although there has been only a slow and painstaking deployment of EHR-S usage throughout the United States to date, presumably this pace of technology infusion will escalate over the next several years, and widespread adoption of the EHR-S will be seen. To continually and rapidly improve human health, it is crucial that the EHR-S be created and deployed in a manner that will not only support individual patient care, but also facilitate clinical research. However, to date, a significant factor limiting the availability of promising new therapies has been the general inability to optimize the utility of electronic information on patients to efficiently capture data for research.

There are many advantages to the reuse of patient care data for research purposes. Observational studies and case series may be much more rapidly

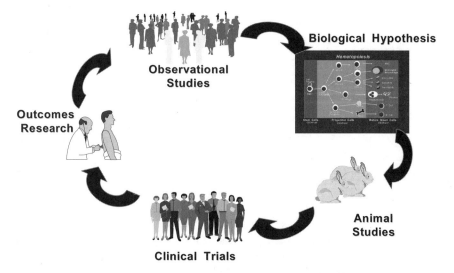

FIGURE 3-1. The study cycle of new treatment discoveries. (From Niland JC. Biostatistical methods in cell transplantation. In: Blume KG, Forman SJ, Appelbaum FR, eds. Thomas' Cell Transplantation. Malden, MA: Blackwell Publishing; 2004.)

conducted to generate new hypotheses for exploration in new interventions. Previously undetected patterns of response or toxicity may be discovered through data mining if a core set of uniformly collected and coded data is available for every patient. Clinical trials may be expedited by screening available patient databases to find potentially eligible subjects. During the conduct of the trial, nonexperimental test results could be imported electronically through the EHR-S and made available for analysis of patients enrolled in the trial. Outcomes research analyses could be fully supported by the encoding of all presenting characteristics, history, comorbidity, interventions, response to treatment, and long-term sequelae and survival.

In discussing the use of EHR-S data to enhance clinical research, the objectives for this chapter are to:

1. Summarize the challenges involved in creating the EHR-S–clinical research interface.
2. Describe several ongoing and future initiatives that will facilitate the creation of this interface.
3. Forecast the future benefits derived from utilizing the EHR-S to speed biomedical research.

Challenges in Reusing EHR-S Data for Clinical Research

Access to EHR-S Data for Research Purposes

The emergence of electronic data within the modern health information infrastructure will provide substantial benefits for medical providers and patients, including enhanced patient autonomy, improved clinical treatment, and advances in health research and public health surveillance.[1] Computerized databases of personally identifiable information may be accessed, changed, viewed, copied, used, disclosed, or deleted more easily and by more people (authorized and unauthorized) than paper-based records. Therefore, this availability of electronic data also presents new legal challenges in terms of confidentiality of identifiable health information, and the reliability and quality of health data.[1] Not only the use of computers, but also other electronic devices such as facsimile transmission of patient information may threaten patient confidentiality and privacy.[2]

Another development that may compromise the confidentiality of medical records is the "team approach" to both medical care as well as a clinical research. It has been reported that as many as 100 different healthcare professionals and administrative personnel may have access to a patient's medical record information within the EHR-S.[3] This could result in confidential EHR-S information being available to people who may not be cognizant of its sanctity, or who may not properly protect the data.[2,3]

These issues are of particular concern when considering usage of EHR-S data for research purposes. Therefore, the first challenge in making the information collected within the EHR-S available for clinical research purposes is protecting the information from inappropriate use. There are three areas of concern when making clinical information available, particularly as Internet deployment of data will be utilized more frequently: Authentication (ensuring that the user is who s/he says s/he is), authorization (ensuring that the user is allowed to do what s/he is requesting to do with the data), and confidentiality (ensuring that the data are given only to the authenticated, authorized user).[4]

Only pertinent data contained within the EHR-S should be released to authorized clinical research team members. Often there is a lack of education and understanding of the privacy, confidentiality, and security issues by patients, providers, payers, and the government.[5] The appropriate protection of EHR-S data to be used for research can be accomplished through a combination of regulatory approval processes, [e.g., institutional review board (IRB) and privacy board for approval of the data to be used and disclosed for the research], and through the application of modern security techniques (e.g., ID/password protection, encryption of the information during transfer, and view restrictions of the type of data that can be seen based on an individual's role).

The challenge of utilizing the EHR-S for clinical research has been made even more complex through the recent passing of the Health Insurance Portability and Accountability Act (HIPAA) with respect to uses and disclosures of protected health information (PHI) for research, in accordance with the Privacy and Security Rules promulgated under HIPAA. PHI consists of individually identifiable health information transmitted by a covered entity through electronic media, maintained in electronic media, or transmitted or maintained in any other form or medium.

Although HIPAA was designed to protect patients from unauthorized use and disclosure of their patient care data, it also applies to data collected by physicians in the process of conducting research, e.g., clinical trials. Therefore, if the EHR-S becomes the source for clinical research information, use and disclosure of this data are subject to the HIPAA regulations. In protecting the confidentiality of PHI, it is important to provide individuals some control regarding their health data, without severely restricting warranted use of the data.[1]

Another key challenge will be the correct identification of patients who may be treated across multiple institutions, or with varying identities within the same institution. Within an organization a patient may inadvertently receive more than one medical record number because of confusion over other key identifiers (e.g., a woman whose medical records in the EHR-S reside under both her maiden and married name.) Medical record numbers are insufficient to identify patients across institutions, because each healthcare facility assigns and maintains independent patient IDs through unrelated medical record number systems that are meaningless outside the organization. Even social security numbers (SSNs) are notoriously unreliable as unique identifiers, with estimates of erroneous numbers possibly ranging up to 10% within a given institution.

Robust methods to correctly identify an individual within and between institutions and correctly link their records across databases will be required to utilize the EHR-S for research purposes. A "Master Patient Index" will need to be in place that can either provide 100% matching on a specified core set of identifiers (e.g., medical record number, SSN, name, birth date, gender, race), or provide an indication that a pair of records may be from the same individual, with some degree of probability. Such suspect pairs would then require further investigation.

Standardization of EHR-S Data for Research

Researchers generally are considered to be among the "secondary" users of the EHR-S, with the primary users being the caregivers who use the EHR-S directly in providing patient care.[6] Additional secondary users include administrators, payers, and regulatory agencies. Secondary users of the EHR-S require standardized coded data fields for virtually every aspect of care to make it possible to search for and gather the necessary information in a usable electronic format. However, it is evident that the primary users of the EHR-S also will derive major benefit from such standardization once fully implemented.

To achieve standardization of EHR-S and research information, standardized terminologies are required, including classifications and nomenclatures for coding data.[7] Currently there is a critical lack of uniformly applied controlled vocabularies in both patient care and clinical research, and a lack of standard metadata ("data about the data," fully describing the type of information to be collected and how). This uneven application of vocabulary standards, along with inconsistent deployment of data services and interfaces, have conspired to create what has been referred to as the "bioinformatics equivalent of neighboring but isolated medieval nation states, each with a different system of weights and measures."[8,9]

A natural harmony exists between the need for standardized vocabularies for clinical applications, administrative needs such as reimbursement groupings, and statistical analysis and reporting. Whereas it is possible to derive the coded data needed for administrative and research needs from the clinical detail of a coded standardized EHR-S, the converse rarely is true.[7] In using standardized vocabularies within the EHR-S, not only will patient care and clinical research be greatly facilitated, but such standardization also will accommodate the data needs of various public health agencies conducting disease surveillance.[10]

Another critical need for standardization to facilitate clinical research as well as care involves the development of a common information model. As biomedical research becomes an increasingly collaborative undertaking, parallel advances in bioinformatics are creating new possibilities for discovery within and across scientific disciplines. However, most existing patient databases have developed independently over time, with tremendous variability in nomenclature, data content, rules, processes, and data structure. The clinical care and research arenas are fraught with examples of this "silo" approach to database development. In short, there has been no unifying information architecture in place to support the desired interoperability between the EHR-S and the clinical research systems.

Quality of EHR-S Data Used for Research

For EHR-S data to be useful for both clinical care and research purposes, the data must be of the highest quality. In addressing both the confidentiality and standardization issues described above, it is quite possible that the quality of the EHR-S data will be enhanced. It has been asserted that providing individuals some control regarding their health data, in conformance with HIPAA regulations, will encourage individuals to allow communal uses of their EHR-S data for societal good, and in the process directly improve the quality and reliability of health research data.[1] Furthermore, the use of controlled vocabularies along with standardized validation rules and data entry controls will greatly improve the integrity of EHR-S data for both healthcare and research purposes.[5]

Initiatives Supporting Integration of the EHR-S with Research

Authorized EHR-S Data Usage under HIPAA

One approach to ensuring appropriate HIPAA-compliant authorized use and disclosure of EHR-S data for the purposes of research is to craft a blanket protocol that outlines the policies, procedures, and the circumstances under which researchers will be approved to use EHR-S data for research. This has been the approach at City of Hope National Medical Center. Such a blanket protocol was written by the Chair of the Division of Information Sciences (the group responsible for providing research support in terms of electronic data management and analysis), and approved through the City of Hope IRB.

The objective of the protocol is to allow for the creation and maintenance of a research data repository (RDR) to provide access to data required for use in any City of Hope clinical research study in a secure and confidential manner. Other major objectives of this RDR is to make it possible to perform required administrative and quality assurance analysis, to conduct prognostic exploratory analyses across all patients, to better understand the association between treatment and response, and to conduct analyses to evaluate the quality of care and outcomes achieved for City of Hope patients.

The protocol describes the procedures for collecting, computerizing, storing, accessing, reporting, and distributing data for individual research studies that have been approved by the City of Hope IRB, including data merged into the repository from the EHR-S. The processes described within the RDR protocol ensure that confidentiality and security are maintained, while making the EHR-S data available to provide further insights into treatment effects, and prognostic and risk factors that may influence development of future protocols and treatment options. However, each individual usage of the data for research purposes requires a separate IRB-approved protocol to be written by the researcher who serves as the study's principal investigator.

Generally, most users of a clinical research data management system such as the RDR are not authorized to access more than one study.[11] Whereas such pan-study usage of data is usually an ancillary form of research within most institutions, it can prove to be quite useful for studying potential associations between risk factors, interventions and outcomes, and generating new hypotheses for future prospective studies. The RDR protocol allows for both access to individual clinical trial data, and the creation of cohorts that may span multiple trials or include patients receiving the standard of care.

Although individual informed consent is obtained for various treatment procedures and these interventions and outcomes are recorded in the EHR-S for patient care, this does not provide the necessary consent for use of these same data for research purposes. Before the enactment of HIPAA, a global patient consent obtained at presentation for patient care could be used to receive permission to use the EHR-S data for any future research purpose. Under HIPAA, this global consent is no longer considered to be sufficient to allow any previously unspecified research to proceed using EHR-S data. Instead, at the City of Hope, typically one of three options needs to occur for HIPAA compliance in obtaining and accessing patient data for research:

1. *Individual Informed Consent or Waiver of Consent:* The first option is to obtain informed consent that includes HIPAA authorization from each patient who is eligible to participate in the research study. This is the case for all clinical trials, and for most other types of prospective research studies. With this approach, the EHR-S data necessary for the research protocol are validly made available to the research team. For studies of an observational nature, it is recognized that obtaining individual informed consent and HIPAA authorization may pose major logistical challenges and may, in fact, be impracticable, and potentially threaten the generalizability of the findings if selection bias occurs.[12] Therefore, researchers conducting low risk observational studies may seek a waiver of informed consent for use of EHR-S information.

2. *Anonymization of Data:* A second option to allow EHR-S data to be provided to an investigator for research purposes (including evaluations preparatory to conducting a larger research study) is that the data are anonymized by an authorized party before distribution to the investigator. This is a viable option in only a limited set of research endeavors, as anonymization includes the removal of identifiers and dates (except for year) of procedures or events. Thus, research looking at specific timelines, requiring IDs for linking of additional data, or needing long-term prospective follow-up is untenable using an anonymized dataset.

3. *Limited Datasets:* A third option is for the investigator to write a protocol requesting the needed EHR-S data in the form of a "limited dataset." The HIPAA regulations have defined 16 fields that need to be eliminated from the dataset to qualify it as a limited dataset (see Table 3-1).[13]

Although the limited dataset excludes key identifiers, the benefit to this form of dataset is that dates of procedures and outcomes may be included. In addition, the investigator can request prospectively collected information from the data source. This makes the data more useful for prognostic

TABLE 3-1. PHI that must be removed to qualify information as a limited dataset

1. Names	9. Account numbers
2. Postal and address information*	10. Certificate/license numbers
3. Telephone numbers	11. Vehicle IDs and serial numbers
4. Fax numbers	12. Device identifiers and serial numbers
5. Electronic mail addresses	13. Web universal resource locators (URLs)
6. Social security numbers	14. Internet protocol (IP) address numbers
7. Medical record numbers	15. Biometric identifiers†
8. Health plan beneficiary numbers	16. Full-face photographs

* Other than town or city, state, and ZIP code.
† Including fingerprints and voiceprints.

evaluations, tests of associations, outcomes research, and any other research that requires the evaluation of time trends, or the impact of time periods or lags on the eventual outcomes. Data will be released to the investigator with a unique patient number (UPN) and no other identifiers; however, there will be an "honest broker" within Information Sciences who holds the link back to the identifiers such as medical record number, should the researcher need to request additional information or follow-up data.

As mentioned above, a key challenge will be accurately matching patient records within and between the EHR-S and the research database. One example of a technological solution for matching patients within and across databases has been developed by the Object Management Group (OMG), an international standards organization that develops technically integrated, commercially viable, and vendor independent specifications for the software industry. The OMG has achieved international consensus on the Common Object Request Broker Architecture (CORBA) to facilitate technical interoperability among disparate information systems. Within medicine and in conjunction with technologists within the healthcare industry, the OMG has created CORBAmed.[14] The CORBAmed objective is to improve healthcare delivery by promoting interoperability among healthcare devices, instruments, and information systems using CORBA.

CORBAmed specifications have been created for a number of "services," including the Patient Identification Services (PIDS). Utilizing Health Level-7 (HL7), PIDS was developed to correlate health records among multiple institutions based on a core set of profile elements, while protecting confidentiality under an array of policies and security mechanisms. This type of service could be used to identify and unite records of information on the same patient stored under multiple IDs within an EHR-S, or to integrate records stemming from the EHR-S with existing data on the same patient within a research data repository.

Recognizing that the issue of data and transmission security is paramount to the implementation of any electronic public health reporting system, the

Centers for Disease Control is developing methods and procedures to address these issues.[10] Such programs use encryption of data, message authentication, and message non-repudiation via a secure data facility to send and receive HL7 messages that meet or exceed current standards for the confidentiality and security of patient information. Such methods to transmit sensitive information electronically should be studied as a model for incorporation into the transmission of required data from the EHR-S to clinical research data repositories.

As another example of an approach to ensure secure access to EHR-S data, the University of California at San Diego (UCSD) has developed PCASSO: Patient-Centered Access to Secure Systems Online.[15] In this model, the UCSD clinical information systems pass data in HL7 messages that are parsed and stored in PCASSO's clinical data repository. At the time of storing, the data are labeled at one of five sensitivity levels: Low, standard, public-deniable, guardian-deniable, and patient-deniable.

Table 3-2 provides the definition and examples for each level of data sensitivity. PCASSO's security mechanisms ensured that patients could only view their own medical data, excluding any data that the patient's primary care provider had specifically labeled "patient-deniable." Individual results and reports can be given this label via a set of rules used by the system's import function. For example, one loading rule states that all notes originating from the psychiatry department would default to the patient-

TABLE 3-2. Sensitivity levels of patient data stored in the PCASSO system

Sensitivity Level	Definition	Examples
Low security data	Data that are not patient-identifiable	Patient data that have been anonymized in accordance with HIPAA rules
Standard data	Routine health information that is identifiable (and does not fall into any of the "deniable" categories)	Vital signs, history and physical, routine laboratory tests
Public-deniable data	Data about conditions specifically addressed by state law	Mental health, HIV/AIDS, abortion, adoption, sexually transmitted diseases, substance abuse
Guardian-deniable data	Data that by law can be withheld from a guardian	Information regarding a teenager's abortion (in some states)
Patient-deniable data	Data that the patient's primary care physician considers capable of causing harm to the patient were it disclosed	Psychotherapy notes, information compiled for use in a legal proceeding, certain test results that are exempted from CLIA*

* Clinical Laboratory Improvements Amendments (CLIA) of 1988.

deniable category. Although PCASSO was designed to provide patients with secure access to their own data, a similar approach could be used for the extraction and storage of EHR-S data for research purposes.

Standardization of EHR-S Data

To optimally meet all the various needs of patient care, clinical research, and public health, it is critical that the controlled vocabularies are capable of describing biomedical concepts in varying levels of detail.[10]

The goals of the National Health Information Infrastructure (NHII) initiated in 2004 include not only the deployment of a standardized EHR-S for every healthcare provider, but also the ability to exchange information across systems and patients, to ensure that all data for a given patient will be available at the point when a medical treatment decision needs to be made.[16,17] This highly integrated approach to data computerization will greatly enhance the ability to extract complete patient information for the purposes of clinical research.

A major step toward standardizing medical vocabularies was achieved when the NHII declared that several standard vocabulary systems would be recommended as the terminologies for the future EHR-S. These are the Systematized Nomenclature of Medicine (SNOMED), the Logical Observation Identifiers Names and Codes (LOINC), and the emerging RxNorm vocabulary system.[18-23]

Other ongoing governmental initiatives also will assist with the development of data standards to support EHR-S and clinical research information. As a major collector and processor of health data, the federal government has engaged in extensive development of minimum datasets and core health data elements,[24] and has helped to identify, define, and implement standardized data for describing morbidity, infectious diseases, and mortality.

Among governmental agencies involved in standards setting for oncologic conditions, the National Cancer Institute (NCI) is a major player in the identification and development of standards. The mission of the NCI Center for Bioinformatics (NCICB) is to provide informatics infrastructure and scientific applications that support advanced translational research in cancer biology and medicine.[8] To help address the lack of data standards in cancer clinical research studies, the NCI developed the Common Data Elements (CDEs) that define the data required for research in oncology.[25,26] When standards such as the CDEs have already been developed for research purposes, it would be ideal for the developers of the EHR-S to incorporate such preexisting standards into their healthcare information systems.

A key component to facilitate the translation of clinical care data in a common manner for reuse as research data is the creation, acceptance, and adoption of a common information model. Achieving this higher level of standardization will allow true exchange of data with both syntactic (formatting for physical exchange of data) and semantic (common meaning for accurate use of the data content) compatability. As a subcomponent of the HL7 Reference Information Model (RIM) initiative within the clinical research domain, the HL7 Regulated Clinical Research Information Model (RCRIM) is evolving a standardized model for research data as well, following the same modeling approaches. The project objectives for RCRIM are to develop a standard structured protocol representation that supports the entire life cycle of clinical research protocols to achieve semantic interoperability among systems and stakeholders. The RCRIM model is going through the HL7 procedure for balloted approval.

Another major nonprofit data modeling initiative that is underway is the Clinical Data Interchange Standards Consortium (CDISC).[27] The CDISC initiative began in 1997 as an open, multidisciplinary, nonprofit organization committed to the development of industry standards to support electronic acquisition, exchange, submission, and archiving of clinical trials data. The CDISC mission is to lead the development of global, vendor-neutral, platform independent data standards to improve data quality and speed product development, facilitating the delivery of new interventions to market more quickly.

Recently the two complementary initiatives have recognized the benefit of collaborating together, and the CDISC clinical research model under development is being taken up by HL7 for balloting and potential adoption under RCRIM. Whereas these modeling initiatives initially involved primarily pharmaceutical and FDA representatives, academic research centers such as City of Hope are now participating in this endeavor, helping to ensure that the final model will meet the needs of institutions conducting clinical research studies.

Clearly, these modeling activities will have far-reaching impact on the entire healthcare community, ranging from large enterprises to individual practices. With the concomitant development and release of the HL7-RCRIM-CDISC model for clinical research, demonstration projects could be conducted to prove the utility and functionality of this domain model for the reuse of EHR-S data for research purposes.

Another NCICB initiative that was launched in 2003 and is closely involved in the HL7-RCRIM-CDISC modeling processes is the Cancer Biomedical Informatics Grid (caBIG) project.[28] The ambitious but critical goal of the NCI caBIG initiative is to create a "virtual web" of interconnected data, individuals, and organizations that will redefine how research is conducted, care is provided, and patients/participants interact with the biomedical research enterprise. This nationwide initiative has engaged approximately 50 NCI-funded cancer centers to assist in providing input into and developing common information management systems for all realms of cancer research.

The "desiderata" being followed within caBIG are to develop open access, open source computer tools, derived from common information models, using standards for data exchange, and following international standards for data and metadata coding.

As one of the funded development sites for the Clinical Trials Management System workspace within caBIG, City of Hope is developing open source shareable clinical trials tools, beginning with an adverse event reporting system. Through this initiative, City of Hope also began participating in the HL7-RCRIM-CDISC modeling initiative. The integration and convergence of these national–international initiatives will help to ensure that future data exchange is possible between EHR-S and clinical research management systems, thus greatly speeding the development and testing of new drugs and therapeutic interventions.

Improving the Quality of Data for Research

Powerful information systems can improve the quality of and reduce errors within clinical data, thereby facilitating not only clinical care but also research.[29] As mentioned above, the labor-intensive act of standardizing the coding and information modeling within the EHR-S is critical to improving the quality and semantic compatibility of these data, thus improving the quality of clinical research conducted based on EHR-S data. Controlling the vocabulary structure for an EHR-S or research database can be achieved through the strict maintenance of a robust "data dictionary." The data stored in the data dictionary afford control over the data in the EHR-S by specifying the naming conventions and standardized data types.[5] The dictionary also stores all of the system profile information that controls data quality including range and error checking, as well as operations scheduling, program access control, menu options, and security.

Accurate and complete research information can best be attained by collecting clinical data directly from caregivers using the EHR-S, and delivering the information back to them in a usable format.[29] It has been demonstrated that data collection will be more accurate and complete when accomplished while the patient is still in the hospital, rather than through retrospective chart review weeks to months later.[30] Real-time (or near real time) data collection by the caregivers themselves through a well-designed EHR-S will ensure that definitions are consistently applied, and missing elements are obtained up front. The daily review of data helps to identify errors of omission or commission, and provides the opportunity for correction immediately while access to the patient and his/her record is still available to the caregiver.

Although such "point-of-care" data collection into the EHR-S by the healthcare team is often the ideal for both clinical care and research, thus far this data capture method has proven to be an elusive goal. Frequently the capture of such standardized coded data at the point-of-care will slow the caregiver–patient session, requiring additional time that can be ill-afforded in a busy clinical practice or academic medical center. However, the downstream payoff of accurate, complete, timely information should be well worth the benefit of continuing to redesign the EHR-S's computer–human interface to make this type of immediate data capture appealing and tenable to the care providers.

Benefits from Integrating the EHR-S with the Clinical Research Data System

Despite the fact that the data being collected are very similar and highly overlapping, at the current time, EHR-S's and clinical research data systems continue to be developed along parallel tracks. There are many reasons for this separation.

The EHR-S has been developed to serve the specific and immediate needs of the primary system users (physicians and other caregivers), whereas the clinical research data systems have been specifically developed to collect research data from multiple electronic and nonelectronic sources, often after the care generating the treatment and outcomes observations has already been rendered. As we have also seen, the data frequently are structured and coded differently within the two systems, or not coded at all within the EHR-S, but entered as text streams, e.g., physician dictations. Therefore, transferring data between the two types of systems often is a difficult task that does not scale easily. In the long-term, it is the ongoing efforts to create and harmonize the various standards (HL7 RIM/RCRIM, CDISC, caBIG, CDEs, etc.), and the enforcement of legislative regulations (HIPAA and 21 CFR Part 11) that will enable integration of data between these two systems.[31]

What will be the benefits of such reuse of patient care data for research that will make these extremely intensive and long-term investments in system standardization and integration worthwhile? As briefly outlined in the introduction, the entire clinical research life cycle depicted in Figure 3-1 stands to benefit from making EHR-S data available for research.

The optimal EHR-S should be designed as a truly comprehensive personal health record, including a birth-to-death, time-oriented dataset of all parameters related to a person's well-being.[5] Through data transferred from the EHR-S, a research data repository can be prospectively amassed and made available under IRB approval for "data mining" of the information. This can lead to new observations within the aggregated data, such as potentially significant associations between certain treatments or patient characteristics and ultimate morbidity, quality-of-life, or survival outcomes. In addition, it is possible to improve patient safety by more rapidly detecting patterns of severe toxicity interventions or dose levels across multiple clinical trials or patients receiving standard care.

Clinical trials could be greatly expedited through the integration of the EHR-S with the Clinical Trials Management System (CTMS). Prerequisites for completion of a successful clinical trial include the accrual of sufficient patients and the ability to generate and collect valid and reliable information regarding the effectiveness of new treatment regimens.[32] The availability of large patient databases derived from the EHR-S will allow for electronic screening to identify potentially eligible subjects.

Additionally, if the data requirements for the protocol are carefully aligned with the coded data within the EHR-S, much of the clinical trial data could be directly transferred to the CTMS from the EHR-S. Only the truly experimental tests or those recorded outside of the EHR-S would then need to be directly entered into the CTMS. Furthermore, electronic decision support could be used to ensure that the milestones and procedures of the trial are being followed according to the protocol, improving the quality of the trial conducted.

Decision support also could be applied against the emerging electronic results, such as laboratory tests, to automatically grade toxicities and detect serious adverse events that require further evaluation and reporting. Thus, patient safety would be enhanced while speeding the completion of the clinical trial. The outcomes for the trial also could be transmitted electronically from the EHR-S to the CTMS, and made available for rapid analysis of the trial results.

By designing the EHR-S to collect coded data in real time, both clinical research and patient care will be enhanced. It has been shown that moving to point-of-care data collection not only provides more accurate complete data for research, but also can have a positive impact on medical services and performance improvement efforts within a healthcare facility.[30]

By integrating data from all medical specialties and modalities, the EHR-S creates a historical view of the health-related course of events in a person's life.[5] This complete longitudinal data view from the EHR-S will provide the necessary data for outcomes research, the investigation of patterns of care, deficiencies in care, and benchmarking for concordance of care with national healthcare guidelines. This form of research can lead to improved care guidelines, performance improvement initiatives within the healthcare institution, and discovery of patterns possibly related to improved medical outcomes, ultimately leading to new clinical trials to test these hypotheses.

Both clinicians and public health officials need access to information about health status, public health risks, and population health issues, including trends in community-centric markers of health.[33] Through integration of the two major health information forces—public health information systems and private EHR-Ss—both areas could greatly benefit from technology solutions that link information about the health of the public with data specific to the care of an individual patient.[33] This data integration would greatly enhance disease surveillance research as well.

Furthermore, both the field of health services research and medical informatics have much to gain from active cultivation of the interface between the two disciplines. Health services researchers will gain access to a wealth of tools, data, and analytic methods, while the medical informaticians will be assisted through the development of new information systems and models and measuring the effects of these and other healthcare processes on both patient care and research.[29]

In summary, it can be seen that, although an extremely challenging goal, all forms of clinical research would be greatly enhanced by integrating EHR-S data with research repositories. The benefits derived form a "two-way street"—not only could EHR-S data be made available to facilitate research, but research results such as graded toxicities could be returned to the electronic health record to improve patient care. If EHR-S information is made available to researchers, patient care potentially will become safer, data will be cleaner and more accurate, performance improvement initiatives will be completed more quickly, and new interventions will be sped from the bench to the bedside more rapidly and effectively. Finally, the benefits of integration with the EHR-S will not be restricted to clinical research, but also will confer great advantages to the conduct of pharmacogenomic, gene therapy, and genotype-phenotype correlative research in the future.

References

1. Hodge JG, Gostin LO, Jacobson PD. Legal issues concerning electronic health information: privacy, quality, and liability. JAMA 1999;282:1466–1471.
2. Dodek DY, Dodek A. From Hippocrates to facsimiles: protecting patient confidentiality is more difficult and more important than ever before. Can Med Assoc J 1997;156(6):847–852.
3. Siegler M. Confidentiality in medicine: a decrepit concept. N Engl J Med 1982; 307:1518–1521.
4. Cimino JJ, Socratous SA, Clayton PD. Internet as clinical information system: application development using the World Wide Web. J Am Med Inform Assoc 1995;2:273–284.
5. Hammond WE, Hales JW, Lobach DF, Straube MJ. Integration of a computer-based patient record system into the primary care setting. Comput Nurs 1997; 15(2) Suppl 1:S61–S68.
6. Carter J. The electronic medical record as a tool for research and patient care. In: Carter J, ed. Electronic Medical Records: A Guide for Clinicians and Administrators. Philadelphia: ACP; 2001:197–212.
7. Chute CC, Cohn SP, Campbell JR. A framework for comprehensive health terminology systems in the United States: development of guidelines, criteria for selection, and public policy implications. J Am Med Inform Assoc 1998;5: 503–510.
8. Covitz PA, Hartel F, Schaefer C, De Coronado S, et al. CaCORE: a common infrastructure for cancer informatics. Bioinformatics 2003;19(18):2404–2412.
9. Stein L. Creating a bioinformatics nation. Nature 2002;417:119–120.

10. White MD, Kolar LM, Steindel SJ. Evaluation of vocabularies for electronic reporting to public health agencies. J Am Med Inform Assoc 1999;6(3):185–194.
11. Deshpande AM, Brandt C, Nadkarni PM. Metadata-driven ad hoc query of patient data: meeting the needs of clinical studies. J Am Med Inform Assoc 2002;9:369–382.
12. Willison DJ, Kashavjee K, Nair K, Goldsmith C, Holbrook AM. Information in practice: patient consent preferences for research uses of information in electronic medical records—interview and survey data. BMJ 2003;326:373–377.
13. http://privacyruleandresearch.nih.gov/pr_08.asp#8d.
14. http://www.acl.lanl.gov/OMG/CORBAmed/mission.htm.
15. Masys D, Baker D, Butros A, Cowles KE. Giving patients access to their medical records via the Internet: the PCASSO experience. J Am Med Inform Assoc 2002;9:181–191.
16. Yasnoff WA, Humphreys BL, Overhage JM, et al. A consensus action agenda for achieving the national health information infrastructure. J Am Med Inform Assoc 2004;11:332–338.
17. http://www.hhs.gov/news/press/2004pres/20040721.html.
18. Cote RA, Rothwell DJ, Palotay JL, Beckett RS, Brochu L, eds. The Systemized Nomenclature of Human and Veterinary Medicine: SNOMED International. Northfield, IL: College of American Pathologists; 1993.
19. Spackman KA, Campbell KE. Compositional concept representation using SNOMED: towards further convergence of clinical terminologies. J Am Med Inform Assoc 1998(Suppl):740–744.
20. http://www.snomed.org/index.html.
21. http://www.cap.org/apps/cap.portal?_nfpb=true&_pageLabel=snomed_page.
22. http://www.loinc.org/background/.
23. http://www.nlm.nih.gov/research/umls/rxnorm_main.html.
24. McCormick D, Renner AL, Mayes R, Regan J, Greenberg M. The federal and private sector roles in the development of minimum data sets and core health data elements. Comput Nurs 1997;15(2) Suppl 1:S23–S32.
25. Chute CG. And data for all: the NCI initiative on clinical infrastructure standards. MD Comput 2000;17:19–21.
26. Silva JS, Ball MJ, Douglas JV. The Cancer Informatics Infrastructure (CII): an architecture for translating clinical research into patient care. Medinformatics 2001;10:114–117.
27. http://www.cdisc.org3.
28. http://cabig.nci.nih.gov.
29. Mandl KD, Lee TH. Integrating medical informatics and health services research: the need for dual training at the clinical health systems and policy levels. J Am Med Inform Assoc 2002;9:127–132.
30. Robertson J. Cardiovascular point of care initiative: enhancements in clinical data management. Qual Manag Health Care, 2003;12(2):115–121.
31. http://www.21cfrpart11.com.
32. Taylor KM, Feldstein ML, Skeel RT, Pandya KJ, Ng P, Carbone PP. Fundamental dilemmas of the randomized clinical trial process: results of a survey of the 1,737 Eastern Cooperative Oncology Group investigators. J Clin Oncol 1994;12: 796–1805.
33. Shiffman RN, Spooner SA, Kwiatkowski K, Brennan PF. Information technology for children's health and healthcare. J Am Med Inform Assoc 2001;8: 546–555.

4
Patients' Needs

RITA KUKAFKA and FRANCES MORRISON

Gaps in Today's Healthcare System

The need for integrated electronic health records (EHRs) is widely acknowledged. The Institute of Medicine has documented the consequences of their absences on the quality and costs of health care. Its 2001 report, *Crossing the Quality Chasm*, stated: "The 21st century will require ... far greater than the current investments in information technology by most health care organizations."[1] The lack of integration arises because individuals' medical data are stored in the warehouses of those who pay for them—providers and insurers—and there is no incentive for overall integration.[2] As will be illustrated in this chapter, patients themselves have a strong incentive for integrated EHRs, and for this reason they are likely to be the best overall drivers for their proliferation.

Many factors are contributing to the shift in the role and self-perception of patients from passive recipients of medical care to active consumers of health services, increasing the demand for health information and other services. As patients become more informed and subsequently empowered in a patient-driven healthcare system, they will demand integrated EHRs as tools to help them manage their health. When patient demands are spoken en mass, our experience tells us that innovative providers and the marketplace will respond.

This consumerism has democratized many systems in the United States. For examples, Intuit, which makes Quicken software, responded to consumer demands for integrated financial records.[3] When consumers demanded better, cheaper cars, they got them: The consumer price index (CPI) for new vehicles did not inflate from 1995 to 1998.[4] When consumers asked for better services and lower costs from retailers, they got them too: The CPI for apparel and house furnishing also remained flat from 1995 to 1998.[4]

Market economies given in these examples are based on the idea that consumers decide what goods and services are desirable, driving the production of both. The healthcare market is different from many other markets in some important respects (e.g., the presence of group purchasers) and the fact that much of healthcare expenditure is paid for through insurance. However, the most critical aspect that distinguishes health care from other markets is that consumers historically have not acted as strong decision makers in their health care. Finally, this paradigm is changing and it has become quite evident that consumerism coupled with a technological revolution is underway, reshaping the way that health care is organized and delivered. A critical feature of this change is the development of information and services that assist consumers in assuming more responsibility for their own health and facilitate active participation in healthcare decisions. As in other consumer-driven markets, consumers who are active in decision making can create a formidable market force. EHRs are so vital to supporting the decision-making process that they will over time be essential to consumers who manage their own health.

While consumerism may enhance the desirability of the EHR, a fundamental gap still exists in the current healthcare system. A lack of integration and continuity of care in general inhibits the development of an integrated EHR, and profoundly disrupts the care process, causing great difficulty for patients and families alike.

The Patient's Need for Integrated Care

From the patient's perspective, the need for integrated care arises because the healthcare system is organized around the providers of care and not around the needs of users of the care.[2] The mismatch often leads to devastating results, especially for those patients with chronic diseases or disabilities and for underserved groups with special needs.

To gain a perspective on this problem, consider patients with chronic diseases. At least 45% of the United States (US) population—nearly 132 million people—suffers from one or more chronic diseases.[5] Chronically ill patients, who typically require the service of many different kinds of healthcare providers, ineffectively struggle to piece together an integrated system of care. More than half of the individuals with asthma, depression, and hypertension who have been surveyed on this topic have complained that they do not have a helping hand, someone to assist them in coordinating care when more than one provider is involved.[6] These problems are also very apparent in the 18 million Americans with diabetes. Now the sixth leading cause of death in America, diabetes is responsible for more than 200,000 deaths each year.[7] The number of US adults with diagnosed diabetes, including women with gestational diabetes (diabetes that develops during pregnancy), has increased 61% since 1991 and is projected to more than double by 2050. Comorbidities are frequent, 46% of those with diabetes also suffer from high blood pressure and 4%–11% depending on the illness, from asthma, heart disease, and behavioral problems.[8] Diabetics require a team of healthcare professionals to help them manage this complex disease. Cardiologists, endocrinologists, nephrologists, dermatologists, podiatrists, case managers, and behavioral support specialists are among the specialists who are needed to encourage patients in the challenging regimens required for the best management of their disease. Where do they find the integrated care they need? Virtually nowhere, and as a result, many get incomplete care.[9]

Successful care for chronic illness reflects a partnership between several parties—the person suffering, their family and support system, and a variety of professionals. So much of good health for those with chronic disease reflects the patient's own ability to moderate behaviors that aggravate their health problems, monitor key health indicators, manage their own medications, and take advantage of appropriate medical services. People with chronic illness need a responsive integrated system of care, a network for support, and a positive sense of their own ability to manage their health. Only 50% believe that their doctor offers them choices, discusses pros and cons, takes their preferences into account, and asks patients for their treatment preferences on a consistent basis.[6] Perhaps most importantly, a feeling of consistent collaboration with their doctor is missing for up to half of all chronically ill people.[6]

Our uncoordinated healthcare system is ineffective not only in the treatment of chronically ill patients; it is equally ill equipped to attend to the needs of patients and health consumers who are well, but engage in poor self-care behaviors that may eventually lead to chronic conditions. The fractured and paternalistic way in which health care is provided thwarts the development of the "patient as partner" concept in which patients and their families take active roles in achieving and maintaining health. The opportunities to engage the patients and families in collaborative decision making on issues such as the adoption of healthy behaviors (i.e., eating right, exercising, quitting smoking, and initiating other self-management behaviors), and preventive care (i.e., screening) must not be missed.

The gap between patients' needs and what is actually delivered in our current fragmented and costly system cannot be fixed by trying harder. According to the Institute of Medicine (IOM) report, *Crossing the Quality Chasm*, "The current care systems cannot do the job."[1] The use of the EHR has been suggested by the IOM as a fundamental requirement for reengineering health care. Many observers have suggested that improved information systems to coordinate care are necessary to enhance the quality of health care.[10] In a recent study, patients in the Department of Veterans Affairs (VA) health system, which has a computerized records system, received more of the recommended care for their conditions than those outside the VA system.[11] VA patients received 67% of recommended care, compared with 51% of non-VA patients, some of whom were uninsured. The study found that the majority of non-VA hospitals, physician offices, HMOs, public health clinics, and other facilities are not as wired as the VA in terms of providing electronic access to patient records. The study looked at 26 conditions, including depression, diabetes, and heart care, in 1588 men over the age of 35.

The Personal Health Record

Although evidence suggests that an integrated health record would be a great benefit to improving patient quality of care, many believe that it would still miss what may be its greatest potential, unless it is also accompanied by a lifelong personal health record (PHR).[12] Connecting for Health, an initiative to address the challenges of mobilizing health information in order to improve quality and empower patients to become full participants in their care, recognizes the PHR as a central element of an integrated national health information system. The Connecting for Health Personal Health Working Group (PHWG) defines the PHR as a single, *person-centered* system designed to track health and support healthcare activities across one's entire life experience.[13] The PHWG's vision is that the PHR is not limited to a single organization or a single healthcare provider, rather as an Internet-based set of tools that allow people to access and coordinate their lifelong health information and make appropriate parts of it available to those who need it. The PHR should offer an integrated and comprehensive view of health information, including information people generate themselves such as symptoms and medication use, information from doctors such as diagnoses and test results, and information from their pharmacies and insurance companies. The working groups' vision is for individuals to access their PHRs via the Internet, using state-of-the-art security and privacy controls, at any time and from any location. Individual PHR users decide who can view their medical record. People can use their PHR as a communications hub: To send e-mail to doctors, transfer information to specialists, receive test results, and access online self-help tools. The PHR will also connect consumers, patients, and families to the incredible potential of modern health care and give them control over their own information. According to the PHWG, the information should include data auto-populated by clinical systems, data received from monitoring devices, and information entered by providers and the individual himself or herself. The goal of the PHR is to help patients and families to be full participants in their own care.

Understanding and incorporating the patient perspective into the design of the PHR will be crucial in the success of such systems to meet patient needs. To that end, the following section summarizes the literature on patient access to and patient demand for EHRs, and briefly describes current research focusing on the results of providing patient access to their EHR. This section is then followed by a discussion of preferred functionality, usability, and comprehension of the health record reported by patients as well as security and confidentiality concerns, all of which have been the focus of research in the last few years.

General Attitudes Toward Direct Patient Access to the EHR

A broad approach to exploring the PHR was reported by the Connecting for Health Working Group on Policies for Electronic Information Sharing Between Doctors and Patients.[14] The main goal of the report by this working group was to assess national attitudes toward the PHR. The researchers came to the conclusion that most people want to access and control their health information, although most had not previously considered the possibility. Results also revealed that the majority of people surveyed believed that having access to their EHR would help them improve their healthcare decision-making process. The respondents preferred the Internet overall as the medium for their record, but preferences varied with age, with older respondents preferring paper over the Internet. In regard to clinician preferences, the report also concluded that clinicians recognize the benefits from using online patient care tools, including increased efficiency, improved patient–provider relationship, and enhanced care.

The Connecting for Health study also touched upon several different models for the PHR. The model in which the patient holds the record independently and maintains the data separate from the clinical encounter has not been demonstrated to be attractive to users or economically viable to commercial vendors.[14] In addition, results published in the Connecting for Health report find people surveyed preferred the provider office as the organization responsible for hosting the PHR.

Current Implementations of Patient Access to EHRs

The creation of the PHR is dependent on access to existing medical records. Previous research on PHRs focused on patients' preferences and attitudes regarding access to medical records in a theoretical sense. Research is now available that reveals the preferences and experiences of individuals who are actually given access to their records. In addition, investigators have been able to evaluate effects of having access to the record on patient outcomes and patient–provider interaction effects. The research illustrates a variety of perspectives related to security, level of patient access, usability, and functionality that occurs in a range of settings. Several existent systems will be reviewed (Table 4.1).

TABLE 4-1. PHR systems

Name	Institution	Reference
PCASSO	Science Applications International Corporation and the University of California, San Diego	15
PatCIS	Columbia University, New York	17
PatientSite	CareGroup Healthcare System, Boston	18
Electronic Record Development and Implementation Programme	UK	20
SPARRO	University of Colorado Health Sciences Center, Aurora, CO	21
MyChart	Geisinger Health System, Danville, PA	22
PAMFOnline	Palo Alto Medical Foundation, CA	23

PCASSO

An early foray into providing patients with their health records is PCASSO, a project that began in 1996.[15] The yearlong evaluation starting in 1999 focused on addressing security issues surrounding patient access to a Web-based system. The system was pilot tested on 41 patients, 26 of whom used the system. The patients had access to laboratories and reports, although clinical notes were not available. Potential problems with patients were handled by referral to the patient's clinician as well as a toll-free hotline staffed by a librarian. Security was addressed by providing user IDs, passwords, a diskette, and a PCASSO card, all of which are required for logon. Researchers concluded that patients were more satisfied than providers with the high level of security.[16] Both patients and providers reported high levels of satisfaction with having access to clinical data on the Internet.

PatCIS

Another project investigating patient access to their own health record was PatCIS at Columbia University.[17] Researchers provided a small number of hospital employees with access to their health records starting in 1999 and offered additional functions including the ability to add data to the record and obtain automated guideline-based health advice. Patients were given access to laboratory and test results, multiple types of reports including radiology and pathology, and discharge summaries. In addition, they were offered a variety of educational resources and advice based on cholesterol and mammogram guidelines. Because the functionality did not exist in the underlying system, patients were not given access to progress or outpatient notes. After approximately 1 year of providing access, researchers concluded that the system had good usability and utility and did not result in negative consequences such as worsened patient–provider interaction.[17] From interviews, researchers did find that patients and physicians believed that use of the system had positive outcomes such as patient understanding of their conditions and improved patient–physician communication.[17]

PatientSite

PatientSite, implemented at CareGroup Healthcare System in Boston, was offered to patients starting in 2000 in order to involve patients in their care.[18] It provided access to the entire available electronic record using a Web site with secure socket layer encryption as well as e-mail access to providers using secure messaging. The system provides patient education using links to resources that may be chosen by the user and/or the provider. These include information about diseases as well as medications. Additional functions such as scheduling, referrals, and viewing bills were also included. Patients were recruited through the providers, and individuals initiated registration online and completed registration using the telephone. Users included 11,000 patients in 40 practices as of February 2003. The median age of the patients using the site was 43 years with 4% over the age of 70. Fifty-seven percent were female. PatientSite physicians came from a number of different specialty practices, including allergy, cardiology, hematology-oncology, nephrology, obstetrics-gynecology, and pulmonology. There are also 225 support staff registered on PatientSite.[18] These include secretarial, nursing, and appointment staff. Although patient-related outcomes have yet to be published in the medical literature, system designers report enthusiastic use by patients and acceptance by providers.[19]

United Kingdom NHS

In the United Kingdom (UK), development of a system to provide national patient access to individual online health records is underway. To determine the effect of this on a small group of patients, first-time access to individual health record was studied in 100 patients.[20] Although this does not technically qualify as a PHR—patients were not given long-term access or allowed to add text—the study gives firsthand insight into patients' reactions to having access. Focus groups and observation demonstrated that patients were generally able to navigate through an EHR that was not modified for their purposes, felt able to understand the information within, and had a generally positive reaction to the experience.[20]

SPPARO

In a longer trial, patients with congestive heart failure were given access to the EHR via a system called SPPARO.[21] The trial lasted 1 year and patients were reevaluated at the end of the year. Outcomes included number of hit-days (number of days that users accessed the system), patient empowerment score, and attitudes toward electronic record access, as well as physician attitudes toward patient access before and after the trial. The researchers used questionnaires and focus groups as assessment tools. Researchers also evaluated health outcomes and found no difference in health status, number of clinic visits, or hospitalizations between patients who did and did not have access to the system. From interviews, researchers identified several benefits that patients reported by having access to their records. Users believed that the system facilitated them in learning more about their condition, coordinating care, learning about medical decision making, reinforcing memory, increasing participation in medical care, streamlining the flow of information, and confirming normal results and the accuracy of the record.[21] Barriers in the use of the online record that were reported by users included the difficulty in understanding medical terms and drawing appropriate conclusions from a complex document. Patient concerns included the potential for clinicians to change the style of documentation with adverse effects on the value of the record.[21]

MyChart

The MyChart project more recently evaluated an additional function of the patient-accessible EHR: Linked Web messaging.[22] This project, which was evaluated in 2002–3 included more than 4000 users, a third of whom completed surveys. The main goal of the project was to assess the effects on patient–provider communication. Patients were allowed to view parts of their EHR such as laboratory results, medications, problem list, and history as well as perform functions including sending messages to providers. Patients were not allowed access to clinical notes. From a questionnaire of 1421 users, researchers concluded that patients had positive attitudes toward Web messaging and online EHR access, although a few had concerns about confidentiality and privacy.[22] Users also expressed concerns about the accuracy of their health information; one third of users believed that their health information was not complete, and one quarter believed that their medical history was not accurate.[22]

PAMFOnline

PAMFOnline is a system developed at the Palo Alto Medical Foundation that allows patients access to secure messaging, health summaries, test results, prescription renewals, appointment requests, and knowledge resources.[23] It was released to the general patient population in January 2002, with an enrollment of 12,000 reported in 2003. In consideration of a lack of reimbursement for e-mail communications with patients, a subscription model was implemented. Patients were charged a nominal fee for the ability to e-mail clinicians. User satisfaction was assessed by questionnaire with reports of high satisfaction with functionality by patients.[23]

After beta testing, participating physicians who responded reported high levels of satisfaction as well as time savings. Clinicians reported a decrease in telephone encounters and office visits after implementation of the system.

Functionality of the Patient-Accessible EHR

Determining the functionality of patient access to the EHR depends on perspective. Functions that are likely to be most useful and acceptable to patients and clinicians will undoubtedly vary. For example, clinicians have demonstrated preferences for certain types of functions to be available to patients but not others. In a recent questionnaire,[24] most physicians responded that medication lists, normal studies, prescription refills, appointments, and referrals should be available to patients, but not progress notes, or abnormal laboratory results. They also strongly felt that care not be given over the Internet.[24] When individuals who do not have access to their EHR were asked what functions they would want from a PHR, the most frequently chosen functions were: e-mailing providers, tracking immunizations, noting mistakes in the record, transferring information to new doctors, and getting test results.[24]

Because of the nature of the systems and studies reviewed earlier, it is difficult to gain a solid and consistent understanding of the most desirable functionality. For example, some systems allow users to view selected portions of their records, whereas others allow users access to all available sections of the record. One system, PCASSO, allowed clinicians to filter specific data as "patient deniable," thus preventing users from viewing it. MyChart, in particular, restricted the patient view, for example restricting laboratory results to certain types of laboratories and not allowing inspection of clinical notes. One third of the users of this system reported feeling that their health information was incomplete.[22] Most of the systems reviewed were overlaid on incomplete EHR systems, therefore core functionality was limited. Furthermore, some functions identified in the previously mentioned national survey as important to patients were not available in any of the systems reviewed. In none of the studies were patients allowed to make comments in their records, although SPPARO users indicated desire for this function in focus groups.[21] Also not available was the ability to transfer information to a specific provider, particularly a provider outside of the healthcare system involved. All systems provided access to at least some test results, several offered access to clinical notes, and a few offered the opportunity to e-mail clinicians in a secure messaging system. How systems approached providing the three functions, laboratory results, clinical notes, and e-mail, will be discussed along with reported patient reactions to the functions when available.

Laboratory Results

Laboratory results proved to be a highly useful function for patients in every system. A central question is whether test results should be available to patients before being discussed with providers. A solution used by PCASSO researchers was to filter "pending" or "interim" test results and only display final results.[16] Patients in the MyChart study did not report concern about having access to laboratory results before seeing the clinician, and wanted more tests available to them online.[22] PatCIS and SPPARO users reported that the ability to follow laboratory results before visiting the clinician was an advantage of the system.[17,21] PCASSO designers reasoned that patients are always made aware of laboratory tests being done, and any definitively diagnostic test, such as a biopsy, would not likely offer a surprise.[16] However, pending results were not provided to patients and a triage information hotline was offered in response to potential clinical questions. The PAMFOnline system allows laboratory results to be available to users after being automatically delayed to allow clinicians to view them first.[23]

Clinical Notes

Access to clinical notes seems to be well received by patients in general, although not all of the systems offered this capability. One system, SPPARO, evaluated the effect of allowing users to view notes over a long period of time. Viewing notes was a widely used function in this system, with the highest number of hit-days overall.[21] A potential effect of allowing patients access to their health records is that clinicians may change the style of documentation. Three of seven clinicians in a focus group felt that they had changed their style of documentation in order to allow patients to understand content, but felt that the difference in time spent documenting was trivial; they even felt that the change was for the better.[21] Clinicians involved in the MyChart project reported discomfort with allowing patients to read notes, particularly about sensitive issues.[22] The PCASSO system allowed viewing of notes, although clinicians were able to assign a status of "patient deniable" to parts of the record, thus preventing the viewing of those sections; psychiatric notes were automatically given this label.[16] The effect of patient access to clinical notes was not evaluated separately in this project, although patients were satisfied overall with the system, the majority feeling that having access was "very valuable."[25]

E-mail

Previous studies have investigated the feasibility and results of offering e-mail capacity to patients and have found high levels of satisfaction by patients and moderately high acceptance by clinicians.[26] Three major issues are involved in providing e-mail to patients: Security, compensation, and the ability to triage messages. Providing e-mail within a patient-accessed EHR is an important function because it provides a higher level of security for communication as well as the ability to automatically triage messages. MyChart took this approach by offering e-mail within the system, offering an additional level of security. Users of MyChart who responded to a questionnaire reported finding the e-mail function within the system easy to use, although level of usage was not reported. Users in this study preferred using e-mail for certain types of communications, such as prescription renewals and obtaining general medical information, but preferred in-person interaction for other communications, such as discussing treatment instructions.[22] To address the potentially overwhelming number of e-mails, PatientSite provides secure messaging through the EHR system with an automated e-mail triage system in place. The provider, who can select specific staff to receive the appropriate type of e-mail, controls this triage. When the patient types a subject line in the e-mail, it is automatically routed to the selected staff. This approach is likely to minimize turnaround time and burden on the clinician, and is consistent with guidelines for use of e-mail by clinicians set forth in 1998.[27] Because compensation to clinicians for e-mailing patients is an issue, PAMFOnline decided to compensate clinicians for using the system by charging a small fee to patients who desire to communicate with their clinicians via e-mail.[23] Another interesting potential use for e-mail was brought up by a focus group participant in the SPPARO project, who suggested having electronic notification when any addition or change was made to their record. However, this would only have utility if it were sent to a patient's regular e-mail account.

Usability of the Patient-Accessible EHR

Overall, users found the systems reviewed to be easy to use. Most of the systems used the Internet to allow access to patients, and users of most systems were given access to a different interface than the clinicians. Users of the PCASSO system reported that the system was "very" or "somewhat" easy, regardless of their computer skill level.[15] In the UK, patients viewed their records with the same system clinicians used; this was a light-pen-based system that was not available on the Internet, but these patients found the system highly usable nevertheless.[20] Formal usability studies of the PHR interface are lacking in the current literature, pointing to a need for further study.

Comprehensibility of the Patient-Accessible EHR

One of the major problems found in providing paper chart access to patients has been illegibility. In one review of patients' responses to accessing their paper charts, only 44% of patients were able to read the clinician's handwriting, and 60% of patients had questions about vocabulary or meaning. Barring increased use of complex medical language or shorthand, legibility is likely to be less of a concern when providing access to the PHR. Vocabulary and meaning, however, are likely to remain an issue. This is supported to some extent by the published studies. One finding of SPPARO was that users found medical jargon difficult to understand.[21] When another set of patients were given one-time access to the EHR, the majority understood most of the content.[20]

In the reviewed studies, how designers handled questions in meaning varied. Users of SPPARO obtained answers to questions about medical meaning by referring to medical dictionaries, online references, friends or family, or by asking medical professionals.[21] Forty percent of respondents to the questionnaire provided by SPPARO researchers reported preferring an edited and more understandable form of the chart.[21] However, because of concern about the data being modified, focus group participants in the SPPARO study preferred an unedited version of the chart that provided links to explanations.[21] In the PCASSO project, potential patient questions were handled by having continuous on-call coverage by a biomedical librarian who had experience in assisting patients with information needs regarding serious diseases. Other implementations included automated links to explanatory information about findings. For example, PatCIS provides informational links called "infobuttons" to assist patients in the interpretation of Pap smear results.[17] PAMFOnline took this solution a step further and provided dynamic hyperlinks for words and phrases found within the record. The researchers found that a single sentence was adequate for explaining most terms found within a Pap smear report.[23] PatientSite provided links on a patient's home page, and these links could be chosen by the user as well as "prescribed" by the provider.[15]

With the potential that legibility and vocabulary will decrease as a barrier, a major issue that will require empirical investigation is the effect of the PHR on patient's ability to comprehend their own medical issues. It is likely that patients will collect data and organize knowledge in a different manner than they would with paper records. This has been shown in clinicians; after using an EHR for several months, they demonstrated evidence of changes in information gathering and reasoning, resulting in different structure and organization of clinical notes.[28] Patients also have demonstrated different cognitive understanding of medical problems than clinicians, maintaining a narrative explanation and structure of explaining illness whereas their clinicians use a pathophysiologic model of understanding disease.[29] One study reported that in focus groups, users identified that having access to their health record aided them in understanding the disease and decision-making process.[21] However, the impact of increased access to records on patients' underlying comprehension of disease is unknown.

Security and Confidentiality Issues

Of the systems presented, the PCASSO project in particular reports rigorous security. The login consisted of a username and password, which were both entered by using a graphical keyboard and mouse; a laminated random number card; and a diskette that contained a private encryption key. Patients who participated in the PCASSO project reported feeling satisfied with the login procedure, which they believed was reasonable and appropriate.[16] PCASSO providers, however, were less satisfied with the safeguards, finding them onerous.[16] Most of the other reviewed systems use a simple username and password, including the PatientSite and PAMF-Online systems. The PCASSO system passed rigorous tests against security breaches, and although none of the other projects reported system breaches thus far, it is unclear what detection or auditing system is being used.

A major issue is whether patients will be satisfied with the level of security provided in these systems. In the Connecting for Health survey, respondents selected their provider as the preferred host for their patient record; this is likely because of an assumption that confidentiality and security concerns will be addressed. Although some systems were met with satisfaction in terms of security, one study in particular demonstrated that security concerns may even increase with exposure to an online system. In the UK, users became more concerned about security after they saw their record than they had been before.[20] Other studies that assessed this issue found that some security concerns remained after having access to their medical record.[22]

Overall, it appears that providing patients with access to their records is feasible and elicits generally favorable response from both patients and clinicians. Several issues remain regarding usability of the systems, comprehensibility of the systems to lay people, and concerns about security. Questions about which functions should be included in PHRs will need to be resolved. The issues of who owns the medical information and whether clinicians will be allowed to conceal certain parts of a patient's records from the individual patient also need to be addressed. Related is the receptivity and consequence of enabling a patient to append his or her health information and the ramification of relinquishing control to the patient regarding who views it. Elucidating the patient's perspective regarding the acceptability of varied solutions to these issues is critical to the design of PHRs, as discussed in the next section.

Future Directions

The assertion in the introductory section of this chapter contends that, as patients become more informed and subsequently empowered in a patient-driven healthcare system, they will demand EHRs as tools to help them manage their health. This assertion is now qualified by one very essential caveat. Patients will demand only those EHRs that are useful to them, and others that do not meet their needs for services, cost, quality, ease of use, etc., will fail. As in other markets, the necessity and benefit of understanding and embracing the needs and demands of the customer is a differentiating business strategy.[2]

A systematic review of the literature on patient utilization of electronic medical records, conducted by Winkelman and Leonard,[30] identified characteristics that enhance or mitigate the influence of medical record structure on patient utilization of an electronic patient record. One finding was that most electronic patient records are designed for physician use for communication among physicians or between physicians and the hospital. This was observed in applications designed for comprehensive, patient-centered disease management programs in which patients are considered to be integral partners in management of their chronic disease. Based on this review, the authors concluded that the structures of prototype electronic patient record systems are constrained by the same organizational, cultural, and environmental influences as paper-based records. The authors go on to suggest that methods currently used in system research and development may not allow the online patient-accessible electronic patient records to reach its full potential as a tool to promote patient self-efficacy, empowerment, and personal responsibility.

Innovative and more patient-centered approaches to the design and evaluation of patient health records are needed to inform breakthrough systems that can best meet patient needs. For example, participatory action research (PAR) is a method to foster participation, collaboration, and mutuality of all stakeholders, and is particularly useful when empowerment is an essential goal. In PAR, the researchers become essentially facilitators, and participants become co-learners; nobody is considered the expert.[31] PAR involves commitment from all participants and requires mutual respect, trust, adaptability, and a holistic approach to problem solving.[32] Listening, dialogue, and negotiating consensus are strategies to achieve mutuality and empowerment. A participatory approach to the development process of an electronic patient health record operationalizes the partnerships among clinicians, patients, and health service providers, and thus more effectively attends to the needs, preferences, and usage behaviors of patients.[30]

The overall impression from published studies of patient health records is that they can improve certain aspects of care, but they are unlikely to substantially improve health status.[33] This perhaps reflects the fundamental limitations of EHRs that focus on information alone: A better-informed patient is not necessarily a healthier patient. Future developments in patient health records should go beyond the provision of information, and focus on enabling patients to become active participants in their care by including services that facilitate behavioral change and self-management skills. This recommendation is based on considerable research that shows the most effective chronic disease programs are those that not only increase patient knowledge about their condition, but also provide opportunities for collaboration.[34] That is, patient-identified problems are acknowledged and recorded along with the physician's medical diagnosis; goal setting and planning functions are provided to enable both patients and the healthcare team to focus on specific problems, set realistic objectives, and develop action plans for attaining those objectives when patients say they are ready to do so; provision of a continuum of self-management training and support services to which patients readily have access and that help them carry out medical regimes. Examples include learning how to use devices, for example, asthma inhalers, quitting smoking, and monitoring tools to help patients make important decisions based on the results of such self-monitoring.

Finally, not all patients are the same and therefore patient needs will vary based on several characteristics. Patients with chronic problems have different needs, for example, when compared with patients with intermittent acute medical problems.[30] Chronic diseases are apt to support long-term partnerships among healthcare providers, patients, and families and may benefit from personal input as well as online tools for decision support.[35] Some novel patient EHRs and systems are now tailoring content and knowledge resources to individual patient characteristics.[36,37]

To meet diverse patient needs, patient health records must address both health and computer literacy. Nearly one of every two US adults has difficulty understanding basic information necessary to make appropriate health decisions. This underscores the importance of simplicity in language and user interface in the patient health record. To be useful for most people in a patient health record, SNOMED and other clinical lexicons need included consumer-friendly terms.[13] Computer literacy skills particularly in older adults presents a challenge too, mainly because the opportunities for the integration of computer use into their daily life is much more difficult than they are for children, college students, and working adults.[38] However, even older adults can improve computer literacy skills when training is guided by self-directed, goal-specific tasks.[39]

President John F. Kennedy may have outlined the essential elements for meeting patient needs in EHRs in a special message to the US Congress on Protecting the Consumer Interest, March 15, 1962. In this message, he outlined the following consumer rights:

1. **The right to safety**—to be protected against products, production processes, and services that are hazardous to health or life.
2. **The right to choose**—to be able to choose from a range of products and services offered at competitive prices.
3. **The right to information**—to be given the facts and information you need to make your own choices.

4. **The right to education**—the right to learn the knowledge and skills you need to make informed and confident choices.
5. **The right to be heard**—the right to have your interests as a consumer represented.

It is perhaps most critical that patient needs be heard and that their needs be incorporated into the development and evaluation of forward-looking patient-centered health records. Meeting patient needs in the EHR sounds to most of us like a good idea. But until we answer some critical first-order questions, and then incorporate our findings to these questions into the design and evaluation of patient health records, it will remain just that—a good idea.

References

1. Institute of Medicine, Crossing the Quality Chasm. Washington, DC: National Academy Press; 2001.
2. Herzlinger RE, ed. Consumer-driven Health Care Implications for Providers, Payers and Policy Makers. Hoboken, NJ: John Wiley & Sons, 2004.
3. Barrett MJ, et al. Personalized Medicine. Cambridge, MA: Forrester Research, 2000.
4. US Census Bureau. Statistical Abstract of the United States. Washington, DC: US Government Printing Office; 2000.
5. Wu Shin-Yi, Green A. Projection of Chronic Illness Prevalence and Cost Inflation. RAND Corporation; October 2000.
6. Bethell C, Lanksy D, Fiorillo J. A Portrait of the Chronically Ill in America. Foundation for Accountability and The Robert Wood Johnson Foundation; 2002.
7. Centers for Disease Control and Prevention. National Diabetes Fact Sheet: General Information and National Estimates on Diabetes in the United States, 2000. Atlanta, GA: US Department of Health and Human Services, Centers for Disease Control and Prevention; 2002.
8. Druss BG, Marcus SC, Olfson M, Tanielian T, Elinson L, Pincus HA. Comparing the national economic burden of five chronic conditions. Health Affairs 2001;20(6):233–241.
9. McGlynn EA, Asch SM, Adams J, et al. The quality of health care delivered to adults in the United States. N Engl J Med 2003:348(26):2635–2645.
10. Steinberg EP. Improving the quality of care—can we practice what we preach? [Editorial]. N Engl J Med 2003;348:2681–2682.
11. Asch SM, McGlynn EA, Hogan MM, et al. Comparison of quality of care for patients in the Veterans Health Administration and patients in a national sample. Ann Intern Med 2004;141(12):938–945.
12. MacStravic. What good is an EMR without a PHR: health? HealthLeaders News, September 3, 2004, www.healthleaders.com. Accessed December 4, 2004.
13. Final Report of the Working Group on Personal Health: Connecting for Health, 2004. Accessed December 4, 2004.

14. Working Group on Policies for Electronic Information Sharing Between Doctors and Patients. Connecting Americans to Their Healthcare: Connecting for Health; 2004.

15. Baker DB, Masys D. PCASSO: vanguard in patient empowerment. In: Nelson R, Ball MJ, eds. Consumer Informatics: Applications and Strategies in Health Care. New York: Springer; 2004:63–74.

16. Masys D, Baker D, Butros A, Cowles KE. Giving patients access to their medical records via the internet: the PCASSO experience. J Am Med Inform Assoc 2002;9(2):181–191.

17. Cimino JJ, Patel VL, Kushniruk AW. The patient clinical information system (PatCIS): technical solutions for and experience with giving patients access to their electronic medical records. Int J Med Inform 2002;68(1–3):113–127.

18. Sands DZ, Halamka JD. PatientSite: Patient-centered communication, services, and access to information. In: Nelson R, Ball MJ, eds. Consumer Informatics: Applications and Strategies in Health Care. New York: Springer; 2004:63–74.

19. Connecting patients and providers via the Web. New England HIMSS, 2002. Available at: http://www.nehimss.org/pubs/pubs.html. Accessed March 10, 2005.

20. Pyper C, Amery J, Watson M, Crook C. Patients' experiences when accessing their on-line electronic patient records in primary care. Br J Gen Pract 2004; 54(498):38–43.

21. Earnest MA, Ross SE, Wittevrongel L, Moore LA, Lin CT. Use of a patient-accessible electronic medical record in a practice for congestive heart failure: patient and physician experiences. J Am Med Inform Assoc 2004;11(5):410–417.

22. Hassol A, Walker JM, Kidder D, et al. Patient experiences and attitudes about access to a patient electronic health care record and linked Web messaging. J Am Med Inform Assoc 2004;11(6):505–513.

23. Tang PC, Black W, Buchanan J, et al. PAMFOnline: integrating EHealth with an electronic medical record system. AMIA Annu Symp Proc 2003:649–653.

24. Dorr DA, Rowan B, Weed M, James B, Clayton P. Physicians' attitudes regarding patient access to electronic medical records. AMIA Annu Symp Proc 2003: 832.

25. Baker DB, Masys D. PCASSO: vanguard in patient empowerment. In: Nelson R, Ball MJ, eds. Consumer Informatics: Applications and Strategies in Health Care. New York: Springer; 2004:63–74.

26. Liederman EM, Morefield CS. Web messaging: a new tool for patient-physician communication. J Am Med Inform Assoc 2003;10(3):260–270.

27. Kane B, Sands DZ. Guidelines for the clinical use of electronic mail with patients. The AMIA Internet Working Group, Task Force on Guidelines for the Use of Clinic-Patient Electronic Mail. J Am Med Inform Assoc 1998;5(1): 104–111.

28. Patel VL, Kushniruk AW, Yang S, Yale JF. Impact of a computer-based patient record system on data collection, knowledge organization, and reasoning. J Am Med Inform Assoc 2000;7(6):569–585.

29. Patel VL, Arocha JF, Kushniruk AW. Patients' and physicians' understanding of health and biomedical concepts: relationship to the design of EMR systems. J Biomed Inform 2002;35(1):8–16.

30. Winkelman WJ, Leonard KJ. Overcoming structural constraints to patient utilization of electronic medical records: a critical review and proposal for an evaluation framework. J Am Med Inform Assoc 2004;11(2):151–161.

31. Walker ML. Participatory action research. Rehab Counseling Bull 1993;37:2–6.
32. Brydon-Miller M. Participatory action research: psychology and social change. J Soc Issues 1997;53:657–666.
33. Ross SE, Moore LA, Earnest MA, Wittevrongel L, Lin CT. Providing a Web-based online medical record with electronic communication capabilities to patients with congestive heart failure: randomized trial. J Med Internet Res 2004;6(2):e12.
34. Von Korff M, Gruman J, Schaefer J, Curry SJ, Wagner EH. Collaborative management of chronic illness. Ann Intern Med 1997;127(12):1097–1102.
35. McKay HG, Feil EG, Glasgow RE, Brown JE. Feasibility and use of an Internet support service for diabetes self-management. Diabet Educ 1998;24: 174–179.
36. Doupi P, van der Lei J. Towards personalized Internet health information: the STEPPS architecture. Med Inform Internet Med 2002;27(3):139–151.
37. Kukafka R, Lussier YA, Eng P, Patel VL, Cimino JJ. Web-based tailoring and its effect on self-efficacy: results from the MI-HEART randomized controlled trial. Proc AMIA Symp 2002;410–414.
38. Poynton TA. Computer literacy across the lifespan: a review with implications for educators. Computers in Human Behavior. In Press.
39. Cody MJ, Dunn D, Hopin S, Wendt P. Silver surfers: training and evaluating Internet use among older adult learners. Commun Educ 1999;48:269–286.

5
The Electronic Health Records System in Population Health[a]

HELGA E. RIPPEN and WILLIAM A. YASNOFF

Population health covers a diverse set of fields ranging from public health to research. Without accurate, valid, and cost-effective collection and dissemination of health information at the point of care, activities in population health cannot be efficient or effective. This chapter (1) discusses how ubiquitous, interoperable, networked, electronic health records systems (EHR-Ss) for healthcare providers and consumers can support population health activities, (2) describes specific functions of the EHR-S relevant to population health, and (3) identifies some challenges that the EHR-S presents to population health.

Population Health and the EHR-Ss

The term population health is defined as organized efforts focused on the health of defined populations in order to promote and maintain or restore health, to reduce the amount of disease, premature death, and disease-produced discomfort and disability.[1] In this context, population health spans several fields such as traditional public health, disease management, research, quality assurance, and policy. Examples of public health activities include surveillance, investigation, intervention, outreach, education, evaluation of infectious, chronic, and emerging diseases, environmental health, and bioterrorism preparedness and response. Research extends beyond clinical research to include topics such as health systems research, metrics on the effects of health information technology, and the dissemination of research findings into practice. Population health also includes best practices and guidelines, health promotion, and disease prevention supporting the delivery of quality health care. Moreover, it includes policy development and implementation as it relates to decisions that influence populations, such as coverage of preventive services.

---

[a] Nothing in this chapter necessarily represents the view or policy of any agency of the United States government.

Traditionally, those working in population health, e.g., public health practitioners, researchers, and policy makers, have depended on various means to obtain and disseminate health information from and to the healthcare delivery system. Many of these approaches have been expensive (such as chart pulls) or of questionable or limited quality and reliability (administrative data).[2] The development of a national health information infrastructure including the implementation of interoperable, networked, EHR-Ss provides an unparalleled opportunity to cost-effectively and appropriately access and disseminate relevant health information.

The EHR-S is a tool for clinicians and consumers to retrieve the information they need to make the best decisions at the point of care. The EHR-S may be defined as an interoperable record of an individual's past and present health status, care received, and plan of care, delivered through secure electronic systems that combine this information with decision support and workflow tools tailored to the context of care delivery.[3] It provides an interoperable system that not only can share information in an appropriate manner but also provide a conduit for delivering new information to providers and consumers. The personal health record (PHR) may also be relevant to population health. It has a broader scope, encompassing the EHR-S and other health information that the consumer deems relevant that are not captured in the clinical setting (see Figure 5-1). In order for EHR-Ss to be effective in the context of public health, they need to be ubiquitous and networked.

Although the EHR-S is focused on the clinical environment, it is critical that the systems be designed, when appropriate, to effectively interface with other systems supporting population health. For example, the EHR-S may automatically forward information on a required reportable disease to a public health system, but it would not provide population level surveillance capabilities (see Table 5-1). The public health service would interface with

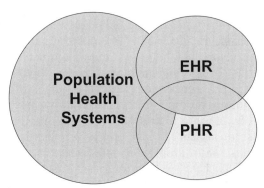

FIGURE 5-1. Systems required to support population health encompass more than what is found in EHRs. EHRs support the delivery of health care and are not designed to support population health. PHRs support the needs of the consumer in managing their health or those of a loved one and have some overlap between EHRs and population health systems.

TABLE 5-1. List of national reportable diseases[17]

Acquired immunodeficiency syndrome (AIDS)
Anthrax
Botulism
   Botulism, foodborne
   Botulism, infant
   Botulism, other (wound and unspecified)
Brucellosis
Chancroid
Chlamydia trachomatis, genital infections
Cholera
Coccidioidomycosis
Cryptosporidiosis
Cyclosporiasis
Diphtheria
Ehrlichiosis
   Ehrlichiosis, human granulocytic
   Ehrlichiosis, human monocytic
   Ehrlichiosis, human, other, or unspecified
      agent
Encephalitis/meningitis, arboviral
   Encephalitis/meningitis, California
      serogroup viral
   Encephalitis/meningitis, eastern equine
   Encephalitis/meningitis, Powassan
   Encephalitis/meningitis, St. Louis
   Encephalitis/meningitis, western equine
   Encephalitis/meningitis, West Nile
Enterohemorrhagic Escherichia coli
   Enterohemorrhagic Escherichia coli,
      O157:H7
   Enterohemorrhagic Escherichia coli, shiga
      toxin positive, serogroup non-O157
   Enterohemorrhagic Escherichia coli shiga
      toxin+ (not serogrouped)
Giardiasis
Gonorrhea
Haemophilus influenzae, invasive disease
Hansen disease (leprosy)
Hantavirus pulmonary syndrome
Hemolytic uremic syndrome, post-diarrheal
Hepatitis, viral, acute
   Hepatitis A, acute
   Hepatitis B, acute
   Hepatitis B virus, perinatal infection
   Hepatitis, C, acute
   Hepatitis, viral, chronic
   Chronic Hepatitis B
   Hepatitis C virus infection (past or present)
HIV infection
   HIV infection, adult($\geq$13 years)
   HIV infection, pediatric (<13 years)
Influenza-associated pediatric mortality
Legionellosis

Listeriosis
Lyme disease
Malaria
Measles
Meningococcal disease
Mumps
Pertussis
Plague
Poliomyelitis, paralytic
Psittacosis
Q fever
Rabies
   Rabies, animal
   Rabies, human
Rocky Mountain spotted fever
Rubella
Rubella, congenital syndrome
Salmonellosis
Severe acute respiratory syndrome-
      associated coronavirus (SARS-CoV)
      disease
Shigellosis
Smallpox
Streptococcal disease, invasive, Group A
Streptococcal toxic-shock syndrome
Streptococcus pneumoniae, drug resistant,
      invasive disease
Streptococcus pneumoniae, invasive in
      children <5 years
Syphilis
   Syphilis, primary
   Syphilis, secondary
   Syphilis, latent
   Syphilis, early latent
   Syphilis, late latent
   Syphilis, latent unknown duration
   Neurosyphilis
   Syphilis, late, non-neurologic
Syphilis, congenital
   Syphilitic stillbirth
Tetanus
Toxic-shock syndrome
Trichinosis
Tuberculosis
Tularemia
Typhoid fever
Vancomycin—intermediate
Staphylococcus aureus (VISA)
Vancomycin-resistant Staphylococcus
      aureus (VRSA)
Varicella (morbidity)
Varicella (deaths only)
Yellow fever

the EHR-S to effectively report any changes to disease patterns, e.g., drug resistant strains that would influence treatment decisions.

EHR-S Functions Relevant to Population Health

It is convenient to divide EHR-S functions into three categories for the purpose of discussing population health components. The first category is direct patient care. Although there has been much discussion and debate in the public health community about this issue, direct patient care remains an ongoing function performed by local health departments across the United States (US). To the extent that public health agencies continue to perform direct care, it should include EHR-S use. The reasons for this are similar to any other clinical environment: EHR-Ss enable more effective and efficient care by helping to assure that available patient information is accessible along with relevant decision support.

The second category is the collection of population data for public health purposes. The general availability and use of EHR-Ss in clinical care provides an unprecedented opportunity for more efficient and effective reporting of information critical to the ongoing monitoring of health status in the community. Whereas not every aspect of such reporting may directly be part of an EHR-S, any EHR-S should have the capability for selective reporting of key health events and indicators to public health. Such reporting should be automatic and electronic, thereby eliminating for all practical purposes the traditional paperwork burden that has historically been placed on providers by public health agencies (typically backed up by legal requirements).

Finally, the third category is the dissemination of population health information to providers (and patients) at the point of care. This would primarily consist of reminders generated from guidelines, typically related to preventive public health interventions. Numerous studies have demonstrated that compliance levels with widely accepted care recommendations increase significantly when patient-specific reminders are generated at the point of care.[4] It might also include general information about ongoing disease patterns and outbreaks in the community that would be helpful to providers. Also, optional patient information that the provider could pass along with public health recommendations would be included here.

Direct Care

Patient care provided by public health agencies should utilize EHR-Ss. The benefits, including better and faster access to available information, elimination of problems related to hard-to-decipher handwriting, coordination of care by all types of providers, and automatic generation of patient recall notices, are all of importance in the public health setting. In addition, the availability of patient-specific reminders to clinicians for preventive care interventions is of particular importance because providing such care is a primary focus in this environment.

Use of the EHR-S can also be helpful in identifying high-risk populations for targeting of specific interventions. For example, patients who have recently arrived from countries where tuberculosis is endemic can be flagged for more extensive testing to determine if they need treatment— before they become overtly symptomatic. The EHR-S can also help to assure that information from home visits is recorded and available to primary care providers in the clinic.

In general, the EHR-S provides the opportunity for consistent application of care guidelines and protocols, including prevention guidelines. By including such guidelines in an EHR-S system, and assuring that they are up-to-date, public health agencies can ensure that they are complying with the most recent treatment recommendations. This also minimizes missed opportunities for delivery of needed care.

A good example of the use of treatment guidelines by public health agencies is the application of childhood immunization recommendations. Each year, the Advisory Committee for Immunization Practice of the Centers for Disease Control (CDC) issues revised recommendations for the timing and sequencing of immunizations that should be given to children, as well as specific guidelines for remediation of deficiencies when vaccines are missed or delivered late. Although the basic recommendations are usually straightforward and easy for clinicians to follow, some aspects can become quite complicated, particularly for children who "fall behind" in receiving vaccines. Using the CDC recommendations in conjunction with a child's immunization history stored electronically in an EHR-S, a report of the immunizations that are needed can be produced at each visit. This allows clinicians to easily follow the recommendations without spending time or energy puzzling over any possible complexities, and reduces the risk of both over- and under-immunization.

It is important to recognize that in the population health context, just as in any other patient care environment, use of the EHR-S alone does not usually result in the availability of complete patient information at the point of care. This is because most patients receive care from multiple providers and at multiple locations in their community. This is particularly true for public health agencies, because their clinics usually provide very specific specialty care (such as diagnosis and treatment of sexually transmitted diseases) and do not typically serve as a comprehensive source of complete care. Therefore, the information about a particular patient is scattered among multiple providers in the community. Integrating this information into a complete record requires the development of community (and ultimately, nationwide) systems for exchanging of health information, so that the various subsets of information from all sites where a patient has received care can be retrieved, combined, and delivered when and where needed. Such systems are being developed in many communities, and public health agencies should participate in these efforts.

Collecting Population Data for Public Health Purposes

Central to the mission of public health is monitoring the health status of populations. It is significant that the first of the three "core functions" of public health is assessment. The Institute of Medicine recommended in 1988 that "every public health agency regularly and systematically collect, assemble, analyze, and make available information on the health of the community, including statistics on health status, community health needs, and epidemiologic and other studies of health problems."[5]

Such assessment activities represent a major portion of the activities of public health agencies. Substantial time and effort are expended in efforts to accomplish this, mostly devoted to data collection. In the context of a healthcare system based on paper records, public health has been forced to create numerous additional paper-based systems to extract information relevant to monitoring the health of the community. These systems are both expensive and inefficient, and inevitably impose an extra work burden on respondents (usually providers or their representatives). Although such systems have been absolutely necessary in the absence of an effective alternative, their inevitable implementation obstacles have resulted in the collection of only a fraction of the desired information.

To organize any intervention on a defined population and to assess the effectiveness of these interventions, information regarding that population is needed. Information on the burden of diseases on the population and their trends help policy makers prioritize interventions and understand the impact of their policies. Information about specific populations and their susceptibility to specific diseases provides researchers the information they need to understand risk factors or assess the viability of a clinical trial. Currently, there are many sources of health information. For example, the CDC collects data from birth and death records, medical records, interview surveys, and through direct physical examinations and laboratory testing so that it can provide credible information to enhance health decisions.[6] What follows are some examples of the types of information needed and how those needs would be relevant to an EHR-S.

The US government publishes *Health, United States* every year highlighting trends relevant to the health of Americans.[7] Much of the data highlighted in the report is from the National Health Interview Survey (NHIS) of the National Center for Health Statistics (NCHS), CDC. This health survey of the civilian, non-institutionalized, household population of the US provides information on the health of the US population, including information on the prevalence and incidence of disease, the extent of disability, and the use of healthcare services. An example is diabetes, which is a focus in the 2003 report. All sampled adults were asked whether a health professional had ever told them they had diabetes. From this information and what is known about the population of the US, the estimated age-adjusted prevalence of diagnosed diabetes increased from 5.3% of the adult population in 1997 to 5.6% in 2002.[7] The ubiquitous use of EHR-Ss will make it possible to assess the true prevalence and incidence of diagnosed diabetes.

The authority to require notification of cases of diseases resides in the respective state legislatures. This means that clinicians are legally required to report any new cases of a reportable disease (see Table 5-1) to their local public health department. Each case requires disease-specific information to be exchanged between the clinician and the public health department. To illustrate, currently clinicians in the state of Virginia are required to report any cases of tuberculosis (confirmed or suspected) "within 24 hours, by the most rapid means possible, preferably that of telecommunications (e.g., telephone, fax, telegraph, teletype) to the local health director."[8] The clinician is required to provide information about the patient's demographics, information about the disease, information about himself/herself, laboratory information, and results.[9] If the patient elects to receive treatment from his/her primary provider, the clinician will be required to keep the public health department informed on the course of treatment, document treatment information, and provide regular follow-up information regarding the patient via paper forms. With EHR-Ss available at the local health department and the clinician offices, appropriate information regarding the patient's relevant health information is accessible. When the public health department is treating the patient for tuberculosis it is critical that the patient's clinicians are able to access treatment information. This sharing of information is very important for assessing potential drug–drug interactions. Moreover, many aspects of the reporting, treatment, and monitoring such as treatment protocols, can be automated, ensuring that the most appropriate treatment is provided.

In the case of clinical trials, the ability to identify and enroll patients with very specific characteristics is often very costly and is critical to the success of the trial. There are several ways that patients are currently recruited by researchers. One method is through disease registries. This approach identifies patients with a specific disease but may not identify other significant aspects of a patient's history to ensure appropriateness for inclusion in the study. The research team contacts the patient directly to inquire whether there is interest in participation. Other approaches for study recruitment include (1) posting online, e.g., ClinicalTrials.gov, which describes open studies that are available and relies on patients finding the information and self-selecting; (2) reaching out to clinicians through education campaigns or advertisements so that they refer patients; or (3) having researchers directly assess hospital medical records and recruit eligible hospital patients.

A ubiquitous EHR-S could enable the identification of consumers with the appropriate characteristics for a study who would benefit most from participation. The consumer could note whether or not they would agree to be notified about clinical trials and, once notified, determine if they want to participate in the study. Another approach would be to have physicians flagged, through their EHR-S, as to which of their patients could be eligible to participate in a clinical trial.

These examples illustrate how the EHR-S can be used by the population health sector. For this to be possible, EHR-Ss need to be ubiquitous, interoperable, and standards-based to facilitate the appropriate transfer of health information for population health purposes as allowed by law. In the case of population health initiatives that require additional information, the EHR-S should allow a seamless interface into other population health applications. For example, clinical research requires that certain information be blinded as well as additional information not typically used for patient care (such as institutional review board approval). If the clinician is treating a patient in a clinical trial, their EHR-S should be able to interface with a clinical trial system to provide any additional needed functionality.

As EHR-Ss are increasingly adopted in health care, most of the health status information needed to monitor the community's health will become electronic. Selection and reuse of this information for public health can potentially be very efficient and inexpensive. To realize this potential, public health reporting ideally should be incorporated into EHR-Ss as they are deployed; retrofitting such capabilities could itself prove prohibitively expensive.

Therefore, public health agencies, led by the CDC, have begun the task of defining the specifics of exactly what items of information are needed under what circumstances, as well as defining standard transactions (e.g., using Health Level-7, or HL7) for electronic transmission to public health. For example, under the leadership of the CDC, HL7 adopted as standards the transactions needed to report childhood immunization events to public health for incorporation in immunization registries.

However, much more work remains in this critical area. Many additional transactions need to be defined for disease and syndrome reporting. Whereas in some circumstances, every event of a particular type would be reportable (e.g., cases of rabies), much of the information of interest to public health would only be reported in selected circumstances (e.g., suspicious rashes in children or young adults after the detection of a case of meningitis). In addition, it would be extremely helpful if the sensitivity and selection criteria for reporting could be dynamically changed by public health authorities when needed for more intense monitoring or investigation of disease outbreaks or other adverse health events.

To accomplish this, specific computer-processable rules defining the circumstances under which electronic health information is to be reported must be developed. Furthermore, standardizing the representation of these rules would greatly aid in their incorporation into EHR-Ss, as well as allowing for dynamic changes when needed.

EHR-Ss should be capable of producing and sending standardized reporting transactions to public health authorities. In addition, they should have the capability to change the selection criteria for those transactions. Ideally, these capacities should be flexible enough to deal with newly defined reporting requirements as they are developed.

Disseminating Health Information to Providers at the Point of Care

A key element in improving population health is communicating to providers and patients about available actions to prevent disease and reduce its impact. Although changing health-related behavior is always challenging, the process cannot even begin without information about the reasons for and benefits of specific changes. Once this groundwork has been laid, it has been repeatedly demonstrated that consistent delivery of preventive care is greatly enhanced when reminders are provided at the point of decision.

Providing health-related information for population health purposes is one clear requirement for the EHR-S. Another requirement is the capability of the EHR-S to help implement public health interventions when appropriate. The success of any such intervention is dependent on its ability to influence the individual consumer. This is true for all areas within population health. The EHR-S can facilitate this in several ways. First, it can provide decision support that enables the implementation of the public health intervention directly to the consumer, through the clinician at the point of care. Second, it can provide a vehicle of communication to clinicians to influence the care they provide to the consumer. Third, it can provide educational information to clinicians, and through them, to the consumer. And fourth, it can reach out directly to consumers, through the EHR-S component of the PHR, providing consumers the information they need to influence their health directly.

The importance of implementing public health interventions through EHR-S is illustrated by the following example. A national public health initiative led by the federal government is Healthy People 2010. It highlights 28 areas (see Table 5-2) and has two main goals for improving health in the US: Increase the quality and years of healthy life and eliminate health disparities. Many of the listed areas can effectively be implemented through EHR-Ss. This is supported by published studies showing that EHR-Ss are effective in increasing the delivery of best practices such as preventive

TABLE 5-2. Healthy people 2010 focus areas[18]

Access to quality health services
Arthritis, osteoporosis, and chronic back conditions
Cancer
Chronic kidney disease
Diabetes
Disability and secondary conditions
Educational and community-based programs
Environmental health
Family planning
Food safety
Health communication
Heart disease and stroke
HIV
Immunization and infectious diseases
Injury and violence prevention
Maternal, infant, and child health
Medical product safety
Mental health and mental disorders
Nutrition and overweight
Occupational safety and health
Oral health
Physical activity and fitness
Public health infrastructure
Respiratory diseases
Sexually transmitted diseases
Substance abuse
Tobacco use
Vision and hearing

health services. For example, the use of reminders in an EHR-S increased the number of mammograms (28.7% to 52.5%), varicella immunizations (29.6% to 55.9%), glycosylated hemoglobin (53.0% to 80.3%), and influenza immunization for persons with diabetes (29.7% to 55.1%).[10] These interventions directly improve the health of the population.

Public health has a long history of producing guidelines for preventive care. CDC has made specific efforts to collect and electronically distribute these guidelines online (see http://www.phppo.cdc.gov/cdcRecommends/AdvSearchV.asp). However, the widespread adoption of EHR-Ss provides a tremendous opportunity for improving population health by incorporating these guidelines into reminder systems at the point of care.

Many of the major benefits of EHR-S use derive from its decision support capability, which has been shown to reduce both errors and costs. Such decision support is implemented with the use of care guidelines that have been encoded for computer processing. For example, one such guideline is "if the patient is age 65 or over, and has not received a pneumovax vaccine to prevent pneumococcal pneumonia, it should be given unless there is a contraindication." Such encoded rules are then used to generate reminders to clinicians—these reminders increase compliance with guidelines.

Public health should take advantage of this opportunity to improve compliance by ensuring that prevention guidelines are encoded and incorporated into EHR-S decision support systems. A first step toward this goal is to create unambiguous flow diagrams that embody the logic of each guideline. This will facilitate efforts by EHR-S vendors and provider organizations to incorporate prevention guidelines in existing systems that have decision support capabilities. Because most guidelines are presented in prose format, there are typically many ambiguities and uncertainties that must be resolved to translate this into a form that is suitable for computer encoding.

Second, the public health community must continue working closely with standards development organizations, such as HL7, to develop and promote adoption of a standard for representation of clinical guidelines within EHR-Ss. Such a standard would allow rapid and inexpensive dissemination of guidelines and facilitate their incorporation into EHR-Ss. It would also greatly ease the task of distributing revised and updated guidelines.

Finally, once a standard for representation of clinical guidelines is adopted, public health should translate all prevention guidelines into this standard format. Also, as new guidelines are developed, their release should include the standard representation so that they can immediately be used in EHR-Ss.

Clinicians should insist that their EHR-Ss have decision support capabilities, and that they support guidelines in the standard format, once it is developed and adopted. Then, through close collaboration with public health agencies, providers can ensure that prevention guidelines are included in their EHR-S's decision support portfolio.

Another potential use for EHR-Ss is to provide a communication channel to providers for public health information, such as treatment protocols during an outbreak. Until the capability for rapid distribution of encoded guidelines is fully implemented, such messages will need to be transmitted through other mechanisms. For example, clinicians need to be alerted about emerging diseases or bioterrorist events. This has been highlighted by the anthrax cases in September of 2001, the severe acute respiratory syndrome (SARS) pandemic, and the monkeypox. To support clinicians in making these diagnoses and providing the best care, they need to know what symptoms to look for and when, as well as the best treatment modalities. For example, informing clinicians of a new SARS case in their region will alert them to watch for the appropriate symptoms, speed diagnosis, limit spread, and save lives.

In the context of clinical research, providing consumers with an opportunity to participate in the latest clinical trials and receive the best care available is important. Moreover, the tools available in an EHR-S can also facilitate the delivery of clinical trial treatments in nonacademic centers allowing more consumers an opportunity to get the most innovative care.

To facilitate this delivery of population health interventions to the consumer, the EHR-S must provide the specific capabilities such as the following:

- Review and update public health interventions appropriate for the clinical setting.
- Implement public health interventions appropriate for the clinical setting (e.g., decision support).
- Tailoring interventions to consumer and clinical practice characteristics (be it for education, prevention, best clinical interventions based on new clinical research, a bioterrorist event, an epidemic, or to ensure best practices).
- Alert clinicians regarding public health events that may influence treatment or practice decisions (e.g., upper respiratory symptoms during a SARS outbreak, how to minimize practice contamination, drug recall).
- Identify clinical trials or other interventions.
- Provide educational information (for the consumer or clinician).

Population Health EHR-S Challenges

The effective use of the EHR-S to promote population health faces a number of challenges. Two key challenges will be highlighted here: (1) privacy, and (2) policy considerations.

Privacy

The ability to aggregate all of an individual's health information across all of their providers over their lifetime and make it available remotely has significant implications for privacy. Moreover, privacy is a major concern to consumers.

The Health Insurance Portability and Accountability Act (HIPAA) privacy rule creates national standards to protect individuals' medical records and other personal health information:

- *It gives patients more control over their health information.*
- *It sets boundaries on the use and release of health records.*
- *It establishes appropriate safeguards that healthcare providers and others must achieve to protect the privacy of health information.*
- *It holds violators accountable, with civil and criminal penalties that can be imposed if they violate patients' privacy rights.*
- *And it strikes a balance when public responsibility supports disclosure of some forms of data—for example, to protect public health.*[11]

In the context of public health,

Balancing the protection of individual health information with the need to protect public health, the Privacy Rule expressly permits disclosures without individual authorization to public health authorities authorized by law to collect or receive the information for the purpose of preventing or controlling disease, injury, or disability, including but not limited to public health surveillance, investigation, and intervention.

Public health practice often requires the acquisition, use, and exchange of protected health information (PHI) to perform public health activities (e.g., public health surveillance, program evaluation, terrorism preparedness, outbreak investigations, direct health services, and public health research). Such information enables public health authorities to implement mandated activities (e.g., identifying, monitoring, and responding to death, disease, and disability among populations) and accomplish public health objectives. Public health authorities have a long history of respecting the confidentiality of PHI, and the majority of states as well as the federal government have laws that govern the use of, and serve to protect, identifiable information collected by public health authorities.[12]

In the context of research, there are several caveats (for details see Clinical Research and the HIPAA Privacy Rule[13]). HIPAA applies and the privacy rule does permit, *"under section 164.512(i)(1)(ii), a covered entity to provide investigators with access to PHI for purposes preparatory to research, such as for purposes of identifying potential human subjects to aid in study recruitment, among other things. Such access is permitted provided that the covered entity receives certain required representations from the researcher and the researcher does not remove any PHI from the covered entity during the course of the review."*[13]

The privacy issue is a critical one for all applications of the EHR-S. Medical information is often extremely sensitive and privacy violations cannot be fully remedied with monetary damages. Citizens are particularly sensitive to medical information collected by the government, including public health agencies that ostensibly are using it for the benefit of the community. Although there is great concern about the adverse consequences of our current paper-based healthcare records, including the challenges it poses to rapid detection of disease outbreaks, there is not a general desire to sacrifice personal privacy any more than absolutely necessary as EHR-Ss are adopted.

The ability of EHR-Ss to capture and aggregate information from all clinicians will remove some of the current strategies used by consumers to maintain confidentiality, such as seeing another doctor. So how will consumers control access? Consumer control over who sees what part of their comprehensive EHR-S is a policy that has been supported by many organizations and countries as they move forward to nationwide implementation of EHR-Ss. For example, Australia has a policy of patient control for access to their EHR-S.[14]

When patients are able to control access to their EHR-S, there are many options with varying effect on population health. Health information sharing required by regulations still must be accomplished. Table 5-3 highlights options and their consequences.

There are also some interesting implications of not sharing the entire EHR-S with clinicians. Is privacy violated if the decision support system does a drug–drug interaction check using controlled-access data? Who should get the notification of a potentially life-threatening event? To what level of granularity is the information controlled? Is it at the clinician, visit, or specific entry level?

From a public health perspective, the ability of consumers to control even de-identified health information would limit the usefulness of the EHR-S in population health. If the sharing of de-identified health information is allowable, it will be important to provide a key to identify an individual when necessary. For example, identified information on those not having had a mumps vaccine during an outbreak in a community is desirable. There can be a targeted intervention of vaccination or care to avoid contact with an infected person.

TABLE 5-3. Implications of consumer or clinician control of information to population health

	Clinician Implication	Population Health Implications	Comments
Control of de-identified data	N/A	Biased sample, smaller sample	Provides minimal protection to the individual while adversely affecting population health
Permission to "profile" for research or public health	May change treatment course for patient, e.g., clinical trials, public health interventions, etc.	Provides targeted interventions and information to consumers and their clinicians	
Emergency access	Able to get basic health information relevant to an emergency for best treatment	Provides re-identification during an emergency (e.g., outbreak)	Specifications regarding when there is a population health emergency need to be codified
Limit access to all or part of EHR	Acceptability and liability issue regarding treatment and "unknown" history	Incomplete or nonparticipant bias concern	
Control of key to re-identify consumer	N/A unless it is the provider that has the key	When there is a legally supported need to know or consumer provided consent	

Healthcare providers are interested in delivering high-quality health care to their patients. These providers have an obligation to use EHR-Ss and to implement population health recommendations when appropriate. However, there are different interpretations of population health and the tension between the providers of health services to an individual versus a population. This is highlighted by the quote, "You cannot practice on the individual and serve the collectivity and be the equivalent servant of both at the same time."[15]

Therefore, population health activities must be very sensitive to the need to maintain the public trust. Measures such as clear and open statements about privacy policies, transparent accountability for information use, and independent review of information practices can all be helpful. In addition, public education about the true nature of risks related to inadvertent release of well-protected electronic information may be useful. The natural tendency of the mass media to focus on sensational examples of improperly released information (often caused by sloppy security and personnel practices) has resulted in an unnecessarily heightened concern about these issues for many people. Finally, well-crafted and consistently enforced personnel policies with respect to privacy (e.g., annual signed confidentiality statements, use of strong passwords, and application of best practices in computer security) will help prevent incidents and reinforce publicly stated goals of protecting information from unauthorized use.

Policy Considerations

In the policy domain, population health faces a number of difficult issues. Clear policies for use of identified, de-identified, and re-identifiable data must be developed. The policy aspects of centralized versus decentralized data repositories must be addressed. The ability of public health authorities to query clinical databases (particularly in an emergency) must be established, while balancing this with the requirement for continued efficient delivery of care. Special agreements may be needed in emergency situations. These should be negotiated in advance; an emergency is not the time to engage in a legal discussion of the implications of access to information, or to work with technical staff to implement an urgently needed new interface or query capability. However, many policy issues remain vexing questions, without clear or easy answers.

There is general agreement that the structure of a national health information infrastructure should not be a centralized database.[16] These issues are the same for population health and an aggregated database from EHR-S extractions.

- A centralized database of all "relevant" clinical information for 280 million plus Americans that spans the course of their life is an enormous database.
- The cost, design, and performance of such a system would be high.

- The risk to consumers would be high in a centralized data model. Once access is obtained, more damage can be done in this type of environment than in a distributed environment.
- It seems to be contrary to what would be acceptable to Americans at this time. People are concerned about inappropriate access to their sensitive health information.

But are databases of aggregated information necessary for population health and, if so, under what circumstances? To answer that question, each aspect of population health needs to be independently assessed. Some examples are highlighted in Table 5-4.

When are studies of the entire population really necessary as opposed to a sample? Is it better to design a study that identifies the information needed as opposed to a study that has limited data around which the study is designed?

Policies for the handling of health information are critical from a consumer's perspective but also from a data ownership angle. Should population health interventions require queries to all EHR-Ss directly or through a distributed query authority? What is the impact of such queries on normal operations? What about in emergencies?

Clinical guidelines and decision support algorithms are one way in which population health interventions can be delivered to the clinical setting. Currently, there are many organizations developing clinical guidelines and algorithms. How will this information be disseminated? Who has the responsibility? How are decision support algorithms encoded into EHR-Ss? Who maintains them?

One of the recurring issues in the evolution of EHR-Ss is the difficulties in correctly identifying individuals so that information is grouped appropriately. Moving forward without a national identifier, many have developed strategies to facilitate the correct matching of personal health information. There is now general consensus that the problem of identification of individuals' data can be adequately addressed without a national identifier.

Another aspect to consider is the long-term storage of these EHR-S records. How long is a provider required to store health information on patients? What if he/she sells the practice, moves, or retires? Should there be a warehouse that can be used to store this information for families or research? After a certain amount of time, should the information on the EHR-S be made available for population health purposes?

As the public health systems interface with EHR-Ss, who has the responsibility to maintain the integrity and operation of the interface? Will the public health savings in data collection be used to develop public health systems or support the implementation of EHR-Ss (or both)?

A nationally networked, interoperable EHR-S will only provide information on populations receiving care. Currently, more than 40 million

TABLE 5-4. Examples of categorizing data needs and questions to consider

Examples	Data Needs	Questions to Consider
Disease surveillance	Disease surveillance, need time trend data to identify changes or shifts over time	What information is necessary? How is it to be used? Limited data with the ability to do time studies later (research query)
Clinical research	Need clinical and demographic information relevant to the trial study. Current statistical software tools require certain data structures for analysis	What data are replicated from the EHR for evaluating the clinical trial? How long will this information be kept? Should the extracted data be de-identified (with key)?
Clinical research—subject identification, recruitment, retrospective studies	Need the ability to identify appropriate subjects and facilitate recruitment for clinical trials or retrospective studies	Are disease registries needed? If EHRs can inform potential subjects, does this change the need? If research queries are possible, how would disease registries operate?
Public health education	Target tailored messaging to the appropriate group	How will the EHR overlap with the PHR? What is the clinician's role as an intermediate?
Immunization	Need immunization prevalence to ensure herd immunity. Identify nonimmunized when intervention is needed	What is the future role of the immunization registry?
Best practices	Determine how well clinicians are following best practices	With decision support, how will clinicians maintain current algorithms? How can clinicians follow their judgment without risk of liability? Who will be responsible for tracking outcomes?

Americans are uninsured. Many individuals use factitious identifying information that may limit population health interventions. There are also consumers that do not receive care frequently enough to allow population health interventions to be realized. Moreover, there are even more people that would not have access to their EHR-S (through their PHR) to gain any direct benefit from those interactions. What strategies can be put in place to minimize the effects of these issues?

Finally, it is also unclear how current population health practices may change in an environment where ubiquitous, interoperable EHR-Ss are present. Some thoughts on the implications of this change in environment are noted in Table 5-5. EHR-Ss may eliminate the need for several public

TABLE 5-5. Comparison of current population health practice and with fully implemented interoperable EHR

Area	Examples of Information and Direction	Current Practice	EHR Potential Practice	Comments
Facilitating care to consumers	Education to consumers regarding a health issue relevant to the population	Print, media outreach	Clinician can disseminate information directly either during a visit or electronically (e-mail). [PHR can be used to reach patient directly outside of the healthcare system]	Given the limited scope of the EHR focused on health care delivered in the clinical setting, direct consumer outreach is more appropriate through a PHR (which could be tied to the EHR)
Clinical prevention guidelines	Dissemination of guidelines to providers and consumers	Print, media, and e-mail outreach to patients and providers. Limited automation into practice environment	Clinical preventive guidelines automated within the EHR	May change the need for things such as immunization registries; can track exceptions instead. May facilitate the development and validation of new prevention guidelines
Best treatment (standard of care)	Dissemination of best practices	Presentations, print, media, e-mail. Limited automation into practice environment	Best practices automated and tailored to patient's condition	May follow acceptance and application of best practices
Identifying of specific populations	Data identifying specific populations with given characteristics and appropriate treatment options from the clinical setting	Surveys, chart review, billing data, targeted clinics, and outreach	Specific populations already seen can be identified at the provider level. Logic can be set to flag for activities such as	May change the need for or future design of disease registries, clinical participation strategies, and efficient public health interventions for high-risk groups

Collecting population health data for public health purposes	Reportable disease reported to public health and recommended treatment back to clinician	Forms, phone call to public health	clinical trial participation, high-risk group targeted health interventions	
	Surveillance to public health	ED admissions (hospital), ICD codes (hospital), laboratory results, over the counter	Automating reporting from the EHR to provide "real-time" reporting	May bring clinicians closer to public health and increase their role in a disease outbreak by providing them with the most appropriate treatment protocols
			Automating reporting of symptoms for all healthcare settings	
	Disease burden to public health	ICD codes, surveys, reporting to disease registries	Automatic reporting from the EHR	
	Immunization rates to public health	Completed forms, Web sites	Automatic reporting or reporting only of those not receiving immunizations (as guidelines are automated)	This capability may provide another way of approaching immunization and may alleviate the tracking of rates in the traditional sense

Note that the EHR is limited to those populations receiving clinical care.

health activities such as immunization registries and significantly change others, for example, the National Health Interview Survey.

Summary

The EHR-S has the potential to enhance population health in direct patient care, health information collection, and more effective implementation of interventions and dissemination of information. Moreover, given the robust information environment in a clinical encounter, it is likely that additional population health needs would not drive a significant number of additional EHR-S requirements. It is likely that population health systems will need to provide a seamless interface with EHR-Ss, when appropriate, to supplement additional functionality or needs.

References

1. Wojtczak A. Glossary of medical education terms. Institute for International Medical Education. Available at: http://www.iime.org/glossary.htm. Accessed October 1, 2004.
2. Wynn A, Wise M, Wright MJ, et al. Accuracy of administrative and trauma registry databases. J Trauma 2001;51(3):464–468.
3. Electronic health record highlights. Acronym glossary and term definition. Available at: http://www.calgaryhealthregion.ca/cio/ci/projects/current/EHR-S/definitions.htm. Accessed August 31, 2004.
4. Garrett N, Yasnoff WA. Disseminating public health practice guidelines in electronic medical record systems. J Public Health Manag Pract 2002;8:1–10.
5. Institute of Medicine (US). Committee for the Study of the Future of Public Health. The Future of Public Health. Washington, DC: National Academy Press; 1988:7.
6. CDC. Data and statistics. Available at: http://www.cdc.gov/node.do/id/0900f3ec8000ec28. Accessed August 30, 2004.
7. National Center for Health Statistics. Health, United States; 2003.
8. 12 VAC 5-90-80 reportable disease list, regulations for disease reporting and control, 32.1–36 and 32.1–37. Available at: http://www.vdh.state.va.us/epi/list.asp.
9. Virginia Tuberculosis Control Laws Guidebook; 2001.
10. Gill J, Ewen E, Nsereko M. Impact of an electronic medical record on quality of care in a primary care office. Del Med J 2001;73(5):187–194.
11. Office for Civil Rights. OCR guidance explaining significant aspects of the Privacy Rule, Department of Health and Human Services. Available at: http://www.hhs.gov/ocr/hipaa. Accessed November 2004.
12. HIPAA privacy rule and public health. MMWR 2003;52:1–12. Available at: http://www.cdc.gov/mmwr/preview/mmwrhtml/m2e411a1.htm.
13. National Institutes of Health. Clinical research and the HIPAA privacy rule. Available at: http://privacyruleandresearch.nih.gov/clin_research.asp. Accessed December 2004.

14. Health Connect. Consent and electronic health records. Available at: http:// www.healthconnect.gov.au/building/Consent.htm. Accessed November 2004.
15. Foubister V. Physicians torn between two loyalties. Am Med News; May 15, 2000.
16. Yasnoff W, Humphreys BL, Overhage JM, et al. A consensus action agenda for achieving the national health information infrastructure. J Am Med Inform Assoc 2004;11(4):332–338.
17. CDC. Nationally notifiable infectious diseases United States 2004, revised. Available at: http://www.cdc.gov/epo/dphsi/phs/infdis2004r.htm. Accessed October 1, 2004.
18. DHHS. Healthy people 2010: a systematic approach to health improvement. Available at: http://www.healthypeople.gov/Document/html/uih/uih_2.htm#obj. Accessed November 2004.

Section 2
Current State

6
Scope and Sites of Electronic Health Record Systems

Joan R. Duke and George H. Bowers

The patient medical record is the primary repository of data about a person's health care. In a January 1991 report, the General Accounting Office[1] concluded that automated medical records offered great potential for improving patient care, increasing efficiency, and reducing costs. In the same year, a book published by the National Academy Press on the computer-based patient record (CPR)[2] identified three ways it would improve healthcare delivery: "First by providing medical personnel with better data access, faster data retrieval, higher quality data, and more versatility in data display. Automated patient records can also support decision making and quality assurance activities and provide clinical reminders to assist in patient care. Second, automated patient records can enhance outcomes of research programs by electronically capturing clinical information for evaluation. Third, automated patient records can increase hospital efficiency by reducing costs and improving staff productivity." All of these conclusions were good reasons, and continue to be good reasons, for adopting the automated patient record, but the actual implementation has proved to be more costly, complex, and difficult for most organizations to accomplish. In addition, for those leading-edge organizations that have fully implemented an electronic patient record, the realization of benefits has been hard to document. Even when the benefits have been documented in these organizations, the benefits are not necessarily seen as transferable to other organizations. Nevertheless, hospitals and other provider organizations are adopting CPRs with more than 50% in some stage of that investment according to the Healthcare Information Management Systems Society (HIMSS) 2003 Leadership Survey.[3]

Building on the explanation of terms in the Introduction (See Chapter 1), CPR, electronic medical record (EMR), electronic health record (EHR), and EHR systems (EHR-Ss) are used synonymously in this chapter. Their use depends on the source of the information referenced.

First, we describe the broad scope of the EHR and then the core underlying technologies. This is followed by a review of different care settings, and the implications of the settings for choices of features. We then discuss the major issues in scoping and setting EHR-Ss, using winners of The Davies Recognition Program[4] as the models for a discussion of management, functionality, evaluation, and value issues.

Scope of EHR

According to the 2003 Institute of Medicine (IOM) letter report[5] on the key capabilities of EHR-Ss, the functions include:

Health information and data: Immediate access to key information that would improve the ability of clinicians to make sound decisions in a timely manner. These data include patients' diagnoses, allergies, and laboratory test results.

Results management: Quick access of new and past test results by all clinicians involved in treating a patient that would ensure that all results are attended to.

Order entry/management: Computerized entry and storage of data on all medications, tests, and other services that would improve the quality and process of providing medical care.

Decision support management: Electronic alerts and reminders that would improve compliance with best practices, would ensure regular screenings and other preventive practices, would identify possible drug interactions, and would facilitate diagnoses and treatments.

Electronic communication and connectivity: Secure and readily accessible communication among clinicians and patients that would increase contacts among care providers involved in the care of the same patient.

Patient support: Tools offering patients access to their medical records, interactive education, and the ability to do home monitoring and self-testing that would increase the degree to which patients are engaged in their own care.

Administrative processes: Tools, including scheduling systems, that would improve administrative efficiencies and patient service.

Reporting and population health: Electronic data storage that uses uniform data standards that would enable physician offices and healthcare organizations to comply with federal, state, and private reporting requirements in a timely manner.

The primary uses cited for the record are for patient care delivery, patient care management, patient care support, patient self-management, financial, and other administrative processes. The secondary uses are education, regulation, research, public health and homeland security, and policy support.

The functional model for the EHR-S, developed under the auspice of Health Level-7 (HL7)[6], further distilled the contents of a patient record into direct care, supportive functions, and information infrastructure. The functional model is just one part of the standards that are needed to provide for the sharing of information across healthcare settings. The model defines the functional content of an EHR but does not address other issues as to the data format, content, context, or dataset. Other standards identified in the 2001 ISO/TC 215 requirements for international standards for EHRs are still needed to allow secure exchange of meaningful healthcare data to allow clinicians to share EHR information that moves with consumers/ patients from one point of care to another.

Technologies

Technologies that support the EHR vary widely in health care. Health care tends to be slower to adopt new technologies than other industries. The range of technology in health care goes from mainframe computers to the very latest in radiofrequency identification technology.

Computing Architectures

The earliest attempts at creating an electronic patient record were done using mainframe computers and dumb terminals. All of the processing occurred on the mainframe and the results were displayed on the dumb terminal. In the mid-1980s, client server architecture was introduced into health care. In this architecture, the "client" is a personal computer or workstation where processing of the data occurs. The server is a central computer that sends data to the client and then stores the resulting data. With the advent of the World Wide Web and browser technology, it became possible to develop applications that could be accessed by a simple browser such as Windows Explorer or Netscape Navigator. In this environment, the application software does not need to reside on every workstation. All three of these architectures are found in health care today.

Human Interface

Even in mainframe environments, the PC workstation has become the most common means of communicating between man and machine. Traditionally, a PC uses a keyboard and a mouse as the human interface. But there is a wide range of other devices that are found in health care for capturing information or displaying it back to the user.

- Printers
- Barcode readers
- Light pens
- Touch screens/touch pads
- Personal digital assistants
- Voice recognition

Operating Systems

The operating system is the software that controls the applications and the use of all of the peripheral equipment such as disk drives, keyboards, and monitors. There are three main operating systems that are used in health care:

- Unix
- Microsoft Windows
- Linux

Data Management Systems

The data management software is usually a separate product from the applications software. Many vendors of the CPR use standard database management systems such as Oracle or Sybase because of the powerful toolsets that come with them.

Another system that combines database management with applications software is MUMPS or M (*M*assachusetts General Hospital *U*tility *M*ulti-*P*rogramming *S*ystem). This language was developed specifically for the healthcare environment and has powerful string processing capabilities. Several vendors have their own versions of MUMPS such as MAGIC® (Meditech).

Application Software

Application software includes programming languages such as C++, HTML, and XML. It also incorporates the programming architecture, such as object-oriented programming.

Networks

The network includes the switches and routers, the cable type such as fiber optic, the network protocol such as TCP-IP, and the network speed such as gigabit. Wireless network technology is also within the scope of networks.

Standards

Standards function at different levels within the EHR, and standard organizations have an important role in specifying the standards and reflecting the needs of the user, developer, and vendor communities. Standards organizations include HL7, which has already been mentioned in reference to the functional model as one of several American National Standards Institutes (ANSI) setting healthcare standards. Other important organizations are the International Standards Organization (ISO), American Society for

Testing and Materials, and DICOM (Digital Imaging and Communication in Medicine), which is responsible for the standard for digital images.

HL7 coordinates a number of standard development bodies that contribute to representation standards needed for the EHR. These include content standards for the EHR itself, the Reference Information Model (RIM), a pictorial representation for representing the relationships among clinical data; the Clinical Document Architecture (CDA) for representing clinical documents, such as progress notes and discharge summaries and enabling their exchange; and the Arden Syntax, for representing rules within health information knowledge bases.

There are also numerous terminology standards. International Classification of Disease (ICD), Healthcare Common Procedure Coding System (HCPCS), and Current Procedural Terminology (CPT) provide a classification of terms grouped by related medical ideas that are used mainly for billing and reporting. SNOMED-CT and LOINC (Logical Observation Identifiers Names and Codes) are the most frequently used ontologies, which are structures that enable medical terms to represent concepts such as clinical findings, parts of the body, procedures, measurements, and other attributes.

Data Storage

Data storage encompasses the hardware and the architecture for actually storing the data. This includes:

- *RAID* (Redundant Array of Inexpensive Disks)
- *SAN* (Storage Area Network)
- *NAS* (Network Attached Storage)
- *DLT* (Digital Linear Tape)
- Optical disk storage

Modalities

"Modalities" is the term used to refer to medical devices that gather diagnostic and treatment information about the patient which becomes part of the CPR. Examples include:

- CT scanners
- MRI scanners
- Direct digital radiography
- Computed radiography
- Ultrasound
- Digital mammography
- Nuclear medicine cameras
- PET scanners
- Bedside monitors

In the last decade, each of these modalities has been made available in digital format, and each has seen the same upswing in adoption as the CPR, making their integration into computer-based records even more compelling.

Settings of CPR

Healthcare provider organizations are many and varied. Beyond hospitals and doctors' offices, direct patient care is increasingly provided in homes, long-term-care facilities, therapeutic centers, ambulatory surgery centers, testing facilities, and other locations. The services provided range from social services to pharmaceuticals and medical equipment, and are provided by many different types of organizations. Each of these organizations has some similar process as well as some different process and content requirements.

The following sections discuss the requirements for the major types of organization delivery care.

Ambulatory Care

In small physician offices, larger group practices, and specialty clinics, there is a need to coordinate care between their own practices and external organizations and testing centers where their patients are seen, such as hospitals, reference laboratories, and imaging centers. Primary care providers deal most often with routine care and managing chronic conditions. Specialists deal with more complex illnesses according to their medical specialty standards. Most ambulatory care is delivered in the physician's office or clinic setting, but providers are also beginning to deliver non-visit-based care through e-mails and electronic monitoring.

Ambulatory systems permit critical diagnostic information to be viewed by the clinician, as well as supporting documentation of the visits, and manipulation of the data for different views and reports. These systems may also include clinical decision support, access to medical knowledge sources, E-prescribing, and ordering of tests and other diagnostic and therapeutic services. Other features include capturing and integrating data from other sources and settings such as laboratories, and communicating with patients and consumers. These systems may also support disease management, clinical trials, and ad hoc querying and reporting.

There are a considerable number of EMR vendor offerings. Differences are in the scope of the offering, from solo practice to multifacility and multispecialty practices. There are also differences among niche products that offer only EMR functions, and products that integrate with the physician's billing systems. Variation is also found in enterprise products that integrate with the acute care record.

Hospitals

Automation of hospitals began in the 1960s with rudimentary tracking and statistical reporting systems. Soon after, financial systems followed, which automated many of the back-office administrative and financial functions. A major driver in the United States for automating financial systems in hospitals was the passage of Medicare legislation in the 1960s which required providers to provide more detail in billing. Clinical systems emerged in the 1970s to automate specific functions within specific departments such as the clinical laboratories and radiology. Later, they were interfaced to the financial systems to provide billing information. With the advent of clinical systems, the need for a patient repository became evident and the building of the patient record began with the attempt to integrate data from different systems and different modalities.

The genesis of the patient record was the clinical data repository, which began to be implemented in the 1980s. The clinical data repository contained the detailed patient data at a transaction level (e.g., admission, discharge, transfer orders, results, clinical documentation) necessary to support patient clinical care. It was environed as a collector of clinical data rather than a complete EMR. The migration of this technology to CPR during the 1990s was driven by the IOM report on the CPR[5] that set the goal for widespread CPR utilization. Progress has been slower than projected, but most hospitals have implemented clinical information systems in major areas of the hospital that contribute or utilize data in the patient records. There are a number of applications that are needed to build the information needed in an electronic patient record. Figure 6-1 is a model of some of the applications that are needed to make up a complete CPR. Replacement of the paper record has been achieved in a few hospitals and provider settings, but is now seen by many organizations as a feasible goal.

The list of vendors of CPR/EHR/EMR-Ss for hospitals appears to be large, but when one addresses the core components of the data repository, the data capture mechanism, and data display, the list narrows to 10–20 major vendors. These systems have applications that address most of the core systems and major ancillary/support department requirements as seen in Figure 6-1.

Hospitals (Rural)

Rural hospitals often benefit from networking with other hospitals and organizations for sharing patient information and services. Technologies for rural facilities include mobile equipment, Internet, telemedicine, teleradiology, and teleconferencing services support to outside centers of expertise. There are a small number of vendors of smaller and affordable application solutions as well as remote application service providers (ASPs) serving this market.

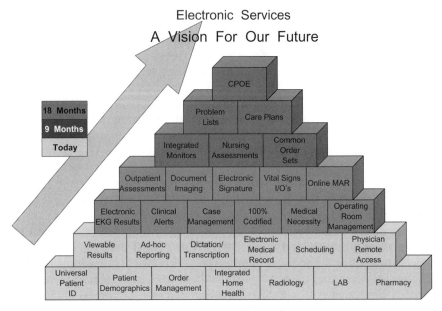

FIGURE 6-1. Building block applications for automation of clinical information in terms of a typical implementation sequence.

Integrated Delivery System

Integrated delivery systems (IDSs) are composed of hospitals, ambulatory care providers, and other related healthcare facilities such as home care, long-term care (LTC), and hospice care. An IDS provides a continuum of care to a particular population, either geographically based or based on a particular population subset or affinity group such as members of a particular HMO or veterans. These health systems were created in response to the desire of payers such as HMOs to deal with a single entity for a wide range of healthcare services.

The IDS faces the challenge of capturing and providing data to multiple types of suborganizations with multiple types of information systems. Key IDS concerns include managing geographically dispersed networks of care; mechanisms for identifying patients across multiple and potentially diverse organizations; enterprise tools for scheduling patients and managing cases; standardization of systems among multiple facilities and providers; and standardizing data within those system so that it is useful for data sharing and population analysis.

IDSs tend to be limited to the larger clinical system vendors, who have the range and depth of application components and integration tools to serve the needs of these diverse environments. Large IDS organizations associated with tertiary care hospitals have tended to be the leaders in the implementation of CPR, such as Latter-Day Saints Hospital (Utah), The Regenstrief Institute (Indiana), Partners Health Care System (Massachusetts), and The Queen's Medical Center (Hawaii).

Emergency/Urgent Care

Emergency departments (EDs) measure their performance on the timely delivery of service to patients who may present with a wide range of acute care requirements. Patients need to be triaged based on their need for care. To manage patient wait times, provide accurate and timely documentation, and reduce costs, there are increasing demands for automation within the ED.

Functions of ED systems include the patient tracking board, patient triage, chart review, nurse and physician charting, patient education and discharge instructions, charge capture, and reporting. ED systems need to be integrated with other clinical systems to send orders and receive results from ancillary systems. An emerging trend in ED systems is the ability to communicate with the emergency response team before the patient's arrival in the ED. Integration of personal digital assistants, wireless computers on wheels, telemedicine, and hands-free input modalities such as voice recognition are also important components.

Vendors for ED systems range from niche vendors to the integrated ED modules from the larger clinical system vendors. In implementing ED systems, consideration must be given to the size, location, and placement of interface devices. Integration with other ancillary systems for orders, tracking order status, receiving results, and receiving images must be taken into account when implementing these systems.

Long-term Care

LTC systems differ from acute care systems in the fact that they usually accumulate significantly more clinical information about a patient because the patient's length of stay is much longer than in an acute environment. These systems focus heavily on clinical documentation of the patient's care, especially for medication administration and nutrition. There is a requirement to maintain the patient's care plan, diet, and the minimum dataset (MDS) which is based on the level of care that sets the reimbursement rate for every LTC patient. The MDS data are used to determine and calculate other scores for payment and quality measures.

Selection of the appropriate LTC software depends on whether the system is for a single facility or for multiple facilities, and whether the facility(ies) is integrated with other care facilities in a continuing care retirement community (CCRC). In a CCRC, facilities may consist of assisted living, independent living, rehabilitation, emergency services, and physician practices. In addition, the systems may be integrated with acute care facilities external to the CCRC enterprise. Technologies in LTC, in addition to information systems, include nurse call system, fall detection and prevention, incontinence, and wander management.

There has been limited development in software packages for the LTC market because the economics (mirroring the LTC reimbursement environment) have not been favorable. LTC vendors have had limited offerings because until recently many single or small LTC facilities have not seen the need or had the money to invest in software. This market is changing with the consolidation of LTC facilities, the aging of the population, and recognition of the linkages needed for sharing of community health information.

Home Care

Home care systems provide the front-end administrative and scheduling functions, as well as clinical functions. These systems provide for the capture of a significant amount of clinical data needed for home care billing (485s), as well as the tools that allow the case workers and nurses to manage the patient. The vendor market has been highly fragmented but consolidation is occurring in the industry as data sharing becomes more important. The home care market is also changing as new services are being provided in the home, including intravenous (IV) therapy, pain control, electronic monitoring of vital signs, and other clinical measurements.

Home care system functions include referral management, administrative reporting, census management, scheduling, care plan capture, and other clinical data needed for payment. Point-of-care functions are mainly deployed on laptop or notebook computers, and include patient assessment, charting, care planning, and progress notes. A challenge with home care systems is the need for the data collected in the field to be remotely communicated to other facilities in order to receive updates such as physician orders from the central office, and to send updates on patient activities, medication profiles, and care plans. These systems are also often used for hospice care. Additional hospice functions include hospice-specific data collection and mailing, and bereavement functions to support the need to communicate with family members.

There are a number of vendors in the home care market including niche vendor products and more integrated products offered by the major EHR vendors.

Behavioral Health

Behavioral healthcare systems have similarities with other healthcare systems in that they need to register patients in ambulatory, inpatient or rehabilitation facilities, schedule appointments, credential staff and providers, document clinical history and treatment, and store data in a repository for reporting and analysis. There are unique requirements that relate to the managed care, regulatory environment, and the nature of the delivery and documentation of services in the behavioral health environment. There are significant data capture requirements from the initial evaluation, development of treatment plans, documentation of treatment, and discharge and termination summaries. In addition, the system needs to support the provider collaboration for mentally ill patients in both inpatient and community settings. It must be capable of tracking counseling and crisis management, tracking legal status and housing requirements, and addressing other human services issues. In addition to the specific functional requirements associated with psychiatric treatment, many state jurisdictions have specific privacy requirements for behavioral health data that go beyond the standard HIPAA (Health Insurance Portability and Accountability Act) privacy requirements. These systems must be capable of maintaining regulatory confidentiality while supporting the delivery of care.

There are very few software vendors that characterize their offering as strictly for behavioral health. More commonly are a number of homegrown efforts or software that has been tailored for behavioral use with a software partner. Recently, some of the larger software vendors have begun offering integrated products targeted for behavioral health (i.e., Meditech). The Indian Health Services under the Department of Health and Human Services has a Web site that has a central repository about the requirements, design, and development of integrated behavioral health applications (http://www.ihs.gov/cio/bh/index.asp).

Sharing Community Health Data

Sharing community-based healthcare information among individual healthcare organizations can enable clinicians to have appropriate and quick access to a patient's medical records. Many healthcare organizations have begun to invest in EHRs that offer connectivity within a particular hospital or a physician group practice, but there is currently no simple way for healthcare systems across a region to share information with one another. In 2001, the National Committee for Vital and Health Statistics recommended a strategy to encourage efficient and secure exchange of health information through a common EHR and through a National Health Information Infrastructure (NHII). More recently, establishment of a national health information system has become a major national priority backed by an executive order.[7]

Although there is a greater degree of interest in sharing clinical information, there are still numerous obstacles that need to be overcome including devising a universal patient identifier, agreeing on data standards, and addressing privacy concerns.

Personal Health Record

In the early 1990s, it was noted that the current healthcare system did not adequately involve the patient in problem solving and managing their own health.[8] Greater emphasis was made on patient education, particularly upon discharge. This interest has evolved into great patient participation in personal health records. A number of vendors and healthcare organizations have been focusing on the personal health record that can be used for the following:

- Help monitor continuity of patients' health care
- Record important health information about the patient
- Help patients better explain any health problems when they meet with their doctor
- Document information that may be useful when filing health insurance claims

Information included in the personal health record can contain the following:

- Personal and family medical history
- Allergies, medications, and other health status information
- Financial and insurance information
- Documentation of recent encounters
- Information about the practitioner participating in the patient's care
- Other information relevant to providers

A standard is being developed by a number of sponsoring organizations including HIMSS, HL7, American Medical Association (AMA), and physician organizations to provide a snapshot in time of the most relevant facts about patients' health care. It may be useful in standardizing the type of information in a personal health record. The continuity of care records (CCRs) is a patient-focused record that allows practitioners from different settings and disciplines to share information and that allows the patient to carry this information with him or her upon referral, transfer, or discharge. The CCR is proposed for the initial implementation of health information exchange networks as well as for the personal health record. Personal health records can help with a better understanding of the patient's role as a partner with their provider and can "overcome (the) EPRs' innate structural limitations as well, thus facilitating EPR utilization by patients."[9] See Chapter 4 for further details.

Major Issues

The Davies Recognition Program, established by the Computer-based Record Institute and continued under the auspices of the HIMSS, began in 1994 to recognize exemplary implementation of EHRs. The rationale for the Davies award was to foster wider adoption in the industry by high-lighting and sharing lessons learned from organizations. The evaluation criteria provide a useful framework for thinking about the process of implementing a CPR/EHR regardless of the setting. The four major areas of evaluation criteria[4] used by the program to assess organizations include:

- Management—the organizational aspect of the EHR strategy, planning, and implementation
- Functionality—the type of support the EHR delivers to meet the objectives of the organization and the user needs
- Technology—the technical design and architecture that enables the EHR to delivery the required functionality and performance
- Value—what the organization has accomplished and how it has measured those accomplishments

In award-winning sites, even great technology and functionality does not ensure CPR success and is frequently the least of the implementation issues. Major issues that separate success from failure are most often organizational. The major differentiators among organizations that succeed or fail are *leadership* and *management*.

Management

Vision and Strategic Direction

Regardless of the setting of the CPR, the organizational vision for electronic records and realistic goals for its implementation must be understood and communicated to the patients, physicians, board members, and others within the organization and outside of it. Executive management must be an active participant with a commitment to the programs that translate the vision into realistic expectations of accomplishment and timing. The effort must be given adequate resources (money and people), and appropriate and involved governance from executive management. Many CPR projects begin with much fanfare and excitement and then drown in the sea of complexity and cultural changes that are required to make them successful.

Goal Setting and Performance Objectives

The next step is to translate the strategic direction into a set of realistic goals that are attainable. Once these goals are articulated, the question is how well the organization measures whether the goals have been achieved. One way is to develop a business plan that addresses the investment decisions and the achievement of a financial goal. This in itself may not be sufficient. The organization must also have performance objectives, whether qualitative or quantitative, that provide measures of the desired change and relate back to the organizational goals. These may include such measures as medication and patient safety, operational efficiency, implementation of standard practices, realization of corporate objectives, staff retention, and customer satisfaction. The following value section describes some measures and results from CPR implementation.

Governance, Prioritization, and Decision Making

A steering committee needs to be active in overseeing the projects, resolving issues, reviewing status, and results. Implementing a CPR is not one project. It consists of implementing a number of integrated clinical projects and applications that collect all of the information needed in a person's longitudinal record of care.

System Selection

There are volumes written on the topic of system selection, but suffice it to say, systems are often selected based on technology bells and whistles and on overconfident vendor promises. The selection of a CPR system must be driven by the organizational priorities, evaluated by an inclusive group based on objective criteria, and verified by installation at similar sites.

Process Redesign

The organization's work or care processes must be redesigned to take advantage of the improved way of accessing and entering data. This change will affect the entire organization, affiliated and nonaffiliated physicians, and the patients. Knowing that the redesign process is traumatic and living through the disruption caused by the vast behavior change is not for the faint at heart. In successful organizations, there is an articulate executive with a long-term vision that leads the charge. There is also a physician champion who is respected, knows how to listen to his colleagues, and is able to demonstrate to his colleagues how electronic records help improve their efficiency and their ability to deliver high quality care. The combination of leadership roles is critical to overall success.

Program Management

Coordinated program management requires that clinical and operational leaders should oversee project teams consisting of clinicians and other operational staffing providing the bulk of the work. The work consists of the redesign of the clinical processes and the configuration of the system to match the clinical flow. The program must be led by a clinical person who can work hand and glove with the technology leader. It is important that the projects be driven by clinicians' needs and implemented as a clinical project rather than a technology project. Each member of the team must be an expert in their area and be able to see larger organizational goals to deal effectively with the ambiguity of such massive changes.

Risk Management

Successful project management requires that organizations look at the various risks associated with the changes associated with the project. Organizations must proactively address the risks including project failure, risks to patient, and risks to the organization. Developing appropriate strategies to deal with each type of risk includes risk identification and tracking, defining principles and rules that guide the change, and identifying ways to handle conflict and misunderstandings. There are frequently unspoken agendas associated with the move toward electronic records. Team member communication skills may be the most important skill needed to address conflict and bridge the gaps among various viewpoints.

Resource Allocation Including Money and People

There are numerous issues with obtaining and justifying the resources required to implement an EHR. HIMSS and other organizations[10] are working to help the industry define return on investment (ROI) and other outcome measures needed to gain approval and understanding from stakeholders, boards, and investors. There is also a need to link incentives for an EHR with reimbursement to the organization that is incurring the costs. Healthcare organizations and the government are aware of this disconnect and are trying to address this through performance-based payments and other incentives.

Training

Training for providers and other users is critical. The training program must be widely available and include computer-based materials that offer the user convenience in learning everything from computer skills to integrating the computer with his or her work processes. Training should also include competency testing and an evaluation form to guide training improvements. The training process goes beyond implementation and includes efforts to train new users, training for new enhancements, reinforcing fundamentals, and providing advanced training for seasoned users.

Implementation

The pace of the implementation depends on the organization and the scope of the applications. Organizations moving to a paperless environment often go "big bang" because of the difficulty of operating in a mixed computer and paper environment. Most often, the approach is to implement the system at a geographic site or a portion of the healthcare organization which operates within a shared information space. In any case, the implementation must provide a way to prove a new concept, learn from experience, and apply lessons learned to the improvement of the system and operational workflow.

Operations

Ongoing management of the CPR system is often not given enough attention. This includes the need to ensure that the data collected are reliable and complete, that security and confidentiality are effectively enabled by the system, and that the users are able to operate the system proficiently and effectively to accomplish their tasks.

Some aspects of a good operating environment include improvement in the support for clinical decisions and a feedback loop to encourage standardization based on best practices. Another focus should be ongoing improvement in the use of the system supported by training and super-users. Changes to the system must be driven by the workflow process changes rather than the special interest of a specific department or user. To ensure that a system continues to deliver effective support and gain user satisfaction, a mechanism for measuring system use and user feedback is critical.

Functionality

The IOM report defined a set of functional areas and established the IOM "Gold Standard."[1] In July of 2004, HL7, a healthcare ANSI standards organization, had put forward a ballot for the EHR Functional Model that has been accepted and can be the framework for EHR requirement documents. Other standards available from HL7[6] to help in construction of an interoperable CPR are the RIM, the CDA, templates, rules, and vocabulary standards.

There are differences in functionality based on the type of care setting and type of provider. Health and Human Services is developing policies, procedures, and criteria for data sharing for ambulatory record certification. There is also collaboration among healthcare industry organizations that recognize the healthcare industry's need for and interest in certification of EHR. This includes the American Health Information Management Association (AHIMA), HIMSS, and National Alliance for Health Information Technology (The Alliance).

There are also a number of initiatives among medical organizations to support the adoption of EHR technology including the AMA (July 2004) and Physicians Electronic Health Record Coalition (PEHRC). These standards, certification processes, and organizational assistance will all help the organizations acquire full-functioned interoperable CPR systems. Along with such initiatives, the aspects identified below present a way to view CPR systems to determine if they contain comprehensive functions for a particular health setting.

- The role of the provider as a system user and as a creator of data collected by the CPR

- The ability to implement and manage the replacement of the paper record with an electronic record
- The outcome or results gained from using the CPR

The most important aspect of a CPR system is the *extent of its use by providers*. Visiting fully automated CPR sites, there is a noticeable difference in that providers are using some type of computation device and there is an absence of paper. This is the best indicator that the CPR system has been successfully integrated into the provider's workflow.

Another difference in successful sites is the *wide access and availability of information*. A fully implemented CPR site contains computing devices used by all types of personnel to view current and historical information about the patient, and offers access to that information at any location including remote sites such as the provider's home or office.

Another key differentiator in CPR systems is the *extent of data capture* and the *availability of all of the necessary patient data in electronic form*. The complexity of capturing multimedia data from many types of testing equipment, various providers, and many locations is a challenge that has baffled vendors and users of information systems. Early systems captured one type of data for a specific operation such as registration, orders, or laboratory data. The difference in fully utilized CPR systems is that all the patient care data are captured and are electronically accessible so that the paper record can be eliminated.

To become paperless, the CPR system must make it easy for providers to enter data into the system and give them added information value. This means that the structure of the information presented and the data collection is made relevant to various settings of care and different medical disciplines. Data not captured within a particular CPR system must be integrated from various external systems. To obtain data from external system sites and different testing modalities, the CPR system may be interfaced, where discrete data elements are transferred electronically. Reports or results may also be scanned and/or sent as text reports. It is much better if the data can be collected as discrete, reusable data elements to enable the reuse of the data for analysis and ad hoc reporting. To do this requires the need for extensive standardization. Organizations that move to reliance on the electronic patient record often have to adopt strategies that are less than ideal in terms of capturing standard or structured data.

An additional factor in becoming paperless is the integration of all of the components of the providers' workflow on a well-designed data capture medium to encourage the use of the CPR. The CPR system must support the provider's workflow so that there is no need for the paper chart. It may appear counterintuitive, but implementing a provider order entry system can facilitate the provider use of computer-assisted documentation.[11]

The third aspect of evaluating CPR systems is how the data collected can influence outcomes. The result of using a CPR at the point of care improves the availability of information and can enhance the clinical decision process. Alerts and rules can be used to identify missing prerequisites, inconsistent therapies, order conflicts, and deviation from policy or standard practice. The alerts can also link to relevant external medical knowledge bases for discipline-specific knowledge and the latest in clinical research. The alerts, prompts, and rules are useful in guiding provider decision. Useful is the key factor. Many attempts have failed because the alerts and rules do not accommodate patient or provider differences and they become annoyances instead of helpful suggestions.

The use of CPR systems can also support clinical practice standardization. CPR systems with standard clinical pathways, data collection templates, order sets, and documentation templates based on specific problems, communicate standards or "best practices" among providers. They also promote operational efficiency through designs that are engineered to reduce process steps and promote patient safety.

Another more subtle outcome measure of CPR use is simply the extent of its use. If the CPR improves the care delivery workflow and the communications needed within and across settings, healthcare professionals will have an incentive to use it. It can transform the care process and lead to more timely completion of the care delivery tasks and more effective sharing of information among healthcare professionals. This is a benefit within itself, and in time may be demonstrated in improved patient outcomes. This is research that still remains to be done.

The ability to use the data collected during care for analysis of variances in care patterns and to recommend improvements in the delivery process is another way the CPR can help achieve better patient outcomes. This can be done within an individual institution or aggregated in studies of practice patterns in a geographic area. There are many secondary uses of the collected data including vital health statistics, population health risks, biosurveillance, and registries.

In considering the ability to influence outcomes, the least studied is the ability to influence health outside of the care facility. This is the opportunity for patients to access the system for educational material and self-management of their care. The patient, as a user of information, can review their own record, communicate with the physician, and use the data to make better decisions about their own care.

Technology

Technology is the utility upon which the CPR resides. In the early days of the CPR, technology was all important because it was frequently the limiting factor in the capabilities of the CPR. As technology has become more powerful, it is important to separate out the information aspects of the CPR from the technology aspects to ensure that the right tools and services are in place for a reliable and responsive system supporting patient care. The technology must support the operational requirements, delivering the required functionality and performance.

System Architecture Including Data Model, Integration, Scalability, New Technologies

In reviewing the system, one can examine the hardware, database management, data storage, multimedia capabilities, and input modalities, but it is more important to identify the service requirements from the technology rather than focusing on the type of technology used. The reason lies with the nature of technology itself. In the 1980s, the lifespan of a particular technology from the time it emerged from the laboratory until the time it was rendered obsolete could be measured in decades. The 88-column punch card as a means of storing and inputting data came into widespread use in the 1950s and was still in use in the 1990s, long after it was considered obsolete. Today, technology moves at a much faster pace. The lifespan of a given technology may be measured in months. Some technologies become obsolete before they have had a chance for widespread adoption. The 100-MB Zip drive is an example of such a technology. But the underlying service requirements are going to be the same. The technology supporting them will be the variable factor.

Rather than describe particular technologies that may become obsolete as this book is printed, it is more important to describe the requirements of the technology as they relate to the CPR. These requirements will be ongoing but ideally newer technology will make it easier, faster, and cheaper to support them.

High Availability

A key requirement is that the CPR data are stored in a safe and secure environment and delivered with high availability. In the past, healthcare organizations developed disaster recovery plans that took into account the type of data by application and the longest period of time the organization could go without access to the application. In the era when the CPR is mission-critical to diagnosis and treatment, any downtime is unacceptable.

An additional factor has been the explosion in healthcare data storage requirements, being driven by large volumes of images as well as voice and data. Adequate storage with immediate recoverability is the goal. Health care has begun using high availability storage architecture that has been in use for many years by the financial and insurance industries. This architecture uses techniques such as data mirroring, multiple redundant servers, and grid computing to meet the high availability requirements.

High Performance

High performance goes hand-in-hand with high availability. The organization that uses the CPR cannot tolerate a slow system. The architecture of the applications must be designed without bottlenecks or single queues for processing data. The data management system must be carefully planned to provide maximum high speed access to data elements. The network must be laid out with redundancy and its capacity must be sufficient to handle the high volumes of information. The hardware must be configured in such a manner as to rule out single points of failure. And collectively, all of the pieces must fit together in a manner in which each of the components complements the others' performance.

Accessibility

A frequently heard complaint about some of the earlier CPR systems was, "I know the system collects the data but I have no way of getting the information back out!". The successful CPR must provide the ability to easily access data from a variety of perspectives:

- The clinician must be able to quickly access all of the pertinent information on a given patient or reference information from knowledge databases. Accessing this information must be a natural part of the clinician workflow. It must be fast and simple to perform.
- The manager must be able to access information on the performance of processes and the productivity of resources through standard reports or through an easy-to-use reporting tool. It must not require knowledge of computer programming to get this information.
- The security administrator needs to have fast access to information on who accessed and used patient information. The system must also be capable of alerting the security administrator to investigate possible violations of security.
- The finance and billing staff need to be able to access clinical information to support coding and billing in a timely manner.
- The system must provide enough security to ensure that the organization's fiduciary responsibility for maintaining the privacy of patient information is maintained.
- The data must not be locked up by the vendor's proprietary operating environment. The data must be transferable for use by standard tools and applications.

Security and Data Integrity

Security and accessibility go hand-in-hand. HIPAA requires that the organization maintain the privacy of protected health information and safeguard the information. Finding the right balance between security and accessibility is critical for a successful CPR. If accessibility is reduced in favor of security, clinicians will probably not use the system. If the system is too accessible, it may be subject to improper disclosure of protected health information or malicious hacking. Another aspect of security is ensuring data integrity. How can we be sure that we have all of the information and that the information has not been corrupted or is incorrect? Data integrity can be achieved through the use of technology as well as analysis and redesign of certain processes.

Integration

Integration and data integrity are closely related. The weakest link in the CPR is the point at which a human being has to enter information into the CPR. The integrity of the data can be compromised if the human makes an error. Technology can help address this by reducing the amounts and type of information that must be manually entered. Data that are integrated between applications can be shared and the risk of errors entering the system is reduced. It will also be more up to date as more people review and revise the data as needed. In many cases, applications need the same data but do not share the same database. In these cases, the applications must be electronically interfaced so that the data elements can be passed between them without risking the integrity of the data.

Integration and Standardization

The use of standards in technology is an absolute requirement. Although there are many vendors with applications that use proprietary software, they all must use standards when communicating with other systems. The major data exchange standards in health care are HL7 which specifies application-level communication and DICOM (Digital Imaging and Communication in Medicine) which specifies the standard for communicating images. HL7 and DICOM have made a significant difference in how systems communicate, but they have not been the perfect solution for systems integration. A joint effort between the Radiological Society of North America (RSNA) and HIMSS was formed called *Integrating the Healthcare Enterprise (IHE)*.

"The IHE initiative is a project designed to advance the state of data integration in health care. Sponsored by the Radiological Society of North America (RSNA) and the HIMSS, it brings together medical professionals and the healthcare information and imaging systems industry to agree upon, document, and demonstrate standards-based methods of sharing information in support of optimal patient care."[12]

Users of the CPR must create continuous pressure on vendors of CPR systems and modalities toward achieving integration through standardization.

Value

The articulation and demonstration of value may be one of most difficult and most important parts of implementing a CPR. Value is key to a realistic understanding and support of what can be achieved, or not, with a CPR. Many leaders in an organization get enthusiastic about technology and system functionality and they see the system implementation as the solution. In such organizations, project goals are expressed in terms of the implementation of the technology instead of the business or medical objectives. Systems are never the end solution. The solution lies with people and how they use the system to accomplish their individual and organization objectives. These objectives give value to a CPR and are the most important factor in having a successful implementation of a CPR.

If the value of a CPR must flow from the strategic objectives of the organization, the role of the CPR in accomplishing business, clinical, and organizational transformation objectives must be understood. The organization must delineate the key strategies necessary to accomplish the objectives to gain the benefits and it must determine the metrics for measuring value. Organizations may take different approaches in framing the value proposition. Some organizations develop business cases with ROI to express the value in dollars. Others may describe anticipated benefits to the organization and patient and then develop quantitative or qualitative measures of success. Key performance indicators may be used, sometimes in concert with a vendor, to measure change, such as decreased claim denials, improved claims adjudication, reduction in cost of medications and supplies, reduction in order turnaround times, compliance with preventative guidelines, and others. Another important measure of success may be bringing about desired changes in work processes which leads to improvements in efficiency or care delivery.

Some examples of goals and outcomes quantified by organizations that have implemented CPRs are listed below. These have been collected from a variety of organizations that have implemented CPRs. Where there is a literature reference documenting these types of improvement, these references have been included.

Improvement in Quality and Patient Safety

Several issues arise in considering the operational definition of "quality." EHR-Ss have the potential to affect each one.

- Overall improved quality of care
  - The study compared the quality of care in the Veterans Administration (VA) healthcare system before and after its reengineering and found that the quality of care improved dramatically in all domains studied. These improvements were evident within 2 years after the system was reengineered and continued through fiscal year 2000. When we compared similar indicators of quality in the VA and Medicare fee-for-service systems during similar time periods, we found that the VA system performed better.[13]

- Medication safety improvements [i.e., reduction of adverse drug events (ADEs), IV to PO conversion, improved allergy data collection and alerts, etc.]
  - Seventy percent reduction in ADEs at Latter-Day Saints Hospital (2001 study by the Agency for Healthcare Research and Quality)[14]
  - Reduced preventable ADES by 62% at Brigham & Women's Hospital (1999 study in JAMIA)[15]
- Improvement in occurrences of preventative screening
- Improved compliance with policies and standard practices (i.e., optimize renal dosing, improved recognition of malnutrition; adherence to Joint Commission on Accreditation of Health Care Organizations restraint protocols)
  - Improved orders that conformed to institutional guidelines at Northwest region of Kaiser Permanente (1999 study JAIMA Symposium)[16]
- Improvement in infection rates
- Improvement in the timeliness, completeness, and quality of documentation (i.e., chart completion time, completion of specific assessments, up-to-date plan of care, availability of patient history, documentation of patient education, documentation of pain assessment, etc.)
  - Reduction of cost for clinical documentation at Heritage Behavioral Health[17]

Improved Availability of Information Wherever and Whenever Needed

Ubiquity and availability affect a number of measurable metrics in hospital settings.

- Reduction or elimination of hardcopy chart deliveries
- Measurements of provider satisfaction
- Reduction in nursing and other staff turnover rates
- Improved communication among care providers
  - Because this information is now guaranteed to be reliable and available to the clinician on the next visit, the provider has incentives to maintain up-to-date problem lists, medication lists, and allergies
- System utilization by providers, percent of adoption of the organization

Enhanced Productivity and Reduction in Costs

Costs are always important. EHR-Ss can affect each of the following economic indicators.

- Return on investment
  - The Davies winners of 2002, Maimonides Medical Center, Brooklyn, NY, and Queens Health Network, Queens, NY, both achieved a documented full return on investment[18]
- Reduced transcription costs
- Reduced printing and form costs

- $200,000 annual savings from reduction in forms and $185,000 annual savings in storage and microfilm at Reid Hospital and Health Care Services[19]
- Reduction in medication costs
  - $2.8 million annual savings from computer-assisted antibiotic dosing program at Bingham and Women's Hospital (2001)[20]
- Reduction in inappropriate and duplicate testing
- Improvements in revenue
  - Increase revenue from electrocardiogram, laboratory, and radiology after the installation of an outpatient EMR at Weill Physician Organization and Cornell University (2002 article in Modern Physician)[21]
- Improved turnaround time for results including medications, laboratory, and interpretation of radiology studies
  - Turnaround for medications, radiology procedures, and laboratory results reporting at Ohio State University Medical Center[22]
- Therapeutic interchanges of certain drugs
  - Computerized provider order entry (CPOE) menus can guide providers to the more cost-efficient test and treatment options by making it easier to choose them[23]
- Time savings and reduced labor costs
  - Time savings for ward clerks, nurses, and pharmacists after CPOE implementation at Montefiore Medical Center[24]
- Reduced billing costs
  - Support of Medicare compliance at Ohio State University Medical Center reduces follow-up billing issues[25]
- Reduction in malpractice claims and self-insurance costs[26]
- Decrease in ambulatory visit time and length of stay
  - Documented a decreased length of stay (LOS) at one of two study hospitals from 3.91 days to 3.71. The LOS at the other hospital did not change and the overall costs did not change (2002 JAMIA study)[27]
- Improvements in performance-based payments

Improved Data for Decision Making

Patients and clinicians should make better decisions, and the process of decision making should be improved.

- Shared access to data by all providers of care
- Improve patient access to medical care and information
- Reduction in emergency incidents for chronic care patients
- Measures of utilization and variance from clinical pathways
- Timely implementation of new safety procedures

The example of benefits included above provides the beginning of a body of knowledge about the utilization of CPR systems to improve patient safety, increase productivity, and reduce costs. Many more benefits, including improvement in patient outcomes, are expected as information becomes more available and useful for patient care and research.

During the implementation of the CPR, all involved in the project must focus their efforts on achieving the potential benefits. Making sure that these benefits are clearly articulated is critical to the success of the project. Measuring and documenting the performance in achieving the goals after implementation often does not happen because it requires effort and organizations assume that they are achieving the benefits, even if they have not measured them. Organizations that put extra effort in establishing the baseline and measuring the changes usually achieve better results. Reviewing key factors[28] from organizations that have successful CPR implementations illustrates that the EHR-S's value can be increased by fine tuning the work processes and articulating clear expectation of the benefits for using the CPR within and outside the organization.

References

1. United States General Accounting Office Report to the Chairman, Committee on Governmental Affairs, U.S. Senate Automated Medical Records Leadership Needed to Expedite Standards Development, April 1993 http://161.203.16.4/t2pbat5/149267.pdf.
2. Dick RS, Steen EB. The Computer Based Patient Record: An Essential Technology for Health Care. Washington, DC: National Academy Press; 1991.
3. Healthcare Information Systems and Management Society. HIMSS 15th Annual Leadership Survey, 2004. Available at: http://www.himss.org/2004survey/ASP/healthcarecio_final.asp. Accessed September 2004.
4. Davies Award of Excellence. A framework for evaluating electronic health records and guidelines for applying to the Davies Recognition Program. Version 5.0, January 2004.
5. Institute of Medicine, Committee on Data Standards for Patient Safety. Key capabilities of an electronic health record—Letter Report, July 31, 2003.
6. Health level 7 electronic health record functional model, July 2004. Available at: http://www.hl7.org/ehr/documents/Documents.asp. Accessed September 2004.
7. The National Committee for Vital and Health Statistics recommended a strategy to encourage efficient and secure exchange of health information through a common electronic health record (EHR) and through a National Health Information Infrastructure (NHII). 2001.
8. Weed LL. Knowledge Coupling. New York: Springer-Verlag; 1991:12.
9. Winkelman WJ, Leonard KJ. Overcoming structural constraints to patient utilization of electronic medical records: a critical review and proposal for an evaluation framework. Am Med Inform Assoc 2004;11(2):151–161.
10. HIMSS, EHR and return on investment. Available at: http://www.himss.org/content/files/EHR-ROI.pdf. Accessed October 2004.
11. Embi PJ, Yackel TR, Logan JR, Bowen JL, Cooney TG, Gorman PN. Impacts of computerized physician documentation in a teaching hospital: perceptions of faculty and resident physicians. J Am Med Inform Assoc 2004;11(4):300–309.

12. Integrating the healthcare enterprise. Available at: www.rsna.org/IHE/index.shtml.
13. Jha AK, Perlin JB, Kizer KW, Dudley RA. Effect of the transformation of the Veterans Affairs Health Care System on the quality of care. N Engl J Med 2003;348:2218–2227.
14. Agency for Healthcare Research and Quality: reducing and preventing adverse drug events to decrease hospital costs. Research in Action, Issue 1, March 2001.
15. Bates DW, Teich JM, Lee J, et al. The impact of computerized physician order entry on medication error prevention. J Am Med Inform Assoc 1999;6(4):313–321.
16. Embedding guidelines into direct physician order entry: simple methods, powerful results. J Am Med Inform Assoc Symp Suppl 1999:221–225.
17. Nicholas E. Davies Symposium Proceedings 2001. Award for behavioral health, Heritage Health Center Inc. Chicago, IL: HIMSS.
18. Nicholas E. Davies Symposium Proceedings 2002. Maimonides Medical Center: Maimonides Medical Center and Queens Health Network. Chicago, IL: HIMSS.
19. Kinyon C. A CFO discovers the power of the automated patient record. HIMSS Proc 2002.
20. Bates DW, Pappius E, Kuperman GJ, et al. Using information systems to measure and improve quality. Int J Med Inform 1999;53:115–124.
21. Cole C. Getting past buzz to buy-in. Modern Physician 2002;6(7):20–22.
22. Mekhjian HS, Kumar RR, Kuehn L, et al. Immediate benefits realized following implementation of physician order entry at an academic medical center. J Am Med Inform Assoc 2002;9:529–539.
23. Birkmeyer J, Birkmeyer C, Wennberg D, et al. Leapfrog safety standards: potential benefits of universal adoption. Washington, DC: Leapfrog Group; 2000.
24. Taylor R, Manzo J, Sinnett M. Quantifying value for physician order-entry systems: a balance of cost and quality. Healthc Financ Manage 2002;56(7):44–48.
25. Nicholas E. Davies Symposium Proceedings 2001. University of Illinois at Chicago Medical Center: The Gemini project. Chicago, IL: HIMSS.
26. Maryland Society of Health Care Information Management Presentation May 21, 3004. Larry J. Smith, MedStar Health. Monetizing quality and patient safety through innovations in risk management. Available at: http://mshism.org/archive.html. Accessed October 2004.
27. Mekhjian HS, Kumar RR, Kuehn L, et al. Immediate Benefits Realized Following Implementation of Physician Order Entry at an Academic Medical Center. JAMIA, Sept/Oct 2002;9:529–539.
28. Ash JS, Stavri PZ, Kuperman GJ. Consensus statement on considerations for a successful CPOE implementation. J Am Med Inform Assoc 2003;10(3):229–234.

7
Patient Safety, Quality of Care, and Computer Provider Order Entry

GILAD J. KUPERMAN

Much of the activity in health care is the result of clinicians' decision making. Clinicians decide to admit patients to the hospital, to order diagnostic studies to gather more information about the patient's physiologic state, and to order medications and other therapeutic procedures. Often, the clinician's decision-making process results in the creation of an order. In a paper-based environment, the order is documented as a handwritten order or perhaps as a verbal order that is transcribed into an order book by another member of the healthcare team. After an order is documented, it is communicated, perhaps through a complex series of steps, to one or more other members of the healthcare team. Diagnostic, therapeutic, and monitoring activities then are set into motion. In a busy inpatient or outpatient clinical environment, the ordering process is repeated thousands of times a day. It has been said that physician decision making is responsible for more than 90% of the cost of health care.

Most of the time, clinicians' decisions are appropriate and the activities that are set into motion are performed correctly. However, recent research has demonstrated that, in a significant fraction of instances, errors may occur in decision making or in execution of those decisions.[1,2] For example, a clinician caring for a patient may decide to order a diagnostic study that in all likelihood will not provide any additional useful findings, or the clinician may order a medication for which there is a less expensive and equivalent alternative. Such decisions lead to inefficient use of resources and the high cost of health care in the United States (in 2003, $1.65 trillion or 15% of the gross domestic product) demands that resources for health care should be expended only when there is clear evidence that the resources will yield some benefit. Inappropriate clinical decision making also may lead to poor quality care.[2] For example, errors in medication ordering can lead to unnecessary patient injuries, and the omission of preventive care activities may be unnecessarily detrimental to a patient's health. Two important reports from the Institute of Medicine (IOM), *To Err Is Human*[1] in 1999 and *Crossing the Quality Chasm*[2] in 2000, documented the nature of quality problems in health care and argued that health information tech-

115

nology in general, and computer provider order entry applications specifically, should be part of any comprehensive approach to quality improvement in health care.

Computer provider order entry (CPOE) applications are software programs that allow clinicians (most often, but not necessarily, physicians) to enter their orders into the computer instead of writing them on paper.* CPOE applications have the opportunity to significantly aid the clinician's decision-making process.[3,4] As will be described in detail, when compared with a paper-based ordering environment, CPOE applications provide an information environment that actively supports the clinician. Examples of features of CPOE that assist the clinician include providing access to relevant patient data and medical reference information, assuring that the order is specified completely and correctly, performing calculations flawlessly, communicating with other systems in a reliable and timely manner, and providing alerts and reminders that guide the physician through the ordering process.[5] Studies of errors in medicine have found that the root causes of the majority of problems (e.g., lack of access to patient data, lack of access to knowledge resources, ordering the wrong drug for a given condition or a drug to which the patient is allergic) can be mitigated with CPOE.[6] All in all, when compared with a paper-based environment, a CPOE application provides a clinician with a much appropriate "cockpit" in which to manage the complexities of modern medicine.

Although CPOE applications have been shown to improve patient safety, improve compliance with guidelines, and reduce much inefficiency in health care, it still is not in widespread use in health care.[7] The main reasons for the slow dissemination of CPOE applications include the large costs involved, the impact of the application on the workflow of the organization's physician staff, the complexity of the implementation, and uncertainty about whether the organization will realize the same benefits that have been documented in academic studies.[8]

This chapter will describe several aspects of a typical CPOE application. Specific topics to be covered include:

---

* The abbreviation CPOE has at times been used to stand for "computer physician order entry" and for "computer provider order entry." The term physician order entry was originally used in recognition of the fact that physicians place most clinical orders—for example, orders for medications, diagnostic studies, and therapeutic and monitoring procedures. However, physicians are not the only users of CPOE applications. For example, medical students, physicians assistants, and nurses (via verbal orders) often will enter data into CPOE applications. Also, entering orders is only one feature of a CPOE application. As will be described, electronic orders often are communicated to ancillary departments, such as nursing, the laboratory, the pharmacy, and radiology, throughout the healthcare enterprise. Thus, all of these departments include non-physician users of CPOE. This chapter takes the latter perspective and will use the abbreviation CPOE to refer to "computer provider order entry."

- The place of CPOE among other information systems' applications in a complex clinical environment
- The functionality most often found in a CPOE application
- The features of a CPOE application that lead to improvements in health-care quality
- Issues encountered in implementing a CPOE application
- Evaluations of CPOE applications

CPOE in the Context of Hospital and Clinical Information Systems

Computer order entry systems are one component of a healthcare organization's information systems environment. The CPOE application must interact well with the other automated systems and, in several instances, is critically dependent on data from these other systems to do its work well.

The information systems of a healthcare organization that are relevant to CPOE are shown in Table 7-1. Registration, appointment, scheduling, bed control, and departmental systems all serve as important data sources for CPOE applications.

Registration Systems

Unambiguous patient identifiers are a critical requirement of any clinical application, and CPOE is no exception. CPOE applications usually use the identifiers that are generated by hospital registration systems. Registration

TABLE 7-1. CPOE in the context of other hospital information system components

Hospital Information System Component	Relationship to CPOE
Registration systems	Provides patient identifiers
Appointment, scheduling, bed control, and credentialing applications	Used to identify who is an inpatient or who is due for a visit. Also, many clinician identifiers come from these systems
Ancillary systems (laboratory, radiology, pharmacy, intensive care unit monitors, etc.)	Primary source of clinical data relevant to CPOE and recipients of electronic orders
Clinical data repository	Receives data from ancillary systems and is accessed directly by CPOE
Electronic medical records and other clinical documentation appointments	If used in conjunction with CPOE, create a more comprehensive work environment
Clinical decision support systems	Some aspects of clinical decision support built into CPOE; others may be separate

systems usually are a robust source of patient identifiers because these same identifiers are used for generating bills to payers.**

Bed Control and Appointment Systems

Hospitals usually have automated bed control systems and many large clinics have appointment and scheduling systems. Bed control systems are used by CPOE to identify who is an inpatient at the current time (therefore, who may have orders entered). Bed control systems also are often the source of information about the patient's location. In the outpatient setting, data from the appointment system are an important part of the workflow. Based on the appointment data, the clinical information system can display the clinician's daily schedule. The schedule display becomes the "launching point" for the clinician to write orders.

CPOE applications also are dependent on a database of providers authorized to write orders. Outpatient scheduling applications often are a good source of provider identifiers in the outpatient setting because only providers authorized to see patients can write orders.*** A robust provider database ideally contains information about the characteristics of the providers and the roles they might play, for example, whether he or she is a physician, nurse, or medical student. The information about the individual's identity can be used by the CPOE application to confer certain authorizations. For example, a medical student's orders may not be active until they are cosigned by a physician, and only attending oncologists may be allowed to sign for certain complex chemotherapy orders.

Ancillary Systems

Ancillary, or departmental, information systems are used to manage a variety of departments often found in a large healthcare organization (e.g., laboratory, pharmacy, radiology, cardiology, pulmonary function, neurophysiology, transcription). In addition to managing the work of the department, these systems also generate clinical data about the patient. In many

---

** As far as the direct relationship between CPOE and billing systems is concerned, CPOE applications usually do not provide billable event data directly to financial systems. This is because an ordered event may not necessarily transpire. For example, a medication or laboratory test may be ordered but not performed (e.g., because the patient is not on the floor). Billing data usually comes from ancillary systems (i.e., the laboratory system, the pharmacy system, etc.).
*** In the inpatient setting, credentialing applications may be a starting point for a registry of the providers who are authorized for the CPOE application. Often, the list of credentialed physicians needs to be modified because credentialing data, which only need to be reviewed every 1–2 years, may not reflect the providers' actual status.

institutions, the data from the ancillary systems are stored in a clinical data repository for easy access by clinicians and other applications.

Clinical patient data must be easily accessible from within the CPOE application in case the clinician has questions about the patient's physiologic state during the ordering process. Laboratory results often are involved in clinical decision support, for example, the CPOE application may detect a drug–laboratory interaction if a potassium preparation is being ordered and the patient already has a high serum potassium level.

In addition to serving as sources of data for a CPOE application, ancillary information systems are also the destination for some automated orders. For example, electronic orders may be routed automatically to laboratory, radiology, and pharmacy systems. The automated communication of orders facilitates the subsequent steps that culminate in the execution of a therapeutic or diagnostic procedure. In some cases at some institutions, the interfaces between CPOE and the ancillary system may not be completely automated; for example, a radiology order might be printed in the radiology department instead of interfaced to the radiology system. Even in these cases, there is some benefit from CPOE (e.g., assured legibility, clearly identified provider), however, the largest gains in efficiency result when the electronic interface has been completed.

Automated Clinical Documentation Applications

There may be automated encounter documentation applications in the clinical setting. Physicians and nurses may electronically document observations and plans; nurses may use an electronic medication administration record. These other documentation applications may interact with CPOE in a variety of ways. For example, automated orders from CPOE may serve an input to an automated encounter note documentation application. Also, the workflow is enhanced if the clinician can order as well as document on the workstation; doing both on paper fragments data and workflow.

Clinical Decision Support

The relationship of CPOE to clinical decision support will be discussed in detail in the section Quality Improvement Features of CPOE.

Summary

CPOE applications are but one component of a complex information environment. The full power of CPOE can only be realized when the interaction with these other components is well understood and well leveraged.

General Overview of CPOE Functionality

Introduction

Most obviously, a CPOE application must allow a clinician to document his or her orders for patients via the computer as opposed to via a paper-based order book. To obtain the benefits of computerization—for example, clinical decision support, having automated data available for research and management purposes, and being able to route orders automatically to appropriate destinations—the CPOE application cannot function merely as a typewriter that captures unstructured text. Rather, the CPOE application must allow orders to be captured in a coded and structured form that can be manipulated by the computer system to yield benefits above and beyond paper-based orders. One of the key challenges for a CPOE application is to be able to capture the richness, diversity, and detail of all of the possible orders that can occur in the clinical setting and still maintain the highest possible degree of coding and structure.

Specific Order Types

Computer-based orders usually are categorized into different types of orders. Commonly identified order categories include medication, laboratory, radiology, nursing, intravenous fluid, total parenteral nutrition (TPN), consults, blood products, and pulmonary orders such as oxygen and ventilators. Most CPOE systems allow the clinician to document important information about the patient such as admitting diagnosis, the patient's condition on admission, and allergy status. Strictly speaking, these are items of documentation and not orders per se; however, documenting these facts in the CPOE application mimics the paper-based workflow used at many institutions.

Each order category has a set of attributes that are filled in ("instantiated") to create any given order. For example, the required attributes of a medication order are the name of the medication, the route of the medication, and the dose and frequency. Optional attributes of a medication order would include a specific stop time, a flag denoting the order as PRN, and textual instructions to be passed along to the nurse and pharmacist. A consult order may have as attributes the name of the service and the reason for the consult request. An order for a laboratory test (or any other diagnostic study) would have the name of the test to be performed and the time for it be performed. Intravenous drip orders are some of the most complex orders because the fluid type must be specified and the amount to be administered may be specified as a defined amount, a defined duration, or an indefinite duration. Intravenous fluids may also contain various additives that would need to be specified. Similarly, TPN orders are exceedingly complex because of the large number of additives that can be included.

Data entry screens facilitate the creation of individual orders. The workflow in some CPOE applications is that the clinician chooses the order category, is taken to a specific screen, and inputs the category-specific order data. In other applications, the physician may simply type the order data, for example, "draw digoxin levels in a.m." and the CPOE application "understands" the order, decides which is the intended order category, and what are the attributes (e.g., laboratory test is digoxin, draw time is tomorrow morning). The approach in which the computer interprets the order is much more complex and the clinician may be taken to a category-specific screen to resolve situations in which the computer cannot fully interpret the entered text.

Order Sessions

At any one sitting, the ordering provider may enter a collection of individual orders. To make the orders "active," the physician needs to "sign" the orders. Clinicians usually type in an electronic identification code that serves as an electronic signature.

Order Sets

Order sets are predefined collections of orders that can be ordered together as a single item. The use of order sets can speed the ordering of large complex collections of orders, for example, an admission order set for a patient being admitted for a bone marrow transplant, or a postoperative order set for a patient who has just had coronary bypass graft surgery. Order sets also can decrease variability in the process of care and thus may increase the quality of health care. Order sets may completely specify every attribute of every order or they may allow the ordering clinicians to make some choices at the time of ordering. For example, an order set for community-acquired pneumonia may include a choice of three antibiotics among all the other orders. Or an order set may include a specific medication, but allow the clinician to specify the dose at the time the set is executed. Several institutions that have implemented CPOE have made the creation and use of order sets a cornerstone of the way they will use CPOE to improve quality.[9] Such institutions may create 50–100 order sets to cover the most common conditions treated at the hospital, or even more. Hospitals must create policy to define which individuals and/or groups in the organization are authorized to create order sets. The CPOE application must contain a feature that allows the library of order sets to be maintained (i.e., browsed, edited, etc.). Some organizations require that a medication safety committee reviews the order sets before they go into production.

Roles in CPOE

Different classes of healthcare providers may have different privileges in the CPOE application. As mentioned previously, many categories of healthcare providers besides physicians may enter orders via CPOE and the application may need to manage each of these situations differently. These rules are set up according to institutional policy. Most often, nurse practitioners and physician's assistants may enter orders with the same privileges as physicians. Orders entered by nurses (usually from verbal orders) become active immediately, but require a cosignature by a physician at some point.**** Orders entered by medical students do not become active until a physician has cosigned them.

In some cases, one physician must cosign another physician's orders before the orders become active. Examples include a senior oncologist cosigning a fellow's orders, an infectious disease physician cosigning an order for an expensive antibiotic, and an attending cardiologist cosigning an order for a cardiac medication. In these instances, the CPOE application must be able to mimic the institutional policies that define these scenarios.

CPOE Functionality Beyond Order Entry

Although CPOE is defined as "order entry," there are features of a complete CPOE system that go beyond the simple documentation of orders by clinicians.

Routing of Orders

As described in the previous section, many types of orders may be routed automatically to the appropriate ancillary system. Other types of orders must be routed to the appropriate healthcare provider. For example, nurses would need to know about nursing care orders and orders for consults likely would be routed to a clerk in the consulting department who would execute the appropriate next steps. In many cases, nurses must be made aware of orders that also are routed to other destinations; for example, nurses must be made aware when medications and imaging studies are ordered.

CPOE applications must create new methods to inform staff when new orders have been entered for a patient. In the paper world, the physician raises a flag on the order book or tells a staff person explicitly when new orders have been written. With a CPOE application, there is no analog of the flag, and telling a staff member would not be possible if the orders have been written from a remote location. To address this need, many CPOE

**** Although CPOE systems decrease the frequency of verbal orders (because physicians can enter orders remotely), it does not eliminate them completely. For example, a physician may need to specify an order when he or she is not near a workstation.

applications include as part of the application a continuously updated screen that informs unit staff when new orders for one of their patients have been written.

Management of Dictionaries

There are several dictionaries that must be maintained to support the CPOE application, for example, medication dictionaries and dictionaries of radiology and laboratory tests. The CPOE application will include features to support management of these dictionaries.

The use of standards in health information technology is important because it facilitates the use and dissemination of such systems. It should be noted that there are few standard dictionaries for use in CPOE systems. Although frequently used standards exist for medications (e.g., the National Drug Codes [NDC] assigned by the Food and Drug Administration) and the LOINC codes for laboratory results, these standards do not represent orderable entities; NDC codes are for dispensable medications and LOINC codes represent results rather than orderable tests. Similarly, there is no clinician-oriented dictionary of orderable radiology tests. The absence of these kinds of dictionaries means that each institution must create its own catalog of orderable items. Usually, the institution begins with the list in the ancillary department and converts it to a form that is "clinician friendly."

Functionality at the Time of Patient Transfer

When patients are transferred from one setting to another (e.g., from an intensive care to an acute care setting), often there is a review and revision of the patient's orders. This is a time when errors are likely to occur because the revision of the orders could be quite substantial (e.g., moving to a post-operative unit) at the same time that a change is occurring in the personnel caring for the patient. For example, at the time of transfer, in some cases, all the medication orders need to be changed but all the other orders will remain the same; in other cases, the medication orders will stay the same but other orders will change. Many CPOE applications contain functionality to assist with these patient transfer situations so the risk of error and preventable injury is minimized.

Orders View

With paper, ascertaining from the order book what are the currently active orders can be arduous. With CPOE, the orders are in a database, so viewing the active orders is much easier. In addition, the orders can be sorted and filtered by a variety of parameters to provide exactly the information the clinician is seeking. For example, the clinician might want to see only currently active medication orders, or orders that were entered in a given date range. Thus, the order view function can be moderately complex.

Differences Between Inpatient and Outpatient CPOE Applications

There are many similarities between the ordering processes in the inpatient and outpatient settings. In each setting, the clinician orders diagnostic studies, therapies, and ongoing monitoring, and in each setting the orders are performed. However, there are also important differences between the two settings and those differences have important implications for CPOE functionality. The differences between the inpatient and outpatient setting that are relevant to CPOE are:

- The kinds of orders that are written
- Routing of the data
- How in the workflow the application is used

Kinds of Orders

Differences in the kinds of orders that are written in the inpatient and outpatient settings stem from differences in patient acuity. Inpatients are much more seriously ill and require more complex interventions. For example, medication orders in both settings require the name of the medication, the route, the dose, and the frequency. Outpatient medication orders result in a prescription and include such outpatient-specific attributes as "number of pills to be dispensed" and "number of refills." However, inpatient CPOE applications need more sophisticated options to manage "holding" a medication, giving additional doses, and handling intravenous fluid and TPN orders. As another example, ventilator orders are not relevant to the outpatient setting.

Routing

Most inpatient orders are routed automatically to the relevant staff or department, and indicate an action (e.g., imaging study, laboratory test) that will be performed as part of the same admission. Many orders in the outpatient setting will be done at some other location at some other time. Large multi-specialty clinics may have routing features similar to those at large hospitals.

How the Application Is Used in the Workflow

The other major difference between the uses of CPOE in the two settings is the workflow for the ordering clinician. In the inpatient setting, the clinician may be using the application on rounds or at other times during the day, and even though there is a general need to be as efficient as possible, there is not a definitive time constraint. In the outpatient setting, however, the application must be used exactly at the end of the visit, before the next patient can be seen. This means that any delays that occur as a result of the use of the application will be felt acutely by the clinician and the subsequent patients. This means that the outpatient systems have a higher requirement for time efficiency.

Quality Improvement Features of CPOE

As mentioned in the introduction to this chapter, many of the current ills of the healthcare system can be traced to problems in the ordering process.[10] CPOE applications can improve the quality of care over paper-based environments in three important ways[5]:

- CPOE is more reliable than paper-based ordering because it automates many manual processes
- The clinician who uses CPOE has easy access to other automated applications that can improve the quality of the ordering decisions
- The CPOE application can have several "knowledge-based" clinical decision support features that embed medical knowledge in the application and actively guide the clinician to make the best ordering decision or point out when an order may be problematic for some reason

This section will give examples of each of the above categories.

Improvements in Care Attributed Simply to Automation

A slew of improvements in the quality and reliability of health care result simply from the automation of the ordering process and associated downstream activities.

Legibility and Identification of the Ordering Provider

All information entered into a CPOE application will be legible. Concerns caused by illegibility are effectively removed. Also, in paper-based systems, the physician signature often is illegible; with CPOE, the identity of the ordering provider is clear and available when needed (e.g., by ancillary departments who may need to contact the provider for clarifications).

Timely and Accurate Communications

Orders can be communicated to the nursing staff, ancillary departments (e.g., laboratory, pharmacy, and radiology) and other automated systems (e.g., automated medication administration record systems) instantly and accurately. Many delays caused by paper-based communication can be eliminated and the accuracy of the communication is not a concern.

Remote Access to Ordering Functionality

With CPOE, orders can be entered or viewed from anywhere in the institution, not just on the patient's unit where the order book resides. With appropriate security and technology, orders can even be viewed and entered from off-site locations. Such functionality decreases the frequency of verbal orders. Also, hospital functions that require access to orders data (for example, utilization review or quality assurance functions) can access orders data without physically visiting the patient's unit.

Required Fields

The application can assure that all fields critical to the complete specification of an order are present. For example, for medication orders, the application can require that the drug name, dose, route, and frequency be specified. In the paper world, many mistakes and inefficiencies result when orders are incompletely or ambiguously specified.

Use of Dictionaries and Pick Lists

CPOE applications offer the clinician predefined "catalogs" of orderable items from which to choose (e.g., formularies of medications, lists of laboratory and radiology tests). Such catalogs reduce confusion by assuring that the orders represent valid items known to the hospital's departments. Pick lists, for example, for lists of acceptable doses for a medication or standard diets, can also constrain the choice of options and help to assure that the clinician makes a suitable choice.

Benefits from Access to Other Computer-based Applications

When a clinician is ordering by using CPOE running on a workstation, often there are other applications available that work synergistically with CPOE to improve the quality of care.

Access to Relevant Patient Data

With CPOE, the ordering clinician can have quick access to data about the physiologic state of the patient, for example, laboratory data, radiology data, and cardiology data. In the paper world, the cumbersome nature of data retrieval might hinder the clinician from obtaining the necessary data.

Access to Medical Reference Information

Many healthcare organizations provide services that allow clinicians to access electronic textbooks, the Internet, and the medical literature from the clinical workstations. Such access, easily available during ordering, increases the likelihood that needed reference information will be obtained.

Access to E-mail

As part of their normal workflow, many clinicians use e-mail to interact with colleagues about clinical matters. Having easy access to e-mail during ordering increases the ease of communications with colleagues and the likelihood that the clinician will obtain needed advice.

Knowledge-based Clinical Decision Support Features in CPOE

One of the most powerful characteristics of a CPOE application is that the orders can be evaluated by expert system software. A high level model of an expert system is shown in Figure 7-1. As new data enter the system, for example, a new medication order, the data are passed to the expert system's inference engine, so called because it "infers" or makes decisions about the data. To make decisions, the expert system uses rules, sometimes stored in a specialized database known as a "rule base," and other data known about the patient.

As an example, there may be a rule that says, "If the patient is on warfarin, and sulfamethoxazole is ordered, inform the provider that the level of warfarin should be monitored closely and may need to be adjusted." When sulfamethoxazole is ordered, the inference engine will identify that this rule needs to be evaluated. The inference engine then will query the patient database for the patient's medication list. If the patient does in fact have a currently active order for warfarin, the rule will evaluate as "true" and the clinician will be presented with a message to be sure to take appropriate action.

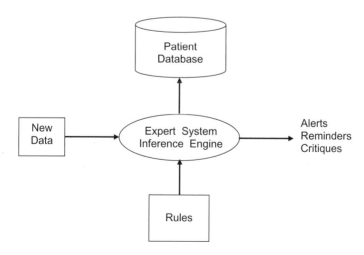

FIGURE 7-1. Model of an expert system.

Expert systems can be used to identify many different kinds of scenarios, from the very simple to the very complex. The design, development, implementation, and evaluation of expert systems still is a very active area of research. Many examples of expert systems have been implemented only at one site by an organization that has a particular interest in that specific kind of functionality. Commercially available CPOE applications may offer only a subset of what follows.

With almost all alerts, the final determination of how best to proceed is left to the provider. The computer uses all available information to decide when to present an alert, but the clinician may well have additional information that would contradict the suggestions of the alert.

Critiquing of Orders

The computer can help assure that often misused or expensive therapies are used only for appropriate purposes. For example, vancomycin is a medication that is often ordered inappropriately. The overuse of vancomycin can lead to increased rates of antibiotic resistance in hospitals. When vancomycin is ordered, the computer can examine the patient database to determine whether the use of vancomycin is warranted.[11] To make its decision, the expert system may need to ask the ordering provider to enter additional information about the patient that is not yet in the patient database. If the expert system determines that vancomycin is inappropriate, it will alert the provider. Another example similar to vancomycin is that radiologic imaging studies often are misused; the CPOE application can help direct the provider to the most appropriate examination.[12]

Similarly, the computer can inform the clinician when an expensive medication is being ordered and there is a less-expensive, therapeutically equivalent alternative.[13]

Corollary Orders

Often in health care, when one clinical action is taken, a second associated action should also be taken. For example, if an aminoglycoside is ordered, drug levels should be ordered at some point in the future; if a diuretic is prescribed, a serum potassium level should be checked; or if the patient is placed on bedrest, some prophylaxis against thrombosis should be ordered. These associated orders are known as corollary orders and the expert system can remind the clinician to order the associated item at the time the primary order is made.[14]

Redundant Order Checking

Certain diagnostic studies, if ordered too frequently, do not add any additional information. For example, a urine culture that is ordered less than 24 hours after a preceding urine culture will add no additional information and would just be a waste of healthcare resources. Subsequent diagnostic studies that would not add additional information are known as redundant tests. Alerts for redundancy are not appropriate for all diagnostic tests. Some healthcare parameters change quite quickly; for example, the oxygenation of blood in response to changes in ventilator settings. In these cases, rapidly repeated tests are appropriate. Even when redundancy is a concern, the time interval within which a follow-up test might be considered redundant is test specific. For example, based on pharmacokinetics, a repeat digoxin level might be appropriate after 24 hours but a repeat phenobarbital level might not be appropriate for 20 days (because it takes that long after a dose change for the drug to equilibrate in the blood).[15,16]

Dosing Decision Support

As mentioned, through the use of pick lists, the computer can guide the clinician to appropriate doses of medications.[13] Advanced functionality can allow the recommendations to be refined based on renal function and age.[17] Some computer applications make dosing recommendations in the pediatric setting; however, this domain is particularly challenging and an area of active research.

Drug-allergy and Drug–Drug Interaction Checking

The computer can alert when a medication order might result in an untoward reaction because of allergies or an interaction with another drug. Allergies must be specified using the same coding scheme as medications. Also, to be useful, the list of drug–drug interactions used by the system must be clinically meaningful and must not overwhelm the user.[18,19]

Alerts for Duplicate Orders

The computer can inform the clinician when an order represents a duplication of an order that is already active. Examples would include alerts for duplicate laboratory tests, radiology studies, or medications. Duplicate medication alerts can represent either exact matches (e.g., two potassium orders) or class-based matches (e.g., two nonsteroidal medications).

Evaluations of CPOE

Beginning in the 1990s, and to some extent before that, a body of evidence in the academic biomedical literature began to emerge that documented the favorable impact of health information technology, and CPOE in particular, on healthcare quality and cost. The IOM reports that documented the problems with healthcare safety and quality and advocated strongly for the use of information systems as a key component of a redesigned healthcare system quoted many of these studies.[1,2] The IOM argued that each of its goals for a redesigned healthcare system (safe, equitable, effective, efficient, timely, and patient centered) required a robust IT infrastructure.

Although it could be argued that the need for CPOE in the current healthcare environment is plainly evident, having studies that document the impact of CPOE on the process and outcome of care is important for several reasons.

First, CPOE is a technology, and it should be evaluated like any technology to determine whether it is safe and effective. Just as other technologies such as medications and surgical procedures need to be evaluated rigorously for their intended and unintended impacts, so should information technologies be evaluated. Second, CPOE projects are costly and compete intensely for scarce capital dollars in the budgets of healthcare organizations. A study in 2002 estimated that the cost of a CPOE project in a 500-bed hospital (assuming no major hardware upgrades were needed) was $8 million and would have incremental ongoing expenses of $1.35 million annually.[20] Objective information about the benefits (financial and clinical) that might be realized is invaluable to a healthcare organization that is deciding whether and when to commit to a CPOE project. Finally, as with any technology, there may be untoward side effects and it is important to know whether and to what extent these are present.

Healthcare organizations vary widely in size and organizational structure and it may not be clear to what extent the impacts of CPOE realized in one kind of organization will apply in another organization. Similarly, CPOE applications and implementations among institutions vary widely and it may not be clear to what extent the impacts measured in one setting will generalize to another setting.

Studies have documented that CPOE can improve the quality of care in the following ways:

- Increase the rates of use of such preventive measures as vaccinations and secondary prevention of myocardial infarction[21]
- Increase compliance with the use of formulary approved drugs[13]
- Improve dosing appropriateness[13,17]
- Improve compliance with medication monitoring guidelines[14]
- Improve the appropriateness of laboratory and radiology test ordering[12,15]
- Reduce the rate of serious medication errors[22,23]
- Improve antibiotic ordering patterns[11,23]
- Reduce total hospital charges and length of stay[24]

Summary

Significant problems with the quality of health care have been identified. Information technology in general, and CPOE in particular, can help address these problems. CPOE applications can improve the quality of care through sheer automation, by allowing the clinician to do his or her work on a computer workstation that might provide access to other automated resources, or by actively guiding the care process with the use of expert systems and medical knowledge embedded directly in the CPOE application.

Implementation Issues

CPOE applications are complex pieces of software and healthcare institutions are complex organizations. Putting the two together, i.e., implementing a CPOE application in a large healthcare organization, presents formidable challenges.

A CPOE project at most healthcare organizations is a multi-year initiative. At a high level, the project usually roughly includes the following steps:

- Strategic planning for the application, culminating in the decision to implement
- Communicating to all key stakeholders in the institution that the decision has been made to implement a CPOE application
- Doing thorough analysis of the workflow and preparing for the changes that the CPOE application will bring
- Doing the requisite hardware planning
- Training the users of the CPOE application, and preparing a plan to support the users after go-live
- Piloting the application, and following up with the complete rollout
- Managing the CPOE application after the rollout is completed

In general, a CPOE implementation project has many of the same characteristics as other large complex projects. For example, CPOE projects need clear sponsorship, adequate resources, strong leadership, and good management. However, many of the project details are specific to CPOE per se.

Strategic Planning and the Decision to Implement CPOE

The decision to implement CPOE typically is made by the organization's senior leadership. Because of the broad changes that will result, and also because of the expense involved, the senior leadership must be able to articulate how implementing CPOE will further the strategic goals of the institution and how the decision not to implement CPOE would severely hamper the institution in its strategic goals. The senior leadership may quote such factors as a desire to improve patient safety and/or otherwise improve the quality of care, a desire to be more efficient, or a vision of CPOE as being necessary to compete in a modern healthcare environment. Discussions about whether and when to implement CPOE will involve the organization's Board of Trustees (who will be involved in the funding discussion), senior administrative leaders, and representatives from the organization's clinical staff, who will act as advocates for the application and communicate to the clinical staff in general why this application is necessary.

After the decision to implement has been made, the organization must determine who will serve as the CPOE project "sponsor," i.e., who in the organization is the key advocate for the project and can help resolve major issues that arise. A project management structure also must be created and a single project leader usually is identified. Regardless of the details of the project organization, strong leaders from both the medical staff and from the information systems department to advance the project must be identified.

Communication Stage

The project leader must engage the relevant constituencies that will be affected by the CPOE application. The list of affected constituencies includes almost all of the hospital departments—medical staffs, nursing staff, the laboratory, pharmacy, radiology, dietary, physical therapy, occupational therapy, respiratory therapy, and others. The project manager must communicate the goals of the CPOE project and as much as is known about the timetable and detailed plans. Even though many of the stakeholder leaders will have been part of the decision to implement CPOE, a broader communication at this time is needed. Such communication will be invaluable at later stages of the project when engagement of the stakeholders will be critical to project success.

Any project that involves a large amount of change will be difficult, even if the eventual state is viewed as better than the current state. CPOE is no exception. CPOE involves a large amount of change in the organization. One key task of the project leader is to keep the involved staff enthused through the early stages of the project when the pain of change is being felt most acutely. Fortunately, the pain does not last forever and once the staff gets used to the new system, the organization has in place a technical platform that can be used to greatly enhance the quality of care.

Analysis and Preparation

As an organization prepares for the implementation of CPOE, it must prepare to automate many processes that are paper-based in their current form. As an organization analyzes the processes that will be impacted by CPOE, it will discover that the actual work that is taking place on the patient care units is much more complex and much more detailed than expected. A high level overview of the key care processes is not sufficient for configuring a CPOE application. The deep details of the care process must be ferreted out and many surprising lessons will be learned.

The organization may discover that its existing paper-based processes are inconsistent across different care units and across different departments. At times, practice may violate stated policies. For example, some organizations may have policies that prohibit "hold" orders (e.g., "hold digoxin today") even though in practice such orders are placed and accepted. Another policy that many organizations enforce inconsistently is the requirement to rewrite certain medication or IV fluid orders on a regular basis. The organization will have to carefully consider whether to change practice to be consistent and aligned with policy, or to allow practice to stay as it is. If practice is allowed to stay as it is, the CPOE application must conform to all the variations in practice. Confusion will result if the CPOE application is designed to support only one method of practice but the requisite practice changes are not put into place in the organization.

A CPOE implementation provides an opportunity for an organization to consider changing the way it conducts certain processes. Indeed, providing a platform that can be the basis for process improvement is one of the goals of a CPOE application. However, the organization must consider carefully which processes it tries to change at the time of the CPOE implementation. Too much change at once can be difficult for the organization to digest.

One key result of the planning phase is an understanding of how the application needs to be customized to meet the requirements of a specific clinical setting. Many CPOE applications provide tools to allow the institution to configure the application for a given clinical environment. The analytic and planning phase provide input to the configuration process.

Hardware and Technical Considerations

A CPOE application will beg such hardware and technical considerations as:

- Server capacity, i.e., do the hardware servers have the capacity to handle the projected transactional load?
- Network capacity, i.e., can the existing network handle the projected increase in traffic?
- Interfaces, i.e., what are the required interfaces to and from other systems (e.g., pharmacy, admitting, laboratory) and will the interfaces be one- or two-way?
- Workstation availability, i.e., are sufficient workstations available to provide access to clinicians, even at peak ordering time?
- Type of device, i.e., will there be fixed workstations, laptops with rolling carts, and/or handheld devices, and for wireless devices, have provisions been made for access points and battery life?

The hardware has to be able to support the needs of the CPOE application and the workflow requirements of the users.

Training and Support

A healthcare organization may have several hundred or even thousands of physicians, nurses, and other staff members that will be users of the CPOE application. Assuring that the application is used properly involves a combination of training and support. Training is the process of educating users about the application in advance of its release. The availability of staff often is limited by the busy schedules of the nursing and physician staff. In addition, the CPOE application is sufficiently complex that not every feature of the application can be taught in the available training time. The goal of training is to give the users a basic understanding of the application's functionality and concepts.

Support is provided after release of the application and is usually intensive in the inpatient environment after go-live (e.g., 24 hours a day for 2 weeks), and tapers off thereafter. A key requirement to a successful rollout is the availability of immediate support (sometimes described as help "at the elbow") during the first several days when users are learning the details of the application. The extensive amount of manpower required to provide the requisite level of support creates a rate-limiting step at which the rollout can proceed. Even though support requirements taper off significantly after the project's early stages, some level of support is always required to address the questions and issues that inevitably arise even after the application is well established.

Rollout

Usually, an organization will pilot the CPOE application in one unit of the hospital to understand how well the application fits in with the workflow of the users and addresses the needs of the institution. Organizations may do a time-limited pilot—i.e., decide in advance to bring down the pilot after a defined period and make adjustments before the full rollout—or simply have the pilot unit be the first unit of the rollout. In the latter case, the organization must be much more confident that the application will be successful in meeting the organization's needs.

Once the organization is confident that the application is ready for broad deployment, a rollout schedule must be devised. As described above, the rate at which the application can be rolled out is determined by the manpower available to provide the support function. Usually the organization wants to proceed as rapidly as possible through the rollout. The main reason for this is that issues arise when one part of the hospital is using paper-based ordering and other units are using computer ordering. For example, if a patient is transferred between units using different ordering modes, orders must be transcribed from paper to computer, or vice versa. This problem sometimes is known as the "straddle issue." Thus, one common approach is for organizations to implement as rapidly as possible collections of units that represent parts of the hospital where transfers usually take place, such as an entire department of medicine or surgery. Units of the hospital that do not exchange patients with other units (e.g., labor and delivery, neonatal intensive care) sometimes are left for last on the implementation schedule.

Postimplementation Management of CPOE

After the implementation is complete, the organization should prepare itself for the ongoing management of the application. Such ongoing management includes the inevitable set of requests for fixes and enhancements.

Summary

CPOE implementations are large, complex, multi-year projects. Commitment from senior leadership is critical. Strong leadership and management are also required for project success. Analyzing the workflow in the organization and adequately planning for the large amount of change that will take place are more critical to project success than is the technical adequacy of the software. Training and support activities can assume a large fraction of the project costs and can create a rate-limiting step at which rollout can occur. A CPOE implementation project shares many of the characteristics as other very large projects.

Appendix

Bibliography of References Relevant to Computer Provider Order Entry Applications

General Articles about CPOE

1. American Hospital Association. AHA Guide to Computerized Order Entry Applications. Washington DC; 2000.
2. Sittig DF, Stead WW. Computer-based physician order entry: the state of the art. J Am Med Inform Assoc 1994;1(2):108–123.
3. Metzger J, Turisco F. Computerized Order Entry: A Look at the Vendor Marketplace and Getting Started. California Healthcare Foundations and First Consulting Group; December 2001.
4. Ash JS, Gorman PN, Hersh WR. Physician order entry in U.S. hospitals. Proc AMIA Symp 1998:235–239.
5. California Healthcare Foundation. A Primer on Physician Order Entry. Oakland, CA; 2000.
6. Payne TH. The transition to automated practitioner order entry in a teaching hospital: the VA Puget Sound experience. Proc AMIA Symp 1999:589–593.
7. Ahmad A, Teater P, Bentley TD, et al. Key attributes of a successful physician order entry system implementation in a multi-hospital environment. J Am Med Inform Assoc 2002;9(1):16–24.
8. Teich JM, Glaser JP, Beckley RF, et al. The Brigham integrated computing system (BICS): advanced clinical systems in an academic hospital environment. Int J Med Inf 1999;54(3):197–208.
9. Computerized Physician Order Entry: Costs, Benefits, and Challenges—A Case Study Approach. First Consulting Group; January 2003.
10. Massaro TA. Introducing physician order entry at a major academic medical center. Impact on organizational culture and behavior. Acad Med 1993;68(1): 20–25.
11. Murff HJ, Kannry J. Physician satisfaction with two order entry systems. J Am Med Inform Assoc 2001;8(5):499–509.
12. Lee F, Teich JM, Spurr CD, Bates DW. Implementation of physician order entry: user satisfaction and self-reported usage patterns. J Am Med Inform Assoc 1996;3(1):42–55.

Impact of CPOE on Clinician Time

1. Lehman ML, Brill JH, Skarulis PC, Keller D, Lee C. Physician order entry impact on drug turn-around times. Proc AMIA Symp 2001:359–363.
2. Overhage JM, Perkins S, Tierney WM, McDonald CJ. Controlled trial of direct physician order entry: effects on physicians' time utilization in ambulatory primary care internal medicine practices. J Am Med Inform Assoc 2001; 8(4):361–371.
3. Bates DW, Boyle DL, Teich JM. Impact of computerized physician order entry on physician time. Proc Annu Symp Comput Appl Med Care 1994:996.
4. Shu K, Boyle D, Spurr C, et al. Comparison of time spent writing orders on paper with computerized physician order entry. Medinfo 2001;10(Pt 2):1207–1211.

Impact of CPOE on Cost and Quality of Health Care

1. Dexter PR, Perkins S, Overhage JM, Maharry K, Kohler RB, McDonald CJ. A computerized reminder system to increase the use of preventive care for hospitalized patients. N Engl J Med 2001;345(13):965–970.
2. Teich JM, Merchia PR, Schmiz JL, Kuperman GJ, Spurr CD, Bates DW. Effects of computerized physician order entry on prescribing practices. Arch Intern Med 2000;160(18):2741–2747.
3. Overhage JM, Tierney WM, Zhou XH, McDonald CJ. A randomized trial of "corollary orders" to prevent errors of omission. J Am Med Inform Assoc 1997;4(5):364–375.
4. Gonzales R, Steiner JF, Lum A, Barrett PH Jr. Decreasing antibiotic use in ambulatory practice: impact of a multidimensional intervention on the treatment of uncomplicated acute bronchitis in adults. JAMA 1999;281(16):1512–1519.
5. Tierney WM, Miller ME, McDonald CJ. The effect on test ordering of informing physicians of the charges for outpatient diagnostic tests. N Engl J Med 1990;322(21):1499–1504.
6. Bates DW, Kuperman GJ, Jha A, et al. Does the computerized display of charges affect inpatient ancillary test utilization? Arch Intern Med 1997;157(21): 2501–2508.
7. Bates DW, Kuperman GJ, Rittenberg E, et al. A randomized trial of a computer-based intervention to reduce utilization of redundant laboratory tests. Am J Med 1999;106(2):144–150.
8. Tierney WM, McDonald CJ, Martin DK, Rogers MP. Computerized display of past test results. Effect on outpatient testing. Ann Intern Med 1987; 107(4):569–574.
9. Tierney WM, McDonald CJ, Hui SL, Martin DK. Computer predictions of abnormal test results. Effects on outpatient testing. JAMA 1988;259(8): 1194–1198.
10. Solomon DH, Shmerling RH, Schur PH, Lew R, Fiskio J, Bates DW. A computer based intervention to reduce unnecessary serologic testing. J Rheumatol 1999;26(12):2578–2584.
11. Shojania KG, Yokoe D, Platt R, Fiskio J, Ma'luf N, Bates DW. Reducing vancomycin use utilizing a computer guideline: results of a randomized controlled trial. J Am Med Inform Assoc 1998;5(6):554–562.
12. Sanders DL, Miller RA. The effects on clinician ordering patterns of a computerized decision support system for neuroradiology imaging studies. Proc AMIA Symp 2001:583–587.
13. Harpole LH, Khorasani R, Fiskio J, Kuperman GJ, Bates DW. Automated evidence-based critiquing of orders for abdominal radiographs: impact on utilization and appropriateness. J Am Med Inform Assoc 1997;4(6):511–521.
14. Bates DW, Cullen DJ, Laird N, et al. Incidence of adverse drug events and potential adverse drug events. Implications for prevention. ADE Prevention Study Group. JAMA 1995;274(1):29–34.
15. Leape LL, Bates DW, Cullen DJ, et al. Systems analysis of adverse drug events. ADE Prevention Study Group. JAMA 1995;274(1):35–43.
16. Bates DW, Leape LL, Cullen DJ, et al. Effect of computerized physician order entry and a team intervention on prevention of serious medication errors. JAMA 1998;280(15):1311–1316.

17. Bates DW, Teich JM, Lee J, et al. The impact of computerized physician order entry on medication error prevention. J Am Med Inform Assoc 1999; 6(4):313–321.
18. Evans RS, Pestotnik SL, Classen DC, et al. A computer-assisted management program for antibiotics and other antiinfective agents. N Engl J Med 1998;338(4):232–238.
19. Kuperman GJ, Teich JM, Gandhi TK, Bates DW. Patient safety and computerized medication ordering at Brigham and Women's Hospital. Jt Comm J Qual Improv 2001;27(10):509–521.
20. Chertow GM, Lee J, Kuperman GJ, et al. Guided medication dosing for inpatients with renal insufficiency. JAMA 2001;286(22):2839–2844.
21. Kuperman GJ, Cooley T, Tremblay J, Teich JM, Churchill W. Decision support for medication use in an inpatient physician order entry application and a pharmacy application. Medinfo 1998;9(Pt 1):467–471.
22. Tierney WM, Miller ME, Overhage JM, McDonald CJ. Physician inpatient order writing on microcomputer workstations. Effects on resource utilization. JAMA 1993;269(3):379–383.
23. Mekhjian HS, Kumar RR, Kuehn L, et al. Immediate benefits realized following implementation of physician order entry at an academic medical center. J Am Med Inform Assoc 2002;9(5):529–539.
24. Chin HL, Wallace P. Embedding guidelines into direct physician order entry: simple methods, powerful results. Proc AMIA Symp 1999:221–225.
25. Hickam DH, Shortliffe EH, Bischoff MB, Scott AC, Jacobs CD. The treatment advice of a computer-based cancer chemotherapy protocol advisor. Ann Intern Med 1985;103(6 Pt 1):928–936.
26. Tierney WM, Overhage JM, Takesue BY, et al. Computerizing guidelines to improve care and patient outcomes: the example of heart failure. J Am Med Inform Assoc 1995;2(5):316–322.

Articles about Quality of Care and Health Information Technology

1. Chassin MR, Galvin RW. The urgent need to improve health care quality. Institute of Medicine National Roundtable on Health Care Quality. JAMA 1998;280(11):1000–1005.
2. Institute of Medicine: Crossing the Quality Chasm—A New Health System for the 21st Century. Washington, DC: National Academy Press; 2000.
3. Institute of Medicine: To Err Is Human: Building a Safer Health System. Washington, DC: National Academy Press; 1999.

References

1. Institute of Medicine: To Err Is Human: Building a Safer Health System. Washington, DC: National Academy Press; 1999.
2. Institute of Medicine: Crossing the Quality Chasm—A New Health System for the 21st Century. Washington, DC: National Academy Press; 2000.
3. Sittig DF, Stead WW. Computer-based physician order entry: the state of the art. J Am Med Inform Assoc 1994;1(2):108–123.

4. Kuperman GJ, Gibson RF. Computer physician order entry: benefits, costs, and issues. Ann Intern Med. 2003;139(1):31–39.
5. Kuperman GJ, Teich JM, Gandhi TK, Bates DW. Patient safety and computerized medication ordering at Brigham and Women's Hospital. Jt Comm J Qual Improv 2001;27(10):509–521.
6. Leape LL, Bates DW, Cullen DJ, et al. Systems analysis of adverse drug events. ADE Prevention Study Group. JAMA 1995;274(1):35–43.
7. Ash JS, Gorman PN, Seshadri V, Hersh WR. Computerized physician order entry in U.S. hospitals: results of a 2002 survey. J Am Med Inform Assoc 2004;11(2):95–99.
8. Poon EG, Blumenthal D, Jaggi T, Honour MM, Bates DW, Kaushal R. Overcoming barriers to adopting and implementing computerized physician order entry systems in U.S. hospitals. Health Aff (Millwood) 2004;23(4):184–190.
9. Payne TH, Hoey PJ, Nichol P, Lovis C. Preparation and use of preconstructed orders, order sets, and order menus in a computerized provider order entry system. J Am Med Inform Assoc 2003;10(4):322–329.
10. Bates DW, Cullen DJ, Laird N, et al. Incidence of adverse drug events and potential adverse drug events. Implications for prevention. ADE Prevention Study Group. JAMA 1995;274(1):29–34.
11. Shojania KG, Yokoe D, Platt R, Fiskio J, Ma'luf N, Bates DW. Reducing vancomycin use utilizing a computer guideline: results of a randomized controlled trial. J Am Med Inform Assoc 1998;5(6):554–562.
12. Sanders DL, Miller RA. The effects on clinician ordering patterns of a computerized decision support system for neuroradiology imaging studies. Proc AMIA Symp 2001:583–587.
13. Teich JM, Merchia PR, Schmiz JL, Kuperman GJ, Spurr CD, Bates DW. Effects of computerized physician order entry on prescribing practices. Arch Intern Med 2000;160(18):2741–2747.
14. Overhage JM, Tierney WM, Zhou XH, McDonald CJ. A randomized trial of "corollary orders" to prevent errors of omission. J Am Med Inform Assoc 1997;4(5):364–375.
15. Bates DW, Kuperman GJ, Rittenberg E, et al. A randomized trial of a computer-based intervention to reduce utilization of redundant laboratory tests. Am J Med 1999;106(2):144–150.
16. Chen P, Tanasijevic MJ, Schoenenberger RA, et al. A computer-based intervention for improving the appropriateness of antiepileptic drug level monitoring. Am J Clin Pathol 2003;119(3):432–438.
17. Chertow GM, Lee J, Kuperman GJ, et al. Guided medication dosing for inpatients with renal insufficiency. JAMA 2001;286(22):2839–2844.
18. Kuperman GJ, Gandhi TK, Bates DW. Effective drug-allergy checking: methodological and operational issues. J Biomed Inform 2003;36(1–2):70–79.
19. Hsieh TC, Kuperman GJ, Jaggi T, et al. Characteristics and consequences of drug allergy alert overrides in a computerized physician order entry system. J Am Med Inform Assoc 2004;11(6):482–491.
20. Computerized Physician Order Entry: Costs, Benefits, and Challenges—A Case Study Approach. First Consulting Group; January 2003.
21. Dexter PR, Perkins S, Overhage JM, Maharry K, Kohler RB, McDonald CJ. A computerized reminder system to increase the use of preventive care for hospitalized patients. N Engl J Med 2001;345(13):965–970.

22. Bates DW, Leape LL, Cullen DJ, et al. Effect of computerized physician order entry and a team intervention on prevention of serious medication errors. JAMA 1998;280(15):1311–1316.
23. Evans RS, Pestotnik SL, Classen DC, et al. A computer-assisted management program for antibiotics and other antiinfective agents. N Engl J Med 1998; 338(4):232–238.
24. Tierney WM, Miller ME, Overhage JM, McDonald CJ. Physician inpatient order writing on microcoputer workstations. Effects on resource utilization. JAMA 1993;269(3):379–383.

8
Public Policy Issues for Computer-based Patient Records, Electronic Health Record Systems, and the National Health Information Network

Don E. Detmer

In 1991, the Institute of Medicine (IOM) called for healthcare professionals and organizations to adopt the computer-based patient record (CPR) as "the standard for medical and all other records related to patient care."[1] Since then, we have embraced the concept of CPRs as more than digitized versions of paper records, strengthened the proof of benefits provided by CPRs and related technologies (e.g., clinical decision support), expanded our thinking about CPRs and other health records, and deepened our understanding of the role that health information technology can have in addressing the shortcomings of the current United States (US) healthcare system.[2] Furthermore, information and communications technologies have advanced, particularly with the advent of the Internet, and provide increasing connectivity and processing power for lower costs. As technological capabilities progressed, many businesses and industries used information technology to better understand and meet consumer needs. As a result, computers are more widely diffused throughout society and both health professionals and the public are accustomed to using computers for a variety of transactions in every day life but alas, too infrequently in healthcare services.

As described elsewhere in this volume, considerable progress has been made in the development and implementation of CPR systems and technologies within individual organizations. Yet 14 years after the IOM's call to action, only an estimated 15% of hospitals and 25% of physician practices in the US use CPR systems.[3,4] Meanwhile, the challenges facing the US health sector continue to grow and the belief that CPRs and related technologies are pivotal to desperately needed changes in the health system continues to spread. Thus, the challenge still facing the health community and policy makers is how to achieve widespread diffusion of this essential technology.

The Policy Milieu

At first glance, the challenge of widespread CPR diffusion may appear to be the same today as it was when the IOM released its report on CPRs in 1991. Although we face some of the same issues now as we did then, several important changes have occurred. Some changes are attributable to the efforts of the health informatics community to address the obstacles to CPRs. Other changes are related to broader developments in the health sector. And yet still other changes that shape the current policy environment for CPRs arose out of an entirely unrelated domain.

From CPRs to Electronic Health Records

In the early 1990s, CPRs were generally understood to be the records used by clinicians either in healthcare organizations or private practice while providing care to patients. CPRs were recognized as being important for improving the ability of clinicians to care for patients. As such, they were seen primarily as being a tool for improving the internal workings of healthcare institutions. Particular emphasis was placed on improving individual patient encounters through improved accuracy, decision support, and elimination of duplicative efforts. The IOM report on CPRs distinguished between primary records (used for delivery of patient care services) and secondary records (used for administration, regulation, quality assurance, and research), but in general, little attention was given to the concept of secondary records or the use of patient data beyond the patient–clinician encounter.

During that period, the concept of CPRs as being more than segregated electronic repositories of patient data (i.e., by including alerts, reminders, clinical decision support, and links to medical knowledge) was gradually moving from the realm of informaticians to the broader healthcare and policy communities. The articulation and widespread acceptance of the vision for CPR systems as interactive rather than a passive tool for clinicians constituted an important advance in the thinking about how the health sector should use computers. It was, however, only a first step and major obstacles to widespread adoption of CPRs remained.

The 1990s were also marked by the deepening and broadening of understanding about the nature of and barriers to quality health care. Important work on the quality of healthcare services by the IOM and others expanded awareness of the factors that contribute to variations in healthcare quality and drew attention to the role of information technology—including CPRs—in addressing the shortcomings of the US healthcare system.[2,5–7] As the decade progressed, the resurgence of cost increases that had been temporarily moderated by managed care, the growing number of uninsured and underinsured Americans, the increasing demand for management of chronic conditions driven by the aging population, and the rapidly expanding base of medical knowledge reinforced the need for a systems approach to addressing challenges in the health sector. As the IOM concluded in *Crossing the Quality Chasm* (page 4):

Health care has safety and quality problems because it relies on outmoded systems of work. Poor designs set the workforce up to fail, regardless of how hard they try. If we want safer, higher-quality care, we will need to have redesigned systems of care, including the use of information technology to support clinical and administrative processes.[2]

Moreover, the emergence of the Internet combined with the societal trend of stronger consumerism to provide citizens with better tools (i.e., access to medical knowledge) has enabled them to be more assertive consumers of health care and more active participants in healthcare decisions. The need to navigate an increasingly complex healthcare system and health insurance plans that increasingly share the costs of healthcare services with patients gives consumers motivation to use these tools.

Finally, there has been growing recognition of the importance of aggregating patient data to create population health databases to support research and public health. As the boundaries between research and the clinical realm have begun to blur, there are new types of data generated and more demands for aggregated patient data. On one hand, the gradual shift of genomics from the research laboratory to clinical setting, accompanied by the concept of personalized medicine (i.e., treatment based on an individual's genetic profile), portends the need for clinicians to manage and analyze more data and more complex data and to apply increasingly sophisticated knowledge in clinical decisions.[8] For example, in early 2005, the Food and Drug Administration approved for the first time the marketing of a genotyping test that will help physicians personalize treatment options for their patients. Specifically, this test detects "certain common genetic mutations that alter the body's ability to break down (metabolize) specific types of drugs" including antidepressants, antipsychotics, beta-blockers, and some chemotherapy drugs. Variations in the gene that is tested can cause a patient to metabolize these drugs too fast, abnormally slow, or not at all and thus cause a dose that is safe for some patients to be toxic for others.[6]

On the other hand, researchers are increasingly using genomic, epigenetic, and clinical data in clinical research. Linking information from personal health records (PHRs) with public health datasets such as ToxNet (i.e., a cluster of databases on toxicology, hazardous chemicals, and related areas) could be extremely helpful in addressing a range of research questions from basic pathogenesis to environmental concerns.[7] Recent concerns over the cost and safety of prescription medications contribute to a growing sense that only a national if not global infrastructure for clinical trial results and biomedical research is needed to mitigate this situation.

Our expanded understanding of the determinants of health and the evolution in thinking about how to improve the quality of healthcare services contributed to our collective thinking about the role of CPRs in strengthening the health sector. Thus, understanding CPRs has expanded to include computer-based patient records, computer-based personal records, and computer-based population records.[11,12] The term electronic health record (EHR) encompasses all three types of records. Further, CPRs and EHRs are now viewed in the context of a national health information infrastructure (NHII). Although the IOM report on CPRs explicitly addressed the need for a national healthcare information system, the concept was not fully developed and articulated until 2001 by the National Committee on Vital and Health Statistics (NCVHS).

More Pronounced Role for the Public Sector

Another important change since the early 1990s has been the shift in thinking about the appropriate role for the federal government in advancing the use of CPRs and EHRs and leading the development of an NHII. The increased visibility of EHRs after the release of the IOM report generated two types of responses. In Europe, Canada, Australia, and New Zealand, governments began to develop national strategies to make EHRs a core feature of their healthcare systems. England, for example, is in the midst of a 10-year project to implement a border-to-border EHR system that connects patients, physicians, and hospitals throughout the country.[8]

Unlike other countries, the US did not have a unified response to CPRs from the federal government. The CPR committee's recommendation to create the Computer-based Patient Record Institute reflects the climate of the time—avoid placing new responsibilities in the hands of the federal government. The Department of Defense (DOD) and the Veterans Administration (VA) did expand efforts to develop CPRs for use in their hospitals and clinics. Non-federal healthcare provider organizations and private practitioners were, however, left to their own devices and only a few major private sector organizations such as the Kaiser health system picked up the challenge of implementing large-scale EHR systems.

The lack of a national response by the US was disappointing, but understandable and perhaps even predictable. In contrast to other nations with single payer systems and a culture of supporting the social good, the structure of the US healthcare sector was at odds with the kind of environment needed to support CPR implementation. In the US, with few exceptions, neither public nor private reimbursement systems rewarded clinicians for managing the total costs of caring for a patient over time. So long as healthcare providers are reimbursed on the basis of separate encounters, there is little incentive to invest in expensive systems that enable clinicians to manage the care of patients over time.

Furthermore, the American culture of emphasis on individual rights and privacy meant that CPRs could not move into widespread use without very robust security and confidentiality protections.[9] Regrettably, appropriate national legislation for secure electronic health systems could not be passed despite bipartisan support early in the process. The resultant HIPAA (i.e., Health Insurance Portability and Accountability Act of 1996) regulations are workable and laudable in all but one key feature—there is not federal preemption of state laws relating to similar data. As discussed below, this must be changed if an NHII is to result because so many US citizens live near the borders of other states (see Privacy).

That is not to say that certain agencies within the federal government have not been active in creating an environment that supports CPRs and EHRs. For example, the National Library of Medicine provided the initial stimulus for the IOM to study the issue of patient records in the late 1980s, has been a world leader in making medical literature available online, and most recently has had a pivotal role in making SNOMED available in the public domain. The Agency for Healthcare Research and Quality (AHRQ) and its predecessors have a long history of supporting research to assess the costs and benefits of information technology in health care. As noted above, DOD and VA were leaders in developing CPRs for their populations.[10,11] But in general, until recently, efforts within the federal government to build the foundation for widespread use of EHRs in the US were fragmented and not led by the department that has the most leverage to influence the behavior of clinicians and healthcare organizations [i.e., the Department of Health and Human Services (DHHS)].

A very important structural change was made during the 1990s to allow the government to better deal with policy debates relating to EHRs. The administrative simplification provisions of HIPAA named the NCVHS to advise the Secretary of Health and Human Services on confidentiality and security, identifiers, and standards for CPRs. The HIPAA legislation restructured the advisory committee that had been focused exclusively on "after-the-fact" vital and health statistics into the nation's health information policy advisory committee. Sensing that there was no national effort to assess the potential of and advocate for an NHII, NCVHS established an NHII working group. This group's initial and subsequent reports have become the template documents for NHII activity in the US.

More recently, EHRs have moved into the foreground at the national level. In April 2004, President Bush called for widespread adoption of interoperable EHRs within 10 years and established the position of National Coordinator for Health Information Technology. The National Coordinator reports directly to the Secretary of Health and Human Services and is charged "to provide leadership for the development and nationwide implementation of an interoperable health information technology infrastructure to improve the quality and efficiency of health care."[12] In June 2004, the President's Information Technology Advisory Committee presented a "framework for a 21st century healthcare information infrastructure that revolutionizes medical records systems."[13] And, in January 2005, Congress charged the federal Commission on Systemic Interoperability to develop a strategy and timeline for implementing an infrastructure that supports interoperable electronic healthcare systems and to report to Congress by October 2005.[14] This work continues through the American Health Information Community (AHIC). Similar interest is evident at the state level. For example, the Massachusetts eHealth Collaborative was established in late 2004 to create a state-wide health information network to improve the quality, safety, and affordability of health care. This coalition includes 34 different institutions with representatives from physicians' and nurses' groups, hospitals, health plans, state government, technology associations, and business, purchaser, and public interest groups. Notably, a major insurer—Blue Cross and Blue Shield of Massachusetts—has pledged $50 million to help fund the first three pilot projects. Each of the demonstration sites will be a "test-bed for universal adoption of EHRs and decision support infrastructure that links together physician office practices, health centers, hospitals, laboratories, pharmacies, and other medical entities."[15]

Moving from Why to How

In the early 1990s, much of the discussion focused on expanding understanding of CPRs and justifying the investment in them. At that time, information technology was just beginning to be used to transform other industries such as banking and travel and there was little evidence that documented the benefits of CPRs or related technologies. Today we have the benefit of seeing how well-designed information systems can support information-intensive processes and numerous studies that demonstrate specific benefits of CPR/EHR and related systems.[16-18]

Furthermore, the need for robust information and knowledge management tools to support all domains of the health sector is widely accepted. Specific weaknesses in healthcare delivery such as safety deficiencies and variation in practice patterns can be remedied through more consistent application of relevant knowledge integrated for clinicians. The bioterrorism event of 2001 highlighted deficiencies in our public health information infrastructure and reinforced the need for a strong health information infrastructure in the US. Researchers seek to make the research process more efficient and reduce the time it takes for new medical knowledge to move from the research bench to the patient.[19]

We still have much to learn about the design of EHR systems that effectively support the work of healthcare professionals and need to continuously refine how we evaluate those systems.[20-22] We have, however, moved from demands for evidence of the need for EHRs to a focus on eliminating barriers to them. As described by one observer, we have reached the tipping point "at which there would be no further need to talk about whether to computerize and the focus would finally shift to the question of how to computerize."[15]

Policy Challenges

Compressing the aspirations for robust information management capabilities for the health sector into a practical clear strategy and then engaging the political will to make the investment in EHRs and the NHII in the face of strong budgetary pressures is the central health information technology challenge for public policy for the remainder of this decade if not longer. This investment of both intellectual and financial capital must be directed to eliminating the most significant stumbling blocks to EHRs and the NHII. Specifically, to advance EHRs, we must focus our efforts on creating and implementing appropriate policies that:

- Provide incentives for and financing of EHRs
- Confront privacy concerns
- Ensure a prepared workforce
- Address the needs of citizens

In addition, the visible progress in the development of standards that enable interoperability of EHR systems must continue and be expanded to assure that global standards emerge.[23]

Incentives and Financing

The old adage "you get what you pay for" is certainly true for the delivery of healthcare services in the US. Clinicians and healthcare delivery organizations are generally paid on the basis of individual encounters with patients. Sometimes they are paid more if a particular technology (e.g., magnetic resonance imaging) is used to diagnose or treat the patient. They have not typically been paid for the use of EHRs.

Nor are they compensated for practices that are made possible through EHRs and related technologies. They are not paid for communication with a patient that eliminates the need for an office visit. They are not paid for assuring that the treatment used is based on the latest medical knowledge. They are not paid to track whether the patient follows the recommended treatment. They are not paid to manage a patient's health over time. And they are not paid for providing data that can be used to assess the effectiveness of specific treatments within specific populations of patients.

Some clinicians and healthcare organizations do follow these practices, but do so at a cost that is not reimbursed. Thus, there is scant if any financial incentive for health professionals and provider organizations to subject themselves to the significant costs associated with acquiring, implementing, and maintaining EHRs—including the temporary reduction in staff productivity as they learn the new system and develop new work flows to accompany the system. Meanwhile, the tangible benefits that are generated accrue to the patient in terms of higher quality care, to the party responsible for paying for the services in terms of potentially lower costs, and to employers and society in terms of healthier and more productive citizens and workers.

Some healthcare provider organizations have recognized that the practice of high quality, effective, efficient care can strengthen their competitiveness and use this strategy as a tool for negotiating with employers and insurers. In turn, employers and insurers have begun to reward healthcare providers who can follow specific practices or achieve certain outcomes. This development may prove to be the most pivotal in creating incentives for physician practices and other healthcare delivery organizations to invest in EHRs.

The Leapfrog Group is one of the leaders in the effort to stimulate healthcare providers and clinicians to adopt practices and technologies that support safe, high-quality, and affordable health care.[24] The large private and public healthcare purchasers that are members of this consortium have agreed to purchase health care on principles that encourage provider quality improvement and consumer involvement. To that end, computer physician order entry (CPOE) is one of four hospital quality and safety practices that are the basis for hospital recognition and reward.

General Electric (GE), which pays more than $2 billion per year in healthcare coverage, is another leader on this front.[25] In 2000, GE began a program to reward physicians for savings achieved through improved care of diabetes and heart disease. GE reports that the average cost of properly caring for diabetics decreased by $350 per year, without factoring in the cost of long-term complications that arise when the disease is left untreated. Taking a more direct approach to encourage physicians to adopt EHRs, GE is paying physician practices up to $15,000 per year for investing in and using computers. The RAND Corporation will conduct a study of the financial impact of this strategy for GE.

As suggested by these examples, there are both direct and indirect incentives that reward the acquisition and use of EHRs. Direct incentives may take the form of insurers (or other large purchasers) providing one-time grants to offset the costs of implementing an EHR system or paying for the use of a specific function offered by EHR or related systems (e.g., CPOE or electronic prescription ordering). Insurers and large purchasers can create indirect incentives for EHRs by paying for performance (i.e., demonstrated quality achieved) or specific practices (e.g., disease management).

The federal government is also taking action in this area. In February 2005, the National Health Information Incentive Act of 2005 was introduced with bipartisan support.[26] This Act authorizes DHHS to provide initial funding through grants, tax credits, or revolving loans to support acquisition of interoperable EHR systems. It also creates incentives for physicians to use technology to improve patient care. For example, it authorizes add-on bonus payments under Medicare office visits supported by EHRs and for e-mail consultations that meet defined standards.

Furthermore, Medicare has recently embarked on a series of pay-for-performance initiatives.[27] In February 2005, the Centers for Medicare and Medicaid announced a pay-for-performance demonstration project that involves 10 of the country's largest physician groups, representing 5000 physicians and more than 200,000 Medicare fee-for-service beneficiaries.[28] Medicare will track how much money these practices save the program and how well they improve healthcare quality. Eighty percent of the savings that exceed the target will go into a pay-for-performance pool to be distributed among the practices that meet predetermined targets.

The development and assessment of various approaches to creating incentives that reward clinicians and organizations for investing in and using EHRs is a critical step on the road to nationwide EHR adoption. Of equal if not greater import is the need to assure that both private and public sectors maintain their current level of interest in and increase their level of investment in EHRs and NHII development. Federal budget and deficit realities in 2005 create a grim picture for increased federal spending on EHR/NHII development in light of the projected costs—almost $600 billion spread over 10 years for rollout of interoperable systems according to one estimate.[29] These admittedly high costs must, however, be weighed against the potential savings to be gained by the health system and the citizens of the nation.

For instance, if differences across regions in per capita spending for Medicare beneficiaries were eliminated with the support of EHRs and practice guidelines, up to 30% of current Medicare spending could be saved for alternative uses such as paying for prescription drug benefits.[30] Alternatively, if CPOE is universally implemented, there could be widespread reduction in preventable medication errors that are estimated to cost up to $2 billion annually in hospitals and $3.6 billion in nursing homes.[5] One analysis concluded that healthcare information exchange and interoperability among providers and between providers and independent laboratories, payers, radiology centers, pharmacies, and public health departments would yield net benefits of $77.8 billion annually.[34] These net benefits do not include the benefits of improved health and life status that accrue to patients whose care would be supported by these systems.

Moreover, these estimates consider the benefits of EHRs and the NHII purely from the perspective of health care. The 2003 outbreak of severe acute respiratory syndrome (SARS) illustrates that robust health information technology systems also contribute to the strength of the total economy. The SARS outbreak in Hong Kong not only impacted the families of individuals who died from the illness, it also disrupted workflow for several weeks, significantly reduced travel to the area, and created panic among residents.[31] This episode of disease is estimated to have cost Hong Kong $1.7 billon.[32]

Hong Kong's experience with SARS could have been much worse had the Hong Kong Hospital Authority not acted quickly to build upon its existing clinical information system to implement a SARS tracking registry. The Hospital Authority moved from a fax-reporting system in February 2003 to a simple database to track cases in March to a Web-based registry called eSARS for reporting and tracking cases in April.[33] This registry was then linked to an electronic system that could track where the SARS patients had been recently to identify other potential cases. The outbreak was over by late June and eSARS has been credited with playing a role in saving lives, shortening the crisis, and managing the economic losses of the outbreak.

A 1999 study concluded the economic costs of an influenza pandemic in the US would range from $71.3 to $166.5 billion.[34] In an era of new global infectious diseases and potential bioterrorism threats, the NHII could be as essential to the economic health of the US as the interstate highway system was in the post-World War II era. Thus, we must broaden our view of the benefits of EHRs and the NHII and fully delineate and begin to quantify the non-health benefits of these technologies.

Privacy

Policy makers still doubt that EHR environments can protect patient privacy, despite a decade of effort.[14] Earning and maintaining trust in the care relationship requires patient confidentiality. Many, if not most, American clinicians and administrators assume that unique personal health identifiers are essential to effective use of interoperable EHRs but many health information policy advocates disagree. Accurate authentication enables tracking of individuals over time and across institutions, assures that the data being viewed belong solely to the desired patient, and ensures providers' having complete patient data available at all times. Algorithms have been developed for accurately identifying individuals without violating privacy and their practicality are being tested, but even after some years of testing, whether it will adequately answer the question for frontier regions of the nation isn't clear to the author at least.

The US differs from other developed countries with regard to authorizing highly reliable personal identifiers for any purpose. Although the issue is nearly frozen here, the entire European Union has committed to a unique personal health identifier for more than 300 million individuals.

According to the eminent philosopher, Onora O'Neill, contemporary societies in the West so much value personal autonomy, that they corrode trust within society. Trust is an absolutely crucial ingredient for any functioning democracy and for a healthy patient–clinician relationship. Privacy, long considered an instrumental good, is thus placed into direct conflict with health, both an intrinsic and instrumental good. Of particular concern is the impact of overly restrictive privacy rules that reduce the ability of researchers to conduct population-based research and long-term medical outcomes research, and that impede the creation of new medical knowledge.[35] The unique personal health identifier seems to have become more a measure of cultural cohesion and social solidarity than a technical issue for EHR development.

Interoperability requires that privacy and confidentiality rules be applied at the national level. Ideally, adjusted HIPAA privacy standards are needed to override state laws. Otherwise, the resulting conflicting rules and standards across the nation will impede the efficient sharing of information and most likely diminish the level of protection desired. America may well lose a golden opportunity to be fully at the table when workable standards are set at the global level.

According to the eminent philosopher, Onora O'Neill, contemporary societies in the West are placing excessive and misplaced weight on personal autonomy, and in so doing are corroding trust within society. Trust is an absolutely crucial ingredient for any functioning society and is essential for a healthy patient–doctor relationship. By elevating privacy to such a high priority, trust suffers. Privacy, long considered an instrumental good, is thus placed into direct conflict with health, which for centuries has been considered both an intrinsic and instrumental good (i.e., health has intrinsic value and also can be instrumental to a host of other good things). The unique personal health identifier seems to have become more a measure of cultural cohesion and social solidarity than a technical issue for EHR development. What remains an open question is whether the power of privacy fundamentalists to advocate successfully in legislative arenas for greater and greater protections of privacy and autonomy will prevent EHRs and indeed other innovations in health care such as personalized care coming from genomics research from becoming mature technologies and part of the infrastructure beneath health care. Of particular concern is the impact of overly restrictive privacy rules that reduce the ability of researchers to conduct population-based research (e.g., epidemiologic, health services, environmental and occupational health) and long-term medical outcomes research, add significant costs to the research process, and impede the creation of new medical knowledge that will benefit current and future generations.[35]

Viewed from a purely pragmatic perspective, many healthcare providers already collect the social security numbers of their patients as part of the registration process. Clearly, a unique personal health identifier that is not readily linked to an individual's financial history would provide greater protection than current practice. Recent thefts of personal financial data highlight the need for a well-developed framework to protect personal information and vigorous enforcement of that framework. Lack of action only provides more opportunities for abuse.

Finally, privacy and confidentiality rules that are adopted must be applied at the national level. HIPAA privacy standards and identifier rules must be implemented as national standards and override state laws. Failure to do so will result in potentially conflicting rules and standards that impede the efficient sharing of information and diminish the level of protection that is actually provided to the data.

Workforce

There are four ways in which we need to strengthen the health professional workforce to assure that we take full advantage of the investment in EHRs and an NHII. First, we need to dramatically increase the number of clinical informaticians in the US. Clinical informaticians are physicians, nurses, and other health professionals trained in integrated computer science with related disciplines including organizational behavior.[36] These individuals work in both healthcare delivery organizations and for vendors of health information technology firms helping to develop EHR and related systems that effectively meet the needs of health professionals and patients and providing leadership in the implementation of EHR systems within organizations. Currently, graduate medical informatics training programs produce fewer than 200 graduates per year. Clearly, we need many more of these experts to participate in the development and support the implementation of EHR systems in the myriad healthcare settings across the nation and to train general users. Generally, clinical informaticians are trained in academic settings. Thus, we must also develop ways to assure that these specialists have sufficient experience in and understanding of the needs of small and rural private practice environments and related networks.

Second, we need to explore an appropriate certification process for applied clinical informaticians in medicine since nursing achieved this some objective some years ago. Such a certification would provide a measure of professional achievement and recognition to those clinicians who invest their personal time and financial resources to become trained in this field. It would also provide health provider organizations seeking to strengthen their informatics capabilities with a means by which to screen candidates. Furthermore, certified applied clinical informaticians would be in a stronger position to negotiate compensation for this expertise.

Third, we must assure that all health professionals—physicians, nurses, pharmacists, therapists, etc.—possess a basic level of competence in the effective use of EHRs and related systems upon graduation from their respective schools. Many health professional schools do not adequately prepare clinicians for the "information-intensive world they will experience."[37] Thus, we must work to expand the time that is allocated to information management in the curricula of these skills and initiate interdisciplinary discussions about what constitutes an acceptable baseline of information management proficiency for all health professionals.

Fourth, we must assure that there are sufficient numbers of health information management professionals who are specifically trained to support EHRs in community practice settings.[37] These individuals will need technical expertise to perform basic general tasks such as data backup, run an office network, maintain reliable Internet connections, and oversee effective security practices. They will also need to be well versed in the practice of medicine and understand the needs of both clinicians and patients.

Citizen Preparedness

Given the increasingly recognized role of individuals as managers of their health and healthcare services and the significant role that PHRs could have in facilitating communication between patients and clinicians, improving accuracy of patient data (e.g., history), and providing new kinds of data that could inform health decisions and support research (e.g., diaries of patient experiences), public policy must also assure that citizens are prepared to use EHRs effectively. There are three key ways that policy can contribute to citizen preparedness.

First, we must address the basic issue of health literacy. Health literacy is

the degree to which individuals have the capacity to obtain, process, and understand basic health information and services needed to make appropriate health decisions.[37]

As identified in the 2004 IOM report, nearly half of all American adults have difficulty understanding and acting upon health information.[37] Research has shown that people with low health literacy get preventative care less frequently, use expensive health services such as the emergency department more frequently, have less knowledge about their illness, and have decreased ability to participate in decision making about their care. Interventions to improve health literacy of the population may address the educational system, health system, or cultural and social factors. DHHS has implemented a research program to increase "understanding of the nature of health literacy and its relationship to healthy behaviors, illness prevention and treatment, chronic disease management, health disparities, risk assessment of environmental factors, and health outcomes including mental and oral health."[38] DHHS further seeks to identify "interventions that can strengthen health literacy and improve the positive health impacts of communications between healthcare and public health professionals (including dentists, healthcare delivery organizations, and public health entities), and consumer or patient audiences that vary in health literacy."[38]

Second, we must support the development of PHR systems that are interoperable and meet the needs of those patients who are ready to use them. PHRs are in their infancy.[39,40] Early experiences suggest that PHRs can help "a significant subset of people understand their health issues, become more engaged in decisions they face, and improve their communication with clinicians."[40] Yet, a 2002 evaluation of the functionality of selected PHR systems found that the systems offered limited functionality and revealed deficiencies that point to the need to clarify intended uses of these applications.[41]

Developmental challenges for PHRs are similar to those for provider record systems. A 2004 study by Connecting for Health concluded that there is a need to develop[39]:

- A common means of correctly identifying each person and ensuring privacy protections
- Common datasets, data exchange standards, and data coding vocabularies
- Policies that "place each person at the center of controlling his or her own information, support the secure storage of both professionally-sourced and patient-sourced data, and promote the portability of the information based on each person's needs and wishes"
- Mechanisms to support physician acceptance and promotion of PHR systems

There is some concern within the health informatics community that demand for PHRs could get ahead of physician adoption of EHRs.[42] There is, however, strong support for PHRs, particularly those that support management of chronic conditions. And some advocates for EHRs and PHRs see patient demand as a potential factor in accelerating adoption and use of these systems.

Third, we must create ways for citizens to become proficient in the maintenance and use of PHRs and related technologies. As a first step, citizens must have basic skills in the use of personal computers to assure that they are able to maintain a secure environment for their personal health information, understand how to use PHRs, and are able to transmit data to and from clinician systems as appropriate. US policy makers may choose to follow the model of the European Union (EU) in developing a certification process for the computer use. The International Computing Driving License (ICDL) is an internationally recognized standard of competence in the form of a certificate that asserts that the holder has the knowledge and skills needed to use the most common computer applications efficiently and productively in the workplace and at home. The ICDL Foundation, a not-for-profit organization, oversees ICDL work in participating countries (including all EU, Scandinavian and Eastern European countries, Zimbabwe, South Africa, Canada, and Australia).[43] Such a model would provide a framework for education of citizens—both school age and adult—and help individuals identify deficiencies in their computer skills.

Conclusion

As we approach the mid-portion of this decade, the policy arguments for CPRs/EHRs and the NHII have shifted. Healthcare costs have continued to increase, baby boomers are approaching retirement with increasing demands on healthcare services, quality and safety issues are seen as serious, and the knowledge base of medicine continues to escalate as a result of research into the human genome as well as other areas of technology. Instead of CPRs/EHRs and the NHII being a development that is essentially a good thing for healthcare delivery, it is seen increasingly as the only opportunity on the horizon with the capacity to seriously impact in a useful way cost, quality, safety, efficiency, effectiveness, access, and timely patient-centered care as well as addressing totally new concerns relating to bioterrorism and public health biosurveillance in the post-September 11 environment, post-Katrina, and potentially an avian flu pandemic.

Since the release of the IOM report in 1991, we have worked to build a foundation for EHRs and the NHII and have made progress in several important areas. We must, however, continue to press forward to address the remaining challenges of creating appropriate incentives, implementing sound standards, assuring security of our systems and confidentiality of patient data, and preparing health professionals and citizens to take full advantage of EHRs and the NHII. We can do so with both broader and deeper support than we have had in the past and thus we can focus our attention on how and when, rather than why and if. As we strive to achieve widespread use of EHRs and implementation of a robust NHII, we must remember that these essential technologies are a means to our ultimate end—improved health for our nation and, indeed, people everywhere.

References

1. Institute of Medicine. The Computer-based Patient Record: An Essential Technology for Health Care. Washington, DC: The National Academy Press; 2001:6.
2. Institute of Medicine. Crossing the Quality Chasm: A New System for Health Care in America. Washington, DC: The National Academy Press; 2001.
3. Cropper CM. Between you, the doctor, and the PC. BusinessWeek Online; January 31, 2005. Available at: http://www.businessweek.com/magazine/content/05_05/b3918155_mz070.html. Accessed April 4, 2005.
4. Versel N. One in five group practices now uses EHRs. Health IT World. January 25, 2005. Available at: http://www.health-it.world.com/enews/01-25-2005_508.html. Accessed January 28, 2005.
5. Institute of Medicine. To Err Is Human: Building a Safer Health System. Washington, DC: National Academy Press; 1999.
6. US Food and Drug Administration. New device clearance: Roche Amplichip Cytochrome P450 Genotyping Test and Affymetric GeneChip Microarry Instrumentation System—K042259. Available at: http://www.fda.gov/cdrh/mda/docs/k042259.html. Accessed March 30, 2005.
7. National Library of Medicine. Specialized Information Services: TOXNET. Available at: http://toxnet.nlm.nih.gov. Accessed April 2, 2005.
8. Baldwin G. Make that fish and chips. HealthLeaders News. February 15, 2005. Available at: http://www.healthleaders.com/news/print.php?contented=64544. Accessed March 3, 2005.
9. Detmer DE, Steen EB. Shoring up protection of personal health data. Issues Sci Technol 1996;4:73–78.
10. Javitt JC. How to succeed in health information technology. Health Affairs Web Exclusive 2004;W4:321–323. Available at: www.healthaffairs.org. Accessed April 3, 2005.

11. Curtis C. A computer-based patient record emerging from the public sector: the Decentralized Hospital Computer Program. In: Steen EB, ed. Proceedings of the First Annual Nicholas E. Davies CPR Recognition Symposium. Schaumburg, IL: Computer-based Patient Record Institute; 1995:53–95.
12. The White House. Executive Order. April 27, 2004. Available at: http://www.whitehouse.gov/news/releases/2004/04/20040427-4.html. Accessed March 25, 2005.
13. President's Information Technology Advisory Committee. Revolutionizing Health Care Through Information Technology. Arlington, VA: National Coordination Office for Information Technology Research and Development; 2004.
14. McGee MK. Commission ready to work on national health record-records systems. InformationWeek; January 11, 2005. Available at: http://information-week.com/story/showarticle.jhtml?articleID-57700565. Accessed January 28, 2005.
15. Massachusetts eHealth Collaborative. News release: Massachusetts eHealth Collaborative launches project to wire health care in the state. December 6, 2004. Available at: www.maehc.org. Accessed March 30, 2005.
16. Bates DW, Leape LL, Cullen DJ, et al. Effect of computerized order entry and a team intervention on prevention of serious medication errors. JAMA 1998; 280:1311–1316.
17. Dexter PR, Perkins S, Overhage JM, et al. A computerized reminder system to increase the use of preventative care for hospitalized patients. N Engl J Med 2001;345:965–970.
18. Mekhjian HS, Kumar RR, Kuehn L, et al. Immediate benefits realized following implementation of physician order entry at an academic medical center. J Am Med Inform Assoc 2002;9:529–539.
19. National Institutes of Health. NIH roadmap: accelerating medical discovery to improve health. Available at: http://nihroadmap.nih.gov. Accessed April 2, 2005.
20. Garg AX, Adhikari NKJ, McDonald H, et al. Effects of computerized clinical decision support systems on practitioner performance and patient outcomes: a systematic review. JAMA 2005;293:1223–1238.
21. Koppel R, Metlay JP, Cohen A, et al. Role of computerized physician order entry systems in facilitating medication errors. JAMA 2005;293:1197–1203.
22. Wears RL, Berg M. Computer technology and clinical work: still waiting for Godot. JAMA 2005;293:1261–1263.
23. Stead WW, Kelly BJ, Kolodner RM. Achievable steps toward building a national health information infrastructure. J Am Med Inform Assoc 2005;12:113–120.
24. The Leapfrog Group. Leapfrog Group fact sheet. Available at: http://www.leapfroggroup.org/about_us/leapfrog-factsheet. Accessed March 25, 2005.
25. Lowenstein R. The quality cure? New York Times. 2005. Available at: http://www.nytimes.com/2005/03/13/magazine/13HEALTH.html?ex=1135141200&en=c0a96da09d89ebf4&ei=5070. Accessed December 16, 2005.
26. US Congress. HR 747. National health information incentive act of 2005. Available at: http://thomas.loc.gov. Accessed March 21, 2005.
27. Department of Health and Human Services. Medicare "Pay for Performance (P4P) Initiatives' Fact Sheet. January 31, 2005. Available at http://www.cms.hhs.gov. Accessed March 29, 2005.

28. McGee MK. Feds unveil Medicare pay-for-performance project. Information-Week. February 1, 2005. Available at: http://informationweek.com. Accessed March 29, 2005.

29. Walker J, Pan E, Johnston D, et al. The value of health care information exchange and interoperability. Health Affairs Web Exclusive 2005;W5:10–18. Available at: http://content.healthaffairs.org/cgi/reprint/hlthaff.w5.10v1.pdf. Accessed April 5, 2005.

30. Berenson RA. Getting serious about excessive Medicare spending: a purchasing model. Health Affairs Web Exclusive 2003;W3:586–602. Available at: http://healthaffairs.org. Accessed April 5, 2005.

31. Wiseman P. Firms in Hong Kong try to ward off virus. USA Today. April 2, 2003. Available at: http://www.usatoday.com/money/world/2003-04-01-hongkong_x.htm. Accessed April 6, 2005.

32. Saywell T, Fowler GA, Crispin SW. The cost of SARS: $11 billion and rising. Far Eastern Economic Review. April 24, 2003. Available at: http://www.feer.com. Accessed April 5, 2005.

33. People's Daily Online (English). IT proves helpful in combating SARS: HK medical official. Available at: http://english.people.com.cn/20030719_120606.shtml. Accessed April 6, 2005.

34. Robertson J. The economic costs of infectious diseases. Parliament of Australia Research Note 36 2002–03. Available at: http://www.aph.gov.au/library/pubs/rn/2002-03/03rn36.htm. Accessed April 6, 2005.

35. Ehringhaus S. Testimony on behalf of the Association of American Medical Colleges before the National Committee on Vital and Health Statistics Subcommittee on Privacy; 2003. Available at: http://www.ncvhs.hhs.gov/031120tr.htm. Accessed April 5, 2005.

36. Safran C. Beyond technology: widespread adoption of EHRs will depend on skilled workforce. Business Briefing: US Healthcare Strategies 2005. Forthcoming.

37. Institute of Medicine. Health Literacy: A Prescription to End the Confusion. Washington, DC: National Academy Press; 2004.

38. Department of Health and Human Services. Understanding and promoting health literacy (R03) PA number: PAR-04-117. 2004. Available at: http://grants2.nih.gov/grants/guide/pa-files/PAR-04-117.html. Accessed April 2, 2005.

39. Connecting for Health. Connecting Americans to their healthcare: final report; 2004. Available at: http://www.connectingforhealth.org/. Accessed April 1, 2005.

40. Sittig DF. Personal health records on the Internet: a snapshot of the pioneers at the end of the 20th century. Int J Med Inform 2002;65:1–6.

41. Kim MI, Johnson KB. Personal health records: evaluation of functionality and utility. J Am Med Inform Assoc 2002;9:171–180.

42. Weiner S. Adoption of personal health records raises questions. IHealthBeat; March 18, 2005. Available at: http://www.ihealthbeat.org. Accessed March 28, 2005.

43. European Computing Driving License. Computer skills for life. Available at: http://www.ecdl.com/main/index.php. Accessed April 4, 2005.

9
"Online, On-demand, and Worldwide . . .": The Department of Defense Electronic Health Record*

Rosemary Nelson, Connie A. Gladding, and David Williams

The Department of Defense (DoD) has a long history of transforming healthcare delivery by using information technology (IT). The DoD recognizes the value of secure and on-demand computerized patient information as a substantive way to enhance patient safety, and the quality of healthcare delivery. Figure 9-1 illustrates the variety of processes and activities conducted in the Military Health System (MHS). In the early 1990s, the DoD placed considerable attention on business process improvement/business process reengineering, geared toward normalizing models of business activities and data, with the goal to standardize all data throughout the MHS defense enterprise. The outcomes of these efforts positioned the DoD to achieve the primary objective of the department's integrated health information systems, which is availability of personal health information at the right time, to the right healthcare team, around the clock, and around the world. The key clinical focus is to enable providers to access beneficiaries' health records at any military healthcare facility around the world, at anytime. Without a doubt, an electronic health record (EHR) is essential for delivery of health care to a service member throughout their military career (active and veteran status), and critical for the capture of empirical data for use in individual planning and management, population management, and disease surveillance.

The MHS acquires, develops, deploys, and maintains superior health technology solutions and services, in support of healthcare delivery provided by the Army, Navy, and Air Force. The DoD executes the TRICARE[1] program which provides worldwide patient care services in military treatment facilities (MTFs), and through purchased care providers, known as managed care support contractors. The global implementation of the Composite Health Care System II (CHCSII)[2]; recently renamed AHLTA, and eHealth initiatives by 2006 will include:

---

* The opinions or assertions in this chapter are the private views of the authors, and are not to be construed as official or representing the views of the Department of the Army or the Department of Defense.

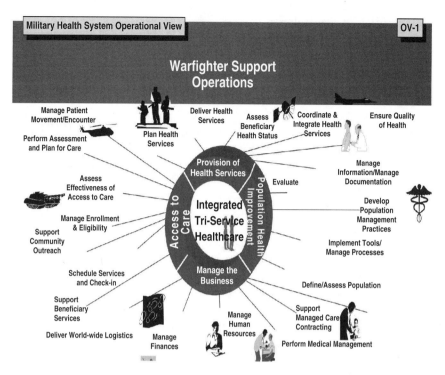

FIGURE 9-1. MHS operational view.

- EHR with structured providers' notes
- Physician orders
- Diagnostic coding
- Electronically access and update patient records
- Order ancillary services such as prescription drugs, diagnostic radiology, and laboratory tests[3]

As of November 2005, the DoDs internet-based EHR was renamed AHLTA. More information about AHLTA can be viewed at http://www.HA.DSD.MiLIAHLTA. As cited by one DoD spokesperson, "For patients, there's no such thing as a lost chart anymore." Providers enter diagnosis and orders for each patient, having access to features that enable providers to program alerts reminding them to schedule mammograms, diabetes tests, or other procedures . . . all in an effort to provide better care, promote wellness, and ensure regular preventive health visits. The mission requirements of the CHCSII support President Bush's Technology Agenda that involve transformation of health care through health IT, resulting in:

- Improved healthcare quality
- Reduced healthcare costs

- Prevention of medical errors
- Improved administrative efficiencies
- Reduced paperwork
- Increased access through innovations in EHRs
- Secured exchange of medical information

A primary driver for the DoD's EHR is making medical and dental records immediately available to providers caring for a highly mobile population that includes 9.1 million beneficiaries, of which 1.4 million are active duty armed service members serving around the globe. By enabling secure electronic access to a beneficiary's comprehensive health record (to include preventative care, illnesses, injuries, exposures, and treatment at any MTF), the AHLTA enables access to any eligible beneficiary's medical/dental record within seconds, from anywhere in the world. Features such as these enable continuation of critical e-business functions, enhance access to care and quality of care, and improve the DoD's ability to efficiently manage the business of the MHS. By streamlining and computerizing business processes and scheduling systems, the AHLTA supports a team-based approach to healthcare delivery, and improves hospitals' and clinics' personnel efficiency in providing timely service to patients. The DoD's direction in the mid-1990s to use commercial-off-the shelf (COTS) software, coupled with advances and maturity in the technology industry, greatly influenced the DoD's direction and drive toward the EHR.

Support to military commanders who must make battlefield decisions was also a key driver for the DoD's EHR. The ability to store health information, access data on disease outbreaks, injuries, and harmful environmental exposures, and cross-reference with the service member's other medical information supports the delivery of health care in field or theater operations. This health information is critical when making decisions related to force readiness and force protection. The ability of providers to detect symptom patterns, and quickly diagnose disease outbreaks, trends, and patterns among troops, is a critical population health requirement. The AHLTA enterprise system also enables provider access to a service member's medical records using laptops, thus providing the portability of information to support treatment decisions in the field. Battlefield providers are able to document service members' injuries and treatment using a pull-down menu application installed on care providers' handheld computers. The DoD' s EHR includes a structured data framework that supports surveillance, population health management, and enables large continental United States medical centers to support providers and patients located in austere war fighting environments.

Legislation and presidential directives are drivers for setting the direction, and executing activities within the DoD healthcare system. There are several critical directives that have influenced the DoD EHR, and have significantly directed both the development and implementation. In reviewing the directives posted below, one can easily see that the core principles are enabling and achieving continuity of information across a service member's life, and improving delivery of health care to all beneficiaries across the DoD enterprise. The next three sections describe the directives that have influenced the DoD's direction. Further sections lay out the genesis, the evolutionary, and the revolutionary periods of development. The last section closes the chapter with a discussion of challenges.

Special Report of the Presidential Advisory Committee on Gulf War Veterans' Illnesses

This report, issued on November 7, 1997, by President Clinton, outlines several bold recommendations to ensure continuity of health and medical record information. This directive formally set in motion the requirement to share health information between the Departments of Defense and Veterans Affairs, to achieve continuity of health across a service member's life. The recommendation mandated ". . . to apply lessons we have learned for the future, I am directing the Departments of Defense and Veterans Affairs to create a new force health protection program. Every soldier, sailor, airman, and marine will have a comprehensive, lifelong medical record of all illnesses and injuries they suffer, the care and inoculations they receive, and their exposure to different hazards. These records will help us prevent illness and identify and cure those that occur."

IT Management Reform Act of 1996

Also known as ITMRA, or the Clinger-Cohen Act, took effect August 8, 1996, and was aimed at ensuring that IT investments directly support the desired business practices, one of which is delivery of military health care around the world. Under this legislation, the CIO must ensure that the criteria below are met before funding any IT solution:

- Solution supports core mission functions, and no alternative private sector or other government source can effectively support the function; solution supports work processes that have been redesigned or otherwise improved
- Solution is consistent with the agency's architecture, and integrates work processes and information flows with the technology to achieve agency's mission and strategic plan
- Agency has a portfolio management approach in which decisions on whether to invest in IT are based on potential return on investment, and decisions to terminate or make additional investments are based

on performance—much like an investment broker is measured and reviewed based on managing risk and achieving results

- Agency reduces risk and enhances manageability by discouraging "grand" information system projects, and encouraging incremental, phased approaches

Compliance with this mandate ensures continued refinement in IT capital investment and portfolio management processes, and also makes sure all proposed IT investments are evaluated against objective and business focused criteria.

Government Act of 2002

The Government Act of 2002 was signed by President Bush on December 17, 2002, and includes a management agenda for making the government more focused on citizens and results, which includes expanding Electronic Government—or E-Government. E-Government uses improved Internet-based technology to make it easy for citizens and businesses to interact with the government, save taxpayer dollars, and streamline citizen-to-government communications. In accordance with this law, the DoD is involved in the Consolidated Health Informatics and the Federal Health Architecture initiative, both of which address adoption of a portfolio of existing health information interoperability standards (health vocabulary and messaging), enabling all agencies in the federal health enterprise to "speak the same language" based on common enterprise-wide business and IT architectures.

The Decade of Health Information Technology

The full title is, The Decade of Health Information Technology: Delivering Consumer-centric and Information-rich Health Care, Framework for Strategic Action, from the Department of Health and Human Services. As the fundamental document for the National Health Information Network, it outlines the need for interoperability and an enterprise architecture that facilitates connectivity between federal healthcare systems and the private sector. The strategies and goals in this publication, issued on July 21, 2004, laid the groundwork for a widespread effort to drive adoption of interoperable health information technology, with the end goal being consumer-centric and information-rich care.

Multiple Standalones 1980 Solutions—Genesis

Since the 1980s, the MHS has recognized the need to apply IT to the problems of delivering cost-effective and safe health care to DoD beneficiaries. Early on, the use of IT by the MHS was focused on improving patient safety, increasing employee productivity, and decreasing the transaction time for laboratory, radiology, pharmacy, appointing, and scheduling functions.

In the 1980s, the MHS partnered with industry to deliver automated standalone systems for laboratory, pharmacy, radiology, and appointment scheduling services in its major medical centers in the continental United States. These initial operating capabilities were *capability* rather than *patient or facility centric*. System user devices were placed primarily in non-clinical care areas, such as in patient administration, laboratories, pharmacies, and radiology departments. The criticality of device placement was quickly realized. Answers to the following types of questions provided guidance:

- Who needs access to the information?
- How many devices are affordable?
- What are maintenance requirements for the devices?
- Where is there room for the device?
- Can unauthorized access be prevented?
- Where is the device most easily used during routine delivery of care?

The number of user devices grew into clinical care areas as the benefits of the system were more understood. The standalone ancillary systems enabled healthcare professionals, such as laboratory technologists and pharmacists, to transcribe provider orders into the system and for these professionals and the patients' providers to retrieve results. Patients quickly recognized the benefits of the systems. The providers, instead of searching for paper laboratory results or scouring laboratory logs, would now call the laboratory and ask the technicians to electronically search and retrieve the most recent laboratory tests, sometimes only having a range of dates and the patient's name. For the patient and laboratory, this translated into fewer "laboratory sticks" or "blood draws" because of misplaced or irretrievable reports.

Quickly following these standalone systems in the major medical centers, were standardized pharmacy, patient administration, and patient appointing and scheduling systems in all of the MHS facilities, regardless of facility size or location. The MHS beneficiary population, as well as its uniformed healthcare professional and provider population, are mobile; both populations quickly became reliant on these automated capabilities, and came to expect them regardless of care location. The MHS, by developing long-term partnerships with industry, learned to "scale," operate, and support its automated systems in the wide range of MTFs of the three services, from medical centers to small remote overseas clinics.

Integrated Intrafacility/Regional 1990 Solutions—Evolutionary

The Composite Health Care System (CHCS), DoD's first-generation EHR, was a hospital-wide integrated information system, primarily supporting ambulatory and outpatient care. Once again, working with a valued industry partner in a long-term contracted relationship, the DoD fielded the CHCS worldwide to more than 500 MHS facilities in the 1990s. This deployment was after several years of extensive testing in a range of healthcare facilities, including overseas locations, and both small and large facilities. The testing ensured user acceptance and effectiveness of the product, as well as training and maintenance strategies and methodologies. The MHS used a mixture of training strategies to reach the needs of its varied users, who were all using one facility-wide, integrated, common system. The training strategies included:

- Classroom instructor-led training
- Computer-based tutorials
- Over the shoulder workspace assistance
- Videotapes for viewing at one's convenience

One tenet that proved necessary to gain user acceptance was role- and scenario-based training. Users needed to be trained in how to apply the system to their specific jobs, using examples they could easily recognize in their day-to-day activities.

Because the CHCS was designed to be used by providers during patient encounters for order entry and results retrieval, devices were placed in clinical care areas. Patients now routinely observed their providers entering information into a system and calling up information on them during their patient visit. No more calls to the laboratory asking for results, because paper records were not in the patients' paper health records—they were in the CHCS! Educating and managing expectations regarding the benefits and safeguards of the information and care patterns were paramount in gaining acceptance by users and care beneficiaries, and in realizing benefits from the system. Congress initially limited the MHS deployment of CHCS to only MTFs that were clearly able to be cost beneficial, and demonstrate a return on investment. Near mid-deployment, Congress recognized the value gained if all MHS facilities and healthcare professionals were using the same tool in the delivery of health care. The mobile patient and provider populations demanded it, requiring the information system worldwide in all MTFs.

The CHCS, a "***hospital or facility centric***" information system, was designed to have all healthcare personnel using the same system, regardless of MTF. All users were linked on a local area network and CHCS delivered a powerful tool, recognized today as "e-mail," improving the quality and timeliness of communications. The fielding of an application for delivery of health care, that was dependent on the local area network, caused a revolution in the network administration arena. Network administrators now had critical applications relying on network availability. Before the CHCS, applications on the network were administrative in nature; users were tolerant of unplanned downtime sometimes for not only hours, but also days. With the CHCS on the network, those days were history. Providers demanded notice of any planned downtime, and expected the CHCS and the network to be reliable and available. The users' expectations made the MHS realize the importance and value of measuring, forecasting, and managing infrastructure and applications availability, reliability, and performance. The MHS also broaden its membership on technical configuration change boards, so as to gain an "end to end" perspective and understanding of the impact of any changes.

Laboratory medical technologists, pharmacists, and radiologists were no longer the "owners" of their standalone systems. The CHCS not only integrated hospital functions, but also interfaced with laboratory instruments, appointment scheduling, pharmacy phone refill systems, and pharmacy dispensing devices. Because changes to either the CHCS or a device interface resulted in impacts to multiple MTF users, DoD leadership needed to consider several IT solution designs before making a decision. For example, the medical record tracking capability was first designed to meet the needs in radiology, but users in health record rooms and clinics quickly recognized the value of this tool, and used it in their daily practices. The MHS rapidly learned the importance and value of diverse team membership for its functional software configuration change control boards, system design reviews, and software tests.

A challenge with implementing the CHCS was the certainty that others would have access to the same information. The CHCS users demanded safeguard features. Various user access levels were created to provide the user access to information commensurate with their job requirements, with system audit logs available for review as needed. Users felt ownership of their data, and wanted the hardware to be physically located within their control. Overcoming the "big brother is watching" and reliance upon "folks in the computer room" took perseverance in gaining users' confidence. Demonstration of the benefits of "expert care and feeding of the systems," and the benefits of this shared view of information, whether laboratory test results, or a provider's appointment calendar and patient visits, was critical to user acceptance. After several costly labor-intensive efforts to "clean up" data, the MHS learned to address adherence to data quality principles in employee performance evaluations, and to highlight the importance of data quality during training. The MHS leadership stressed that the information was "shared information," and many would be dependent on it for making patient care decisions to include providers making patient care decisions and administrators making resource decisions.

In some geographical areas, the MHS consists of Army, Navy, and Air Force MTFs with a shared patient population, such as, Tidewater, Puget Sound, San Antonio, Guam, Hawaii, and New England. These shared patient environments presented other complexities that needed to be addressed such as Service-specific business rules and vocabularies, and individual MTF nuances. In several geographical areas, because of cost, close proximity, and shared patient populations, one CHCS platform was installed to support several hospitals and clinics. At the time, the hurdle was thought to be the technical capacity of the computing and communications infrastructure. It became clear very quickly that the largest hurdle was gaining concurrence among the MTFs to a common set of business rules and vocabulary. The MHS had learned the scope and variance among the MTFs' care and administrative processes, as well as vocabularies.

To reap the benefits of an IT product implemented worldwide in diverse healthcare facilities, the MHS recognized the need to reengineer common processes, with a common vocabulary supporting common business rules. In the areas with shared patient populations, the CHCS was dependent on a regional area network, as well as the local facility area networks. The DoD healthcare IT community learned to work closely with the remainder of DoD to ensure the regional network administrations remembered that critical healthcare applications were reliant upon their networks. This caused dramatic changes in operating procedures, as well as downtime and maintenance notifications for computing and communications centers. Before making any change to the networks, impact analyses were conducted on the critical applications riding over the network. In deploying the CHCS in this regional configuration, the MHS learned to support Tri-Service MTFs with one CHCS. The CHCS served to help standardize healthcare delivery practices across the three services, and highlighted the necessity of interoperability with non-healthcare networks and medical equipment. The MHS learned the importance of the use of standards, the need to plan for emerging standards, and the growing demands for computing power and infrastructure bandwidth to support critical applications.

One Patient, One Record Enterprise 2000 Solution—Revolutionary

In early 2000, the MHS transitioned from the *facility centric information system* which centered on provider order entry and results retrieval, to its first *patient centric information system*. This was achieved with deployment of the CHCSII and eHealth portal and applications, which has one Clinical Data Repository (CDR) that stores all beneficiaries' health records. Regardless of when and where the patient is seen, the provider can access securely the patient's record, 24 by 7, in real time. The CHCSII provides structured clinical documentation tools, a unique beneficiary health identifier, a standard healthcare lexicon, and consolidates health, dental, inpatient, and outpatient records into one EHR. The eHealth portal and applications enable the rich CHCSII data content to securely reach across the globe via the Internet.

To gain user acceptance, the MHS's initial EHR, the CHCS, was designed to accommodate local or regional business rules and vocabulary, with each CHCS location building its own set of "files and tables." Examples of this file and table flexibility in the CHCS design included:

- Nomenclature of outpatient clinics
- List of providers
- Nomenclature of laboratory or radiology tests
- Pharmaceutical drug lists

These files and tables were clearly understood by local CHCS users, but limited the transportability and understandability of the data to other CHCS locations. When answers were needed to an inquiry across the enterprise, queries were made to each of the CHCS locations, vice one query to one system; this was a time- and resource-intensive activity to query, normalize, and aggregate data across enterprise facilities. Additionally, when patients moved to another region or location, the electronic records did not transfer across the CHCS locations, because of the uniqueness of the data and terminology in each system. These functional issues contributed significantly in the technical design of the CHCSII.

The CHCSII technical design was driven by the functional "to be" MHS healthcare delivery business process. After the functional "to be" business process was fully defined, functional requirements were developed and approved by the stakeholders, and technical requirements analysis and design began. The MHS draws upon a robust and repeatable requirements management and investment portfolio management methodology to determine the steps the DoD will take in modernizing a system. An overview of the methodology is as follows:

- Functional proponents/business owners rank well-defined functional capability descriptions against the organization's business process priorities, using a risk/value matrix. The outcome of this step is a prioritized listing of functional capabilities, composed of functional requirements.
- Stakeholders "rack and stack" prioritized capabilities based on available funding, resulting in the highest ranked capabilities being funded before the lower ranked items, until the funding is exhausted. The outcome of this step is a prioritized investment portfolio.
- The funded capabilities listing or investment portfolio is provided to the IT program manager to finalize requirements analysis, develop acquisi-

tion strategies, procure or design/develop products, and integrate, test, deploy, train, and sustain the IT solutions. The outcome of this step is a list of expected IT capabilities, constrained by the budget.

The MHS Requirements Development Process (RDP) consists of five phases, each depicted with their primary responsibility in Figure 9-2.[4] The process includes configuration management, metrics collection, and reporting activities to help ensure the rigor and quality of process products. A critical guiding principle throughout this process is continuous communication and feedback with the user and stakeholder community. This communications loop provides answers to frequently asked questions, such as:

- Has the requested change been received and analyzed?
- What is the disposition of the change requested?
- Was the requested change funded?
- When will work begin to fix the identified problem?

Phase 1, Initial Submission/Preliminary Assessment, includes activities to identify or propose changes to MHS information systems and the resulting preliminary assessment of those changes.

Phase 2, Functional Requirements Development, includes activities necessary to develop functional requirements related to changes or enhancements to MHS systems as proposed in Phase 1. Various types of requirements documents are developed, with related cost and schedule estimates.

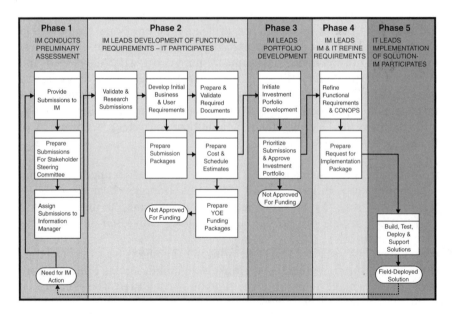

FIGURE 9-2. Summary view of information management requirements development process (RDP) activities.

Phase 3, Information Management/Information Technology (IM/IT) Investment Portfolio Development, includes activities to assemble, prioritize, and approve the IM/IT investment portfolio.

Phase 4, Functional Requirements Refinement, includes activities to validate and refine requirements and submission packages developed in Phase 2 and funded in Phase 3. Once a package has been validated, it is submitted to the IT program manager, for implementation.

Phase 5, Solution Implementation, includes activities that provide completed requirements descriptions and necessary funding to the IT program manager for solution implementation.

The RDP provides a structured, sequential, and outcomes-oriented pathway to a finished IT product. The MHS uses the RDP for all IM/IT initiatives. As an example, this focused business priority approach resulted in the MHS's decision to design an enterprise CDR for the CHCSII.

Why one CDR? The military family is very mobile, the uniformed providers are mobile, and team-based care is practiced. So the technical solution needed to be *patient or beneficiary centric*, vice *provider or facility centric*. Organizations with a more stationary patient population or fewer healthcare facilities in a more regional or local area may be better suited with a different technical solution. With this technical design, the CHCSII operations are very dependent on a robust wide area network. The MHS has learned to work effectively with numerous infrastructure providers for local, regional, and wide area networks to provide clinical automated systems to network users. Service level agreements with visible performance management metrics were a necessity.

The CHCSII CDR has proven very valuable in supporting homeland defense, medical surveillance, and medical readiness. With a single central database, it is possible to easily identify clusters of symptoms or signs that may be attributed to a biological or chemical attack, or an epidemic or bioterrorism event. Having a comprehensive record of a service member's history of immunizations, treatments, allergies, problem lists, encounter notes, current medications, eye examinations, dental examinations, and family history, enables a clinician to quickly determine a service member's readiness for deployment to support military operations, whether humanitarian or war. Ability to make this pre-deployment assessment saves critical time, labor, and dollars. The pre-deployment assessment serves as a baseline assessment, and may prove critical if a service member develops post-deployment symptoms, illness, or impaired health.

Applying the lessons learned during the 1980s on scalability and supportability, and the 1990s lessons learned on interoperability and data sharing, has resulted in today's AHLTA being available to DoD providers and patients regardless of where the care is being provided. If the care is delivered in a tent, in the midst of a desert, onboard a ship at sea, in a major medical center, or a small clinic, there is an AHLTA version that has been designed and tested to meet the need. The product can scale up or down, function with a communications link or an environment with no communications, and is capable of operating in very austere conditions, while always capturing the healthcare encounter data to support continuity of care for United States service members.

The MHS decided early on that continuous functional stakeholder and provider involvement is critical to user acceptance of AHLTA. The MHS involved providers in the requirements definition, design and development processes, selection of COTS products, and in determination of training and implementation strategies. Among the more challenging AHLTA design issues for the system integrators, was design of an effective user interface. To meet this challenge, the MHS empowered a group of providers to work with the system developer to design the computer screen "look and feel." Most frequently cited benefits include:

- Universal records availability and legibility
- Automated coding done as a byproduct of documenting the patient encounter

Surprisingly, the most frequently cited challenges were usually about people, organization, and processes, rather than technical matters. Understanding these lessons learned helped to prioritize focus areas for successful implementation of transformational technology solutions.

Throughout the 1990s, the MHS continued to seek enterprise-wide solutions that would facilitate providing the highest quality of health care in the most effective and efficient manner possible. The Internet was viewed as such a solution; it afforded profound opportunities to rapidly extend the reach of current systems and significantly reduce time and costs for deploying additional systems and applications enterprise wide. The MHS established an eHealth Office to ensure that attributes of the Internet were fully leveraged. The mission of the eHealth Office includes:

- Develop a unifying MHS corporate Internet strategy
- Work across government and industry organizations
- Identify and advocate enterprise policies
- Use of open architectural standards
- Serve as the clearing house for eHealth functional requirements
- Manage information requirements for the MHS

The importance of a central office in establishing common services such as single sign-on, context management, data standards, role-based security protocols and same "look and feel" across Web-base applications cannot be overstated. One example of the eHealth Office efficiencies is that in less than 45 days congressionally mandated pre- and post-deployment survey forms were built, integrated, and deployed for worldwide use.

Currently, there are numerous examples of eHealth initiatives across the MHS. These initiatives are on the critical path to transform the delivery of health care through applications in disease management, clinical care, administrative and financial transactions, professional education, and remote medical consultation. The TRICARE Online (TOL) is a good example of one such initiative; TOL's keys to improve health care via the Internet include:

- Improve patient access to services and benefits
- Improve population health and disease management
- Provide a platform for Health Information Portability and Accountability Act compliance for required transactions and code sets
- Optimize the business management aspects of the direct and purchased care systems, specifically claims, enrollments, eligibility, appointments, and pharmacy transactions
- Provide a common, MHS-wide, secure Internet-based platform for telemedicine and future eHealth initiatives
- Provide a common environment for coordination and reuse of software capabilities across the enterprise
- Deliver provider-to-provider, and patient-to-patient secure e-mail

The TOL provides a portal to the MHS eHealth applications and systems. The eHealth online appointing application enables DoD beneficiaries to book an appointment online, and have the transaction automatically reflect in AHLTA. The TOL portal provides a common secure Internet platform, and allows beneficiaries access to numerous eHealth applications. One feature of the TOL application is the ability for DoD beneficiaries to create their own personal healthcare homepage. The beneficiary can access information on their healthcare team, and store medical information and resources in a secure environment. The beneficiary can also customize their TOL homepage to:

- Create a personal health journal
- Store favorite links to health or wellness sites
- Access disease tracking and management tools

Beneficiaries are able to access a wellness center for a comprehensive collection of features, factoids, and news to keep them and their families informed about health issues. They can obtain answers, learn more about symptoms, medications, treatment options, and check drug/drug, and drug/food combinations for possible harmful interactions. The TOL includes access to an eHealth application for children that allows access to age-appropriate tools that help them learn more about themselves and the world around them. Additionally, beneficiaries can make appointments online with their primary care provider, and select specialty clinics in accordance with MTF business rules.

The Internet is an ideal tool for achieving implementation of enterprise-wide solutions. A central tenet of the eHealth Office is to coordinate across the three services, looking for opportunities and reuse of software capabilities across the enterprise.

Challenges Ahead

AHLTA and eHealth portal and applications are transformational products, and are designed to support reengineered healthcare business practices (identified in 2001 and 2002), including focusing on preventative care and team healthcare delivery. The MHS leveraged previous IT investments, and is sequentially building additional automated capabilities. AHLTA and eHealth portal and applications truly enable rapid revolutionary changes in the enterprise wide delivery and quality of health care. It supports a holistic team approach to providing health care, enabling workflow improvements and efficiencies.

With the integration of COTS applications, the MHS intends to maximize the opportunity to adopt industry best practices. With the lexicon and data repository, the MHS anticipates better patient and population management opportunities, as well as increased data sharing with other healthcare organizations, such as Department of Veterans Affairs. Remaining to be addressed is the data sharing between the MTFs and the network of managed care support contractors. As infrastructure and EHRs become more available in private sector doctors' offices and physician practices, and as interoperability standards are agreed upon by the healthcare community, the MHS expects to incorporate the electronic documentation on beneficiary care delivered outside of the MTFs, thus achieving a comprehensive EHR.

The healthcare communities of administrators, patients, providers, industry, and standards development organizations, have high hopes for healthcare IT. The MHS believes innovation stimulated by IT and the use of COTS in leveraging best practices in the delivery of health care will continue to improve care, lower costs, improve quality, and empower beneficiaries. The MHS leadership faces with balancing high expectations and technology performance capabilities, while addressing user and beneficiary fears regarding privacy matters.

A health system's ability to rapidly leverage IT solutions depends on the readiness of its beneficiaries, providers, IT staff, and existing infrastructure. One of the most significant challenges for management innovation through IT is managing organizational change, and determining the magnitude and pace of change an organization can handle. Preparing an institution and its people for change is at the core of success. Minimizing the difficulty of transitioning may build false expectations and create disillusionment when difficulties are encountered. The MHS has learned the necessity to perform readiness assessments of both user community and infrastructure. Periodic assessments have proven invaluable before implementation, during implementation, and post-implementation. Additionally, the MHS has chosen to field functionality incrementally, starting small and building on earlier successes.

Yet another challenge is managing expectations across many stakeholders, to include expectations regarding the value and benefits of the IT product. Communicating effectively inside and outside of the organization is central to managing stakeholders' expectations. The use of clinical champions is an effective strategy in strengthening communications and managing expectations. Acknowledging successes and failures builds credibility. Clinical process reengineering is a large hurdle, and requires the full participation of providers and the beneficiaries.

The MHS has learned the value in providing role and scenario-based training, with both classroom and "over the shoulder" training in the workspaces. Flexibility in training strategies is vital. Depending on the user, training in groups may be most effective, whereas in other instances, one-on-one training may be the only alternative. Having learned in the 1980s to train all users regarding the importance of data quality and integrity, a challenge remains to hold all levels in the organization accountable for good quality data, especially when there is one database, shared by many. The MHS has learned that fixing data quality problems is more than a technology issue, but also requires repeatable business processes that must be addressed very early in IT implementations, rather than later, and especially at the point of data creation, rather than at an aggregated level.

Lastly, an organization must recognize the cost/risk tradeoff needed to select and field a technology solution even as newer and better technology breakthroughs are occurring. Healthcare executives face the daunting task of balancing risks against the costs and benefits of implementing new technology for tomorrow, while simultaneously conducting today's business, as both healthcare practice and technology evolve, similar to a race car driver having tires changed in the course of speeding around the racetrack. For healthcare organizations to capitalize on technological advancements, leadership must drive the organization to realize the benefits, rather than drift into benefits accrual. Targeted benefit assessment should consider the impact on operations, budgets, personnel, beneficiaries, and processes.

In closing, high-level lessons learned that span the IT lifecycle include:

- Identification of the "as is" and "to be" healthcare delivery processes
- Identification of the "as is" and "to be" technical standards framework
- Identification of the "as is" and "to be" systems solutions
- Requirements analysis, acquisition, design, development, integration, testing, implementation, training, operations, and maintenance of the IT product

Specific lessons learned are grouped into three categories: Right Aligning Business Processes and Information Requirements; Manage and Sustain Successful Organizational Change; and Manage to Cost, Schedule, and Performance Objectives for Information Technology Investments.

TABLE 9-1. Right aligning business processes and information requirements

Define "as is" and "to be" business processes
Correct data errors at the source of data entry
Acknowledge the magnitude, difficulty, and necessity of clinical process reengineering
Consider along with cost, technical performance, and space requirements, the workflow, information visibility, and patient/provider interactions when determining user device placement
Define IT product functional requirements of the "to be" business process
Gain stakeholder concurrence of the "to be" concept of operations
Manage functional requirements and software changes with a multidisciplined, diverse functional representation software configuration control board
Restrict information access levels to job needs
Engage users/clinicians in requirements definition, solution design and development, product testing, and in determining implementation strategies
Instantiate data quality principles into capability training and product implementations
Drive toward benefits realization

The Right Aligning Business Processes and Information Requirements (Table 9-1) lessons learned includes proven strategies and measures related to defining information management requirements, ensuring user/stakeholder acceptance of IT capabilities, and designing IT solutions that support the business processes of healthcare delivery.

The Manage and Sustain Successful Organizational Change (Table 9-2) lessons learned focuses on change management, and process improvement activities that have proven effective in gaining widespread use of new IT products.

The Schedule and Performance Objectives for Information Technology Investments (Table 9-3) lessons learned focuses on actions proven to be critical to providing IT products meeting cost, technical, and performance parameters.

TABLE 9-2. Manage and sustain successful organizational change

Manage users', stakeholders', and beneficiaries' expectations
Assess user, organization, and infrastructure readiness for change
Influence and gain commitment by executive leadership
Identify and empower clinical champions
Conduct pre- and post-implementation product reviews
Enable employees and beneficiaries to understand and directly support IT initiatives
Seek and deliver consistent communications to beneficiaries, stakeholders, and users
Use role- and scenario-based training
Implement capabilities that show immediate benefits to providers
Offer "over the shoulder" assistance in the work centers
Plan for and accommodate different learning styles in training strategies
Identify and empower clinical champions to assist in training and user acceptance
Routinely publish progress, benefits realized, and lessons learned
Implement capability in small increments
Ensure training strategies accommodate different learning styles

TABLE 9-3. Manage cost, schedule, and performance objectives for information technology investments

Leverage existing computing and communications capacity
Test in a near real production environment
Build a long-term contractual relationship with industry partners
Engage users/clinicians in solution design and development, especially the user interface (human/computer interface)
Hold industry partners accountable for the performance of their products
Manage technical requirements and computing and communications infrastructure changes with a multidisciplinary configuration control board
Perform operating and maintenance tradeoff analyses when considering design alternatives
Standardize vocabulary to support comparative analyses
Adopt data, communications, security, and computing standards to enable interoperability
Anticipate and plan for emerging standards
Recognize the benefits and tradeoffs of integrating COTS products
Consider privacy and security capabilities in the product during design and development
Measure, forecast, and manage infrastructure and applications performance

References

1. http://www.tricare.osd.mil/. Accessed June 23, 2005.
2. http://www-nmcp.med.navy.mil/chcsii/. Accessed June 23, 2005.
3. Office of the Assistant Secretary of Defense (Health Affairs), Concept of Operations for the Composite Health Care System II, ACAT Level IAM, August 2003.
4. Information Management Decision Information Management, Technology, and Reengineering TRICARE Management Activity; Information Management Requirements Development Process (RDP), June 2005, version 2.1.

10
The Global Perspective

WALTER W. WIENERS, ZAKIR BICKHAN, DENNIS GIOKAS,
PAUL FITZGERALD, and AYSHA OSBORNE

An evaluation of existing electronic health record systems (EHR-Ss) in nations that have advanced to broad-scale implementation offers an ideal opportunity to consider carefully each nation's program, and in turn, to learn from various nations' experiences. However, to benefit from the lessons learned from operating programs, assessments must be thought through carefully and thoroughly.

Marion J. Ball, EdD, Fellow, Global Leadership Initiative, clarifies the broad issues that call for careful scrutiny of international EHRs. Dr. Ball stated: "What works in one country may not be politically or culturally acceptable in another. There may be differences in the decision-making process or in the funding model, etc. Nations with comprehensive social welfare state apparatuses may be facing broad healthcare funding issues that may have negative implications in other countries."[1]

To date, there have been few cross-national studies about EHR initiatives or fully developed programs. Additionally, independent, rigorous evaluation of both government- and industry-driven EHR projects has yet to occur. To address these limitations in global knowledge sharing, we sought to conduct a collaborative observational study designed to contribute to a more in-depth understanding of the benefits of EHR innovations within the healthcare arena across borders and to offer a summary of lessons learned from selected countries.

This chapter probes the factors that influence successful EHR programs in three countries—Canada, Australia, and the United Kingdom (UK)—that lead in this area within the context of their healthcare systems and their broader national healthcare information technology (IT) strategies. After establishing the context of the healthcare system in which each program operates, we describe EHR program formation, structure, model, investments, and plans in detail. Based on collaboration by coauthors representing EHR executives and implementation vendor management, and a review of independent studies of these countries' programs, we begin to draw upon useful lessons learned that can serve to inform all countries planning large-scale EHR programs.

The concept of EHRs began about 40 years ago but the first implementations did not really begin until the 1980s; today, with the exception of a few countries, the use of EHRs internationally is still very low. This is beginning to change rapidly, however. With the emergence of purpose-built EHR-Ss to underpin multidisciplinary integrated shared care in a number of countries, a whole new dimension to the field is being added.[2] With this perspective in mind, we assess the three nations that lead in this field, Canada, Australia, and the United Kingdom.

Canada is a leader in the field because its pan-Canadian initiative is bringing together various regional initiatives that are poised for subsequent national implementation. Australia's EHR program was selected because of the significant implementation that is in progress. The UK, especially in England, is an ideal third nation to assess because its EHR program is progressing within the context of the largest healthcare IT modernization ever undertaken by a country. We will examine these three countries' EHR projects beginning with an introduction to the health systems in which each EHR project operates.

Canada

We describe the Canadian experience, first in terms of the country's health system, then in terms of the formation of their EHR-S solution, Infoway, followed by its strategy, architecture, and a delineation of achievements and challenges.

Overview of Single Payer, Publicly Funded System

Since 1968, Canada's healthcare system has been predominantly publicly financed. Its national health insurance program is fulfilled through 14 interlocking federal, provincial, and territorial plans, with each of these jurisdictions also acting as payer and linked through adherence to five national principles set by the federal government in the Canada Health Act: public administration, comprehensiveness, universality, portability, and accessibility.[3] These principles are prerequisites for receiving federal funding for insured services. The Canada Health Act also establishes standards related to insured healthcare and extended healthcare services. However, it is the responsibility of Canada's jurisdictional governments to organize and deliver these health services, including hospital care, physician services, public health, and some aspects of prescription and diagnostic testing.

The aim of Medicare is to ensure that all eligible residents of Canada have reasonable access to medically necessary insured services on a prepaid basis, without direct charges at the point of service. What was originally designed as a single-payer, publicly funded system actually operates as a hybrid model of public–private funding, with mostly private delivery.

Canadian Medicare covers virtually all hospitals' and doctors' services. However, fiscal restraint and an ambulatory shift in services have forced reconsideration of how Medicare operates and is funded. Most of the services are delivered through public entities. But there has been an increase in the delivery of services by the private sector such as laboratory and diagnostic imaging services. In 2004, approximately two-thirds of healthcare spending was publicly funded, and one-third was privately paid. The total budget was $121 billion (all dollars in Canadian) and represented 10% of gross domestic product (GDP).

Growth in private spending has significantly outpaced growth in public spending, however, resulting in the public share declining. The sectors of care that have expanded with restructuring and with reducing acute care, many of which are now in the community, operate within a hybrid of public, private, and other financing arrangements.[4]

The Formation of Canada Health Infoway Inc. (Infoway)

The Political Impetus

By the late 1990s, several provincial federal reports advocated the need for a compatible, integrated system of health records to be developed on a priority basis. For instance, the Fyke Commission stated: "The electronic health record is the cornerstone of an efficient and responsive healthcare delivery system, quality improvement and accountability."[5] The reports also recognized that the few electronic information initiatives that were in place were standalone investments, with each attempting to solve one problem, at one time, in one place.

Against this backdrop, in September 2000, the First Ministers unanimously agreed to work together to strengthen a Canada-wide health IT structure. In turn, they committed to developing EHRs and common data standards to ensure compatibility of health information. In doing so, they acknowledged the dramatic benefits that flow from timely access to current, accurate, and complete information.

Extensive consultation and negotiation ensued and the result was the creation in 2000 of an independent, not-for-profit corporation with a Board of Directors called Canada Health Infoway, Inc., a new type of entity for Canada at that time. Launched with an initial investment of $500 million, the memorandum of understanding between the federal government and *Infoway*—along with the business plan that was approved in June 2002—set the framework for how money would be invested toward developing the EHR.[6]

Clear, simple governance structures are crucial to any transformation at the business or industry level. With the creation of *Infoway*, one entity has the national mandate to accelerate the implementation of EHRs and a better chance of focusing the health system stakeholders and investors and the end goal. Before *Infoway*, there was a plethora of advisory committees, organizations, and entities that believed they had a mandate to implement components of EHRs with no single vision or implementation focus.

In February 2003, during the 2003 First Ministers Health Accord meetings, the First Ministers recognized *Infoway's* success to date and expanded *Infoway's* mandate to include Telehealth. It was agreed that *Infoway* should receive an additional $100 million for Telehealth and $500 million to acceler- ate investments in the EHR; the later recommendation is part of a report on the future of health care in Canada. In March 2004, recognizing the need for better systems to support Public Health Surveillance, *Infoway* was funded with an addition $100 million to bring its total capitalization to $1.2 billion.[7]

Susan J. Hyatt, the first *Infoway* Vice President, Portfolio Manager, and General Manager (Toronto) and current Global Healthcare, Independent Advisor, Initiate Systems, Inc., observed that, "the collaboration, negotia- tion and support of executive champions that is required at both the politi- cal and bureaucratic levels of government is critical to the success of these entities both in the formative stages and as they progress. Developing and executing the strategy to obtain additional funding that resulted in the $600 million took many months of effort by the *Infoway* Board and management in discussions leading up to the First Ministers Health Accord 2003."

Infoway's Mandate and Organizational Structure

Infoway has a unique mandate: 1) to bring tangible benefits to Canadians by fostering and accelerating the development and adoption of electronic health information systems with compatible standards and communication technologies on a pan-Canadian basis, 2) to build on existing initiatives, and 3) to pursue collaborative relationships in pursuit of this mission. This mandate represents a formidable technical challenge as well as an organi- zational one, because, as mentioned previously, the responsibility for health- care delivery in Canada is managed by the 14 Canadian federal, provincial, and territorial jurisdictions.

To address this challenge, a partnership between the 14 Deputy Minis- ters of Health from all jurisdictions was established. To be effective, each member has an economic and vested interest in supporting *Infoway's* success by ensuring the corporation's federally provided funds are best leveraged across their individual jurisdictions. The structure of *Infoway* reflects a deliberate attempt to create an entity responsible for implement- ing the common goal held by the various levels of government in a collab- orative, cost-effective, and timely manner.

Accountability

Infoway is equally accountable to its 14 jurisdictions. In addition to stan- dard reporting requirements such as financial audits and annual reports, several measures of accountability have been added:

- An annual general meeting is held to review progress and approve the annual business plan
- At least every 5 years, an independent third-party evaluation will be conducted to measure overall performance in achieving the outcomes identified in the funding agreement
- An annual compliance audit will be undertaken specific to the terms and conditions of the funding agreement with the government of Canada, with the findings reported to all *Infoway* members
- Under the terms of the funding agreement, project default provisions have been established, including a reimbursement requirement
- *Infoway* has adopted a "gated funding" approach usually found in private enterprise; this means funds are only dispersed once preestablished milestones are met

Investment, Model, and Strategy

Infoway's corporate objective is to have the basic elements of interoperable EHR solutions in place in half of the country (by population) by the end of 2009. This section outlines the business strategy and operational approach *Infoway* has developed to meet this objective.

Business Strategy

Infoway's strategy consists of seven complementary elements:

1. *Target strategic investment programs. Infoway* has identified nine program areas for investment. These include the first six key building blocks of EHR solutions: registries, interoperable EHR (clinical data across the continuum of care), Drug Information Systems, Diagnostic Imaging Systems, Laboratory Information Systems, and Public Health. The seventh program is Telehealth (a channel for healthcare delivery) with a focus on Tele-medicine, Tele-homecare, Tele-learning, and Tele-triage. The eighth program is Infostructure (architecture and standards), which along with registries, are foundational programs. Without them, interoperable EHR solutions and seamless sharing of information would be impossible. The ninth program is Innovation and Adoption, which focuses on end users and technical innovations that are complementary to *Infoway's* mandate. Each investment program will have many projects, the sum of which will provide *Infoway* with a balanced portfolio.

Infoway's success will be measured by the extent to which it leverages its investments to maximize benefits to its member jurisdictions. One aspect of this, to reuse and replicate solutions across the country, will be supported by Knowledge Transfer activities that are embedded in all *Infoway* investments in order to facilitate the identification, capture and dissemination of project artifacts and best practices. Facilitating knowledge sharing with those involved in the design, implementation, and use of EHR solutions also accelerates overall progress.

2. *Collaborate with health ministries and other partners.* Acceleration of EHR solution development is a true collaborative effort. This is because *Infoway's* investments have been closely aligned with the priorities and objectives of health ministries and other public sector partners, stakeholders who are the builders and implementers of technology solutions.

3. *Develop strategic alliances with the private sector.* Infoway's emphasis on interoperability and vendor-neutral architecture and standards ensures a more inclusive marketplace for potential IT partners. In this way, it influences market dynamics and creates mutually beneficial arrangements. Effective alliances with the private sector also will help *Infoway* to better leverage its investments and to better align its strategies and the business directions of the IT industry.

4. *Focus on end-user acceptance.* Giving healthcare professionals the tools and information they require to provide quality care is not enough: To provide optimal quality of care, they first need support to integrate technology into their regular provider–patient care activities. Consequently, to promote a better understanding of the organizational and behavioral changes required for the successful introduction of new technology, *Infoway*—through its partners and investments—engages healthcare professionals during both the design and implementation of EHR solutions.

5. *Measure benefits and make adjustments.* Every initiative must generate real value—measurable benefits—for the end-user, the healthcare client, and the healthcare system. To ensure this is true of all *Infoway* projects, a formal benefits evaluation is built into every program. At a minimum, solutions should deliver healthcare efficiencies (better use of resources and of provider's time); improve accessibility to patients; improve the quality of care and healthcare outcomes (through services such as computerized physician order entry, access to relevant clinical data, and decision support); and ensure patient safety (through services such as drug utilization review).

6. *Invest with public sector sponsors.* All *Infoway* investment projects must have a public sector sponsor that contributes financially to the project. This approach encourages accountability and success by ensuring that both *Infoway* and its partners jointly share project risks and rewards. It also allows *Infoway* to maximize its investment capital and reward early adoption through tiered funding. The public sponsor leads the development and implementation, with *Infoway* playing the role of Strategic Investor.

7. *Operational model.* Figure 10-1 illustrates *Infoway* as a strategic investor that seeks out best-of-breed solutions and other opportunities that can be leveraged to support a more efficient and sustainable healthcare system. The investments must be in alignment with *Infoway's* program strategies, solution architecture, and interoperability standards. *Infoway* works in partnership with health ministries, regional authorities, other

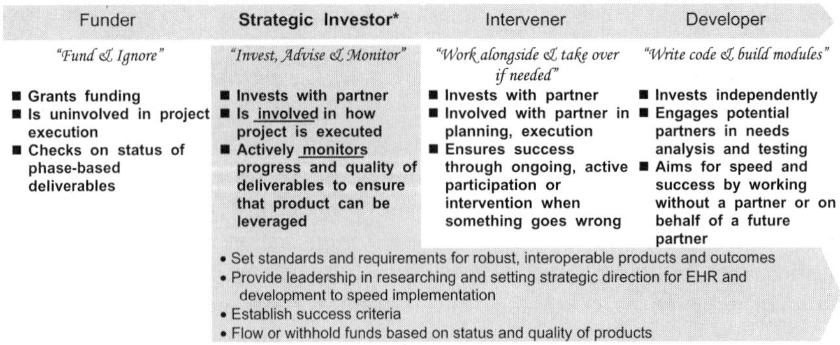

Funder	Strategic Investor*	Intervener	Developer
"Fund & Ignore"	*"Invest, Advise & Monitor"*	*"Work alongside & take over if needed"*	*"Write code & build modules"*
■ Grants funding ■ Is uninvolved in project execution ■ Checks on status of phase-based deliverables	■ Invests with partner ■ Is _involved_ in how project is executed ■ Actively _monitors_ progress and quality of deliverables to ensure that product can be leveraged	■ Invests with partner ■ Involved with partner in planning, execution ■ Ensures success through ongoing, active participation or intervention when something goes wrong	■ Invests independently ■ Engages potential partners in needs analysis and testing ■ Aims for speed and success by working without a partner or on behalf of a future partner

- Set standards and requirements for robust, interoperable products and outcomes
- Provide leadership in researching and setting strategic direction for EHR and development to speed implementation
- Establish success criteria
- Flow or withhold funds based on status and quality of products

FIGURE 10-1. *Infoway's* role as strategic investor. (*Source:* Building Momentum: 2003/04 Business Plan. Montreal: Canada Health Infoway, Inc.; 2003.)

healthcare organizations, as well as with IT vendors and suppliers. Collaboration with health ministries and other partners allows *Infoway* to: (a) align priorities; (b) plan associated technology and required adoption activities (such as Change Management and Knowledge Transfer) and effectively deploy new solutions; and (c) determine overall costs, including *Infoway's* required contribution, as well as implementation schedules.

As a strategic investor, *Infoway* focuses on both investing in an initial solution and in its development for reuse and subsequent deployment. *Infoway's* specific responsibilities include:

- Setting standards and requirements for robust, interoperable, replicable product solutions
- Providing leadership in researching and setting strategic direction for EHR development to speed implementation
- Establishing success criteria
- Releasing or withholding funds based on status and quality of project results using a gating methodology

Given its inherent structure, *Infoway*, by itself, does not build, directly implement, or hold proprietary EHR solution components. It also is not a granting agency; instead, it has an active role in monitoring the progress and quality of deliverables for each funded project. Rather, *Infoway's* role as strategic investor focuses on initial investment in a solution and its deployment. At the same time, this collaborative and highly engaged approach requires that *Infoway* provides timely guidance and advice to support project continuation throughout the project's lifecycle.

EHR Solution Architecture

The specification of a common framework and set of standards for designing, developing, and deploying interoperable, reusable EHR solutions is the key to achieving *Infoway's* mandate. Without such a specification, healthcare solutions across Canada would be a patchwork of incompatible systems and technologies.

Infoway developed its Electronic Health Record Solution (EHRS) Architecture Blueprint based on domestic and international best practices that have been confirmed through extensive consultations across Canada that examined:

- Methods to identify the actors in a healthcare encounter. This was particularly challenging given that multiple jurisdictions and healthcare delivery organization all had their own mechanisms for identity management
- The optimal way of making data available to authorized providers from multiple systems
- Mechanisms to make data semantically consistent
- Mechanisms to make systems scalable and high performing
- Mechanisms to make systems secure and private
- Approaches for adoption of the IT systems by healthcare providers
- Mechanisms to make systems portable and configurable to a diverse set of requirements
- Approaches to integrate systems in a loosely coupled manner[8]

The result was a Blueprint, a fully validated architectural framework, which lays out the business and technical considerations and approaches that will ultimately guide the development and implementation of sustainable EHR solutions in Canada. It provides a valuable framework from which individual jurisdictions can develop their own cost-effective EHR solutions while at the same time deliver reusable solutions to other jurisdictions.

The Solution

The *Infoway* EHRS Blueprint is a peer-to-peer network of message-based interoperable EHRSs deployed across Canada as shown in Figure 10-2.

Figure 10-2 presents a high-level view of the components of any EHRS and its interrelationships. Specifically, it depicts two EHRS deployments that are interconnected with one another through services grouped in a layer called the Health Information Access Layer (HIAL). The HIAL also allows for an abstraction layer for applications (EHRi) that create or use EHR content. This network of interconnected EHRS across the country

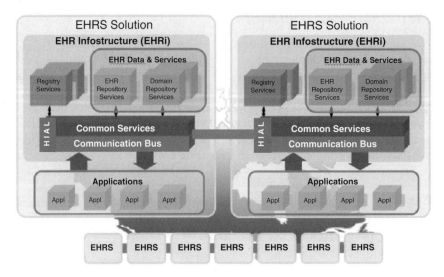

FIGURE 10-2. The solution: Distributed network of EHRS systems. (*Source:* Electronic Health Record Blueprint Solution Architecture. Version 1.0. Canada Health Infoway, Inc.; July 31, 2003.)

delivers the vision of a peer-to-peer, distributed network of interoperable systems. These interoperated systems could exist at the local, regional, provincial, or even national level to meet requirements of particular healthcare organizations (military, veterans, Aboriginal, or other). Each EHRS would enable communication with a given set of applications that cover a defined geography of points of care. These points of care also include applications used by patients or healthcare providers from homes or business offices. Connecting to one of the EHRS entry points provides secure validated and audited access to all information available across the network.

Components

Within one EHRS, an EHRi will store, maintain, and provide access to EHR data about persons who have had access to the healthcare system in the given jurisdiction. This EHRi will receive data from operational systems used in healthcare organizations or directly by care providers and patients. Conversely, it will also provide data back to the same operational systems for use by care providers involved in the continuum of care for any given patient.

The EHRi is composed of multiple systems that need to participate and interact with one another, including the following:

- The *EHR Data and Services* container highlights the fact that a combination of both the EHR repository and the domain repository systems are required to have a complete set of clinical data for a person. Information from the EHR is combined with other clinical data from one or more domain repositories to provide a person's complete longitudinal health record.
- *EHR Repository* situated at the center of the EHRi that maintains the clinical picture and history of all persons. The EHR contains information about healthcare encounters for each person and often stores detailed clinical data replicated from point of service applications. For example, these data include clinical referral notes, discharge summaries, health profiles, and immunizations.
- *Domain Repositories* store, maintain, and provide subsets of clinical information pertinent to the clinical picture of a person, such as drugs or medication profiles, laboratory test results, and diagnostic images. These data are typically stored at a jurisdictional level and are not replicated in the EHR. With the information that is provided by the domain repositories, the EHRi service can offer a complete longitudinal view of all EHR data to users and client applications.
- *Registry Systems* provide identification resolution services for key entities that need to be identified in the context of any transaction (such as patients, providers, system users, locations where services are provided, consent policies that apply to a transaction's context).

The HIAL is an interface specification for the EHR Infostructure (OSI Layer 7) that defines service components, service roles, an information model, and messaging standards required for the exchange of EHR data and execution of interoperability profiles between EHR services. The HIAL could be implemented in a variety of ways. The EHRS Blueprint depicts it as an independent system solution acting as a gateway between operational systems and jurisdictional level systems participating in the EHR Infostructure. This architecture provides independence, an application abstraction layer, between the tens of thousands of operational systems that need to be connected to the EHR Infostructure. Providing for this application abstraction layer is a key objective, given each jurisdiction in Canada will have different physical deployment models of systems. The HIAL thus provides a consistent view of the enterprise, and ultimately the EHR, to all operational systems.

Operational systems represent all the applications used by healthcare organizations or care providers that store, manage, and/or provide access to clinical data for persons. Operational systems also generically called *applications* interact with one EHRi in a given jurisdiction. This interaction is instantiated by way of message exchanges between applications and the HIAL.

Key Features

The key features delivered by the proposed solution are:

- Harmonization of definitions and standards between all EHRS for full interoperability:
  —EHRi's are able to communicate by exchanging messages across any number of jurisdictions
  —Applications communicate by exchanging messages with an EHRi within a given jurisdiction
  —Regardless of a jurisdiction's EHRi configuration, all applications view the EHRi in one consistent way everywhere in the country
  —Semantic, security, privacy, transactional, policy, and administrative metadata are exchanged and interpreted similarly between EHRi's
- Interoperability is instantiated between the core components of an EHRi (EHR, registries, and domain repositories)
- Standards are established so all system users agree on the semantic meaning of the information stored and accessed from the EHRS
- Policies and agreements are established between all jurisdictions that maintain and operate an EHRS

Interoperation

At its most basic level, the EHRS can be described as a collection of client applications for updating and accessing EHR data. The solution element that actually makes it possible for these systems to interoperate is the common interface specification called the Health Information and Access Layer (HIAL), which defines the various service roles, and the information model and messaging standards required for the exchange of EHR data and the execution of interoperability profiles between EHR services and client applications. For simplicity, these service components can be grouped into two key categories: Common services and communication bus.

Common services is the set of basic software service components used by EHRi application interfaces to process message exchanges with other applications according to the HIAL specification; these include auditing, security, and privacy services. Communication bus represents the set of basic software service components that provide support for network and application protocols, low-level message assembly, routing, and delivery between EHRi systems.

The System in Action

The EHRS interacts with other healthcare applications to deliver a seamless, interoperable view of clinical data for use across the continuum of care and jurisdictional health delivery authorities. The following highlights ways in which it works:

- The information stored in the EHR and in domain repositories is person-centric and longitudinal. Logically, it forms a lifetime health history for each individual. Clinical data for any encounter are stored in only one EHR, located in the person's home province or territory, or wherever he or she receives care.
- Information may be organized into multidimensional categories such as time, clinical data type (laboratory, drugs, clinical notes), practice area, and disease class. All data clinically relevant over time and for use across the continuum of care are retained.
- Applications and source systems are key elements of the solution. Authorized healthcare providers use applications to view and navigate a person's EHR. These include applications at the point of care that a provider is interacting with a patient. In this solution, data are pushed or published into the EHR from applications or source systems.
- The same applications read and use data out of the EHR. EHR data are viewed from applications that providers use in their daily activities. These applications are responsible for visualization of data. For example, a primary care doctor using a physician management system may view four sets of data on their system—one from the person's EHR, another from the physician management system's physician order entry module (i.e., for a new prescription or laboratory test).
- An EHR is not an online transaction-processing (OLTP) store for any clinical system used in points of service; rather, applications will store data in the OLTP data store of the application. In near real-time, the clinical data pertaining to that encounter are replicated into the EHR via the EHRi.
- The interface between applications and EHRi is message-based. Most of the messaging will be for the purposes of reading and writing clinical information in and out of the EHR. As such, messages will be based on industry standards such as HL7 and DICOM. Applications may also use the value-added services of the EHRi, remotely invoking a service method. These may be supported via mechanisms such as SOAP and remote call protocols such as RMI and DCOM.

Accomplishments and Current Challenges

There has already been enough experience to have accumulated accomplishments and to understand what challenges remain.

Accomplishments

Maintained national leadership. Leadership and formal commitment to the interoperable EHR by high-level government leaders has been in place for the last four years. This is a critical success factor, because national commitment and support are required to drive a successful program. As a result,

Infoway and jurisdictions are well underway in aligning their strategies and investments toward implementation of an interoperable EHR across 50% of Canada by the end of 2009.

Became fully operational. It has taken *Infoway* 2.5 years to be fully operational and for it to fully develop its program strategies. Various factors contributed to this success. In its first year, *Infoway* was in startup mode, with a keen interest in obtaining investments and early project wins. In the meantime, the mandate was expanded twice and infused with additional capital by the federal government. Strategic planning sessions with jurisdictions (resulting in multi-year planning and budgeting) and refinements to the business plan (moving from a tactical focus to a strategic one with defined investment programs) also contributed to a slower than desired start. By the end of fiscal year 2005, *Infoway* will be at a point where all jurisdictions are actively engaged in one or more of its investment programs.

Established technology replication and re-use. By the end of fiscal year 2005, the replication of client registry and provider registry solutions, as well as the shared-services model is driving economies of scale, cost-savings, and accelerated deployment. Additionally, cost avoidance and knowledge transfer across jurisdictions through "How-to Toolkits" that contain a broad range of project artifacts that are leveraged by others enable faster project startup.

Implemented standards-based solutions. Infoway is moving the private and public sectors toward implementing standards-based solutions. For the first time in Canada, standards for interoperability are adopted, adapted, or developed and endorsed on a pan-Canadian basis. For the public sector, this creates an environment for true interoperability and choice, while lowering overall cost. For the private sector, it creates a larger marketplace for its products and services, rather than the fractured marketplace that previously existed in Canada.

Protected privacy. At the same time, privacy remains a top priority in all project investments. Each project has a requirement for a privacy impact assessment, which provides a framework to ensure that privacy is considered throughout the design or redesign of programs or services. The assessments identify the extent to which projects comply with all appropriate statutes. In turn, assessments assist managers and decision makers in avoiding or mitigating privacy risks; at the same time, they promote fully informed policy, program, and system design choices.[9] In addition, each project requires a privacy audit to ensure that business and systems privacy policies and procedures are implemented correctly.[10]

Current Challenges

Sustaining investments. Infoway has identified a number of challenges that have affected its pace, progress, overall success, and adoption by end-users of its project investments. One reason progress has been slower than planned is that *Infoway's* investment ratios are considered by some jurisdictions to be too low. They currently stand at 25% to 50% of total capital costs. These are lower than shown in the business plan because a number of elements in an investment project are not eligible for investment, such as networking infrastructure, end-user workstations, and end-user clinical information systems. These, coupled with the monies jurisdictions must budget for ongoing systems operations, maintenance, and support, decrease the *Infoway* investment percentage even more, when looked at over a 10-year period. Related to this is the fact that jurisdictional budget approval for projects can take between 12–18 months. Finally, procurements are done by each jurisdiction, versus being coordinated across multiple jurisdictions; this is compounded by a long cycle of between 6–24 months.

Increasing capitalization. Infoway capitalization is insufficient to achieve objectives. In late 2004, *Infoway* commissioned a study on the overall cost to complete its mandate of an interoperable EHR across Canada. This cost projection did not include infrastructure—such as networking and data centers—but does include other costs that are currently not eligible for funding, namely, clinical information systems. The cost estimate is in excess of $10 billion (Canadian) of capital investment in Canada. The existing $1.2 billion matched by over another $1.2 billion from the jurisdictions is not enough to accomplish the goals and objectives.

Increasing user acceptance. Another significant challenge *Infoway* and its partners face is the adoption and acceptance by healthcare professionals of the interoperable EHR. In Canada, there is a low level of physician automation, particularly in the primary care sector; conversely, acute care settings have clinical systems. Until the family physician is automated and clinical data that need to be shared across the continuum of care are truly interoperable, *Infoway* will continue to be challenged to meet its objectives.

Funding physician systems. Infoway cannot fund the networking, computer systems, or software in physicians' offices. Compounding the situation is the fact that most jurisdictions lack a plan or funding to completely automate this sector.

Australia

We describe the Australian experience in the same steps as the Canadian section.

Overview of Large Public and Private Sector System

Australia, with a population of approximately 20 million people, has a complex federal system of government, consisting of three key levels: The national parliament; six state and two territory parliaments; and a range of local government organizations.[11] Australia's total health sector expenditure in 2001–2002 was $66.6 billion (all in Australian dollars), representing 9.3% of the GDP.[12] The Australian government is the largest contributor of health funding, providing 46.3% of total health expenditure, with the state, territory, and local government contribution accounting for 22.3%.[13] Other sources of health funding in Australia come from private health insurance funds, individual (self-funded) payments, workers' compensation, and compulsory motor vehicle third-party insurance funds.[14] A key component of the Australian government's contribution to health funding is providing approximately 50% of the cost for the state and territory governments to run public hospitals. This funding is provided under the Australian Health Care Agreements ($42 billion under the current 2003–2008 agreements).

The Australian government's other main funding roles in the healthcare arena are the Medicare Benefits Scheme (Medicare) and the Pharmaceutical Benefits Scheme (PBS). Medicare supports access to health care for Australian citizens and residents by providing subsidies for medical services such as a general practitioner's (GP) consultation, public hospital accommodation and treatment, as well as some specialist, pathology, and diagnostic imaging services.[15] The PBS provides subsidized access to listed prescription medicines (approximately 80% of prescription medications available at pharmacies) at a cost of more than $5.1 billion per annum.[16]

Although the Australian government is the largest provider of health funding, it does not have a large role in delivery of health services. Instead, most services are delivered by the states, territories, other providers, or take the form of direct subsidies to individuals via private health insurance rebates, Medicare, and the PBS.[17] The Australian government also has a leadership role in devising and influencing national policy.

The state and territory governments are traditionally responsible for public hospital service provision and funding, nursing home services, community health and community mental health services, public health promotion and education programs, and child and family health services. Additionally, they regulate registration of health professionals, private hospitals, and day surgery centers.[18]

Private health insurance is a key feature of the Australian system. Although Medicare provides Australian citizens and residents with free treatment as public patients in public hospitals, individuals can also purchase private health insurance to cover all or some of the costs of health care as a private patient (Australia has virtually no employer-based health insurance schemes). Private health insurance allows patients to be treated at the hospital of their choice by the doctor of their choice and covers services generally not covered by Medicare, including dental and optical treatment, ambulance transport, physiotherapy, and occupational therapy.

There are two types of private health insurance coverage available in Australia: Hospital coverage, which covers all or some of the costs of hospital treatment as a private patient, and ancillary coverage, which helps cover the cost of services such as physiotherapy, dental, and optical treatment. Patients may elect to take out either hospital or ancillary coverage or both.

In response to decreasing private health insurance membership in the 1990s, the Australian government introduced incentives to encourage enrollment and retention of private health insurance. These included a 30% rebate on membership fees and Lifetime Health Cover, which means that people who take out insurance before 30 years of age pay lower premiums throughout their life.[19] As a result of these incentives, approximately 49% of the Australian population today is covered by private health insurance.

*The Formation of Health*Connect

The e-Health Initiative Context

Since the late 1990s, the e-health agenda has been organized at a national level in Australia. Health Online, which provided an initial blueprint for national action, was published in 1999 and updated in 2001. A review of Australia's e-health initiative has led to a new governance structure with the creation of the Australian Health Information Council (AHIC, for strategic agenda setting) and the National Health Information Group (NHIG, for implementation). Notwithstanding the development of a national agenda, in a recent report prepared for the NHIG and the AHIC, the Boston Consulting Group identified more than 360 current or planned information management and information communication technology activities in Australia. The three largest areas of e-health investment were identified as clinical information systems, patient administration systems, and EHR projects, with a projected expenditure over 2 years that would equal $720 million.[20] The mixture of public and private health funding and provision of health services, coupled with the multiple levels of a federal system of government, presents challenges for nation-wide implementation of any electronic health initiative.

Health*Connect*

The largest Australian e-health project at the national level is Health-*Connect*, Australia's EHR service. A joint Australian, state and territory government project, Health*Connect* involves the collection, storage, and exchange of consumer health information in summary format via a secure network and within strict privacy safeguards. The aim of Health*Connect* is to improve the delivery of health care, to provide better quality of care, and to improve patient safety and health outcomes.

The Health*Connect* project grew out of a recommendation in 2000 by the National Electronic Health Records Taskforce to create a national health information network.[21] The recommendation was supported by all Australian Health Ministers (Australian government, state and territory) who agreed to jointly fund a 2-year research and development program to examine Health*Connect's* value and feasibility. The research and development program began with a mixture of research, design, and development work and live trials, with the first trials of Health*Connect* commencing during October 2002 in Tasmania and the Northern Territory.[22]

Organizational Structure

The Health*Connect* Program Office was established at the outset of the project to manage the research and development work and is staffed by Australian, state and territory government employees. The majority of Program Office staff is located in Canberra, the nation's capital city, with other members in each state and territory.

A Health*Connect* board also was established to guide the development of Health*Connect*. The board membership includes representatives from all governments as well as provider, consumer, and industry representatives. The Health*Connect* board reports to the Australian Health Ministers' Advisory Council (AHMAC) via the NHIG.

Program Activity in Four Phases

Health*Connect* is currently progressing through four overlapping phases of activity, the first of which commenced with the research and development program in 2001.

Phase I (2001–2003) included 2 years of research and development to test the feasibility and value of the Health*Connect* concept, and served as a basis for deciding whether to implement it on a national scale. Trials of Health*Connect* began in discrete regions within the states of Tasmania, Queensland, and the Northern Territory, while work also began on developing the business and systems architectures and data components of Health*Connect*, such as event summaries and data standards.

At the same time, Medi*Connect* was under development as a separate project from Health*Connect*. Medi*Connect*—an electronic medication record system—focused on reducing the incidence of adverse drug events by improving consumer and healthcare professionals' access to more complete medication information. The Medi*Connect* Development Group, a ministerial advisory group composed of medical, pharmacy, consumer, and software vendor representatives, guided its development. A field test of the system commenced in early 2003 and concluded in December 2004.

Phase II (2003–2005) saw the continuation of research and development with an emphasis on preparing to implement Health*Connect* nationally. During this phase, existing trials and tests continued, with preplanned, additional trials to be implemented and tested in Queensland and New South Wales. Parallel to the Health*Connect* trials, work continued on the architectural design, system, and data components. This work led to the development of a multitiered architecture, composed of a national coordination layer, a number of Health*Connect* Records Systems (data storage services), and a user access layer. The user layer provides linkages between the Health*Connect* Records Systems and general practices, hospitals, allied and community health services, and private specialist services.

Phase III (2004–2008) began with a shift in the Health*Connect* project from research and development to actual implementation on a national level. In 2004, the Australian government announced the national implementation of Health*Connect*. Initially, a strategically planned implementation of Health*Connect* will occur in three states—Tasmania, South Australia, and the Northern Territory—with expansion to the other states and territories in the future. Phase III also includes incorporation of Medi*Connect* functionality into Health*Connect*.

During 2004, the Australian Health Ministers established the National e-Health Transition Authority (NEHTA) to drive national information management and information communication technology priorities.[23] NEHTA is a non-government organization whose work program is focused on the priority areas of clinical data standards, identification standards, consumer and provider directories, supply chain procurement standards, consent models, secure messaging and information transfer, and technical integration standards. During 2005, the Health*Connect* Program Office was divided into a design function that is operating within the NEHTA and an implementation function that is under the control of the new Director of National e-Health Implementation.

Phase IV (2006–2008) will occur as the remaining states and territories participate in implementation of Health*Connect*.

Investment, Model, and Strategy

Investment

The Health*Connect* Indicative Benefits Report conservatively estimated cost offsets of $396 million per annum should there be a 100% enrollment by consumers and providers.[24] Although 100% enrollment is not anticipated for many years, this provides an indication of the level of benefits that could be achieved. The report concluded that when fully implemented, additional direct financial benefits could accrue, giving a total indicative benefits range of $554 million to $604 million per annum.

Cost modeling of Health*Connect* shows that the overall cost is highly dependent on the registration process and to a lesser extent on the technical solution adopted. The major establishment components outside registration are expected to be infrastructure deployment, change management programs, and system integration. These costs would be spread over a number of years and are estimated to be $30 million per annum over 10 years. A more complete analysis of the cost of Health*Connect* is contained in the Health*Connect* Interim Research Report (2003).[25]

Annual recurrent costs, including registration, are anticipated to be in the order of $160 million. There are also indirect costs associated with the development of privacy, security, and identification arrangements; IT and data standards; computing infrastructure within participating organizations; workflow changes; and telecommunications infrastructure. Although these costs are substantial ($2–3 billion), they will be incurred whether or not Health*Connect* is implemented.

The Australian government has committed $128 million over 4 years toward national funding for Health*Connect's* implementation. This is in addition to previous funding of $23 million for Health*Connect* and $35 million for Medi*Connect*. In addition, state and territory governments are expected to make substantial investments in their computing infrastructure and clinical information systems.

Key areas of work guiding the current implementation of Health*Connect* include: Analysis of the potential benefits of Health*Connect*; creating an implementation guide; reaching agreement on the business rules and clinical data terminologies; analysis of legal issues; and creation of an evaluation strategy. Two of the key documents arising from this work are the Benefits Realization Framework and the Implementation Approach.

Benefits Realization Framework

The implementation of Health*Connect* is being driven by a benefits realization approach. The approach is guided by a Benefits Realization Framework identifying priority groups and settings for Health*Connect* implementation and includes governance suggestions and evaluation arrangements required for achieving and measuring benefits from Health-*Connect*.[26] The key features of the framework include the following:

- Obtaining high enrollment rates by healthcare providers and medical consumers with a focus on increasing the efficiency of the processes underpinning episodes of care
- Increasing the usefulness of information to clinicians with a focus on information flow between providers and among healthcare facilities to increase patient safety by decreasing the impact of adverse events (including adverse drug events)
- Implementing full-cycle governance to ensure ongoing management of Health*Connect*
- Focusing on initial Health*Connect* registration, enrollment, and communication processes in areas where there are high healthcare expenditures.

Implementation Approach

Together with the Benefits Realization Framework, the Implementation Approach forms the backbone of Health*Connect* implementation planning work.[27] As discussed earlier, states and territories are progressing with implementation of Health*Connect* at different rates. The Implementation Approach focuses on national alignment of the individual state, territory implementations of Health*Connect* by providers and consumers. Compliance with specified capabilities will enable states and territories to implement their individual strategies at different rates while ensuring national consistency; at the same time, a targeted enrollment strategy aims to achieve a "critical mass" of participants in order to maximize the benefits of Health*Connect*.

The Implementation Approach identifies key provider types that form the core care team for most medical consumers. The provider types—including GPs, community pharmacists, hospitals (including accident, emergency, and outpatients), pathology and radiology—will be targeted for enrollment. It is also expected that this group will expand to include provider types that are key to targeted consumer groups.

The priority groups for consumer enrollment are those that will be the major recipients of benefits from Health*Connect*. As recommended in the Benefits Realization Framework, these will include the very young (0–4 years), particularly newborns and their parents, and patients with chronic and complex conditions and comorbidities, such as cardiovascular disease and diabetes. The complex conditions occur in a higher proportion in older Australians (55+ years) and Aboriginal and Torres Strait Islander peoples.

As indicated by the Health*Connect* Benefits Realization Framework, implementation of Health*Connect* is expected to deliver broad benefits for consumers, providers, and the health sector.[28] By improving access to consumer health information across the healthcare sector, Health*Connect* will deliver health outcome benefits through increased coordination of care, better quality of care, and a reduction in the number of adverse reactions. Health*Connect* will also reduce the amount of time providers spend finding consumer information, enabling their business to become more efficient.

Solution Architecture for HealthConnect

Background

Health*Connect* is a repository for consumers' lifetime records.

A Health*Connect* record consists of a series of event summaries, which contain key information about a specific healthcare event (e.g., a GP consultation, hospital admission or discharge, or pathology test). Therefore, it is not a complete record and does not replace providers' own clinical records or clinical information systems. Providers will continue to maintain their own consumer health records but may choose to incorporate information from Health*Connect* into their own records.

Creation of event summaries will be a simple process in order to minimize the impact on provider work practices. Health*Connect* will generate event summaries by drawing on information already collected by the provider in their own clinical information system. The information within the event summaries will be structured as data groups. Some key data groups will be stored as Health*Connect* "lists" which are collections of similar Health*Connect* items describing key aspects of a consumer's health formed to serve a specific purpose.

Examples of lists, which Health*Connect* will automatically derive from event summary information, are prescribing and dispensing history, procedure and treatment history, and recent health services. The lists, which are maintained by a provider, are current medications, active problems and diagnoses, adverse reactions, and warnings.

Participation in Health*Connect* is voluntary for both consumers and healthcare providers and is open to all Australian citizens and residents. The Health*Connect* record is primarily designed to support the provision of healthcare services and improve health outcomes primarily through a reduction in adverse reactions. Health*Connect* will also assist the decision support ability of provider clinical information systems by ensuring that information about the consumer being treated is more complete than otherwise possible.

Consumers control access to the Health*Connect* record and they nominate service provider organizations that can access their Health*Connect* record. Consumers will be able to change their access control arrangements, for example, changing their general practice or adding a specialist group to their list. Organizations not identified on the consumer's list will not be able to access the consumer's record, other than using the emergency override facility. This emergency override facility can be used only in an emergency in which the consumer is unable to give consent to access their Health-*Connect* record. It should be noted that once a provider downloads Health-*Connect* information into his or her own systems and records, it becomes the responsibility of that organization to control access to the downloaded information.

Model

Over time, the Health*Connect* repository will also become a highly valuable national information resource supporting important national initiatives and activities including clinical research, policy making, and planning health outcomes evaluation. These uses are collectively referred to as secondary uses. Access to Health*Connect* information for secondary purposes will only occur in line with strict protocols and with ethics committee approval. Figure 10-3 illustrates the business design of Health*Connect*.[29]

The core of Health*Connect* is a national system of shareable EHRs that is able to receive, store, retrieve, and deliver consumers' summary EHR information via secure e-health communications and with strict privacy safeguards for use in the delivery of health care.

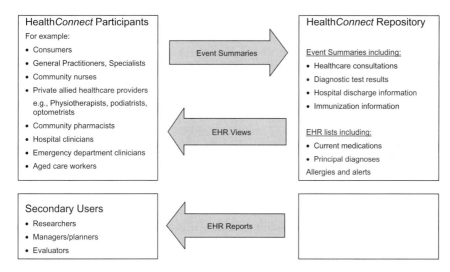

FIGURE 10-3. Key components of Health*Connect*. (*Source:* Health*Connect* Business Architecture. Version 1.9. Commonwealth of Australia.)

The Health*Connect* Business Architecture provides the business rules for security and access control, privacy, consent, identification, registration, information storage, processing, and messaging.[30] The initial implementation of Health*Connect* will be compliant with version 1.9 of the Business Architecture, whereas version 2.0 is expected to include major changes and define a workable and achievable solution for the next stage of Health-*Connect* implementation.

Consumer participation in Health*Connect* is voluntary and nondiscriminatory and does not limit availability of health services to consumers. Although Health*Connect* is available to all citizens and residents of Australia, early implementation focuses on those likely to get the greatest long-term benefit—those with chronic diseases, infants, and populations with high morbidity.

Provider participation in Health*Connect* is available to all providers involved in the chain of healthcare delivery. Whereas the initial focus is on medical practices, pharmacies, hospitals, diagnostic services, health and aged care facilities, this scope will be extended through arrangements with each provider group.

Data Considerations

A consumer's Health*Connect* record is made up of a collection of event summaries, which provide summarized information about healthcare events that are relevant to the ongoing care of a consumer. These event summaries will be produced according to defined metadata covering format, data items, and allowable code sets.

Users access data from the stored event summaries for an individual consumer through a series of predefined Health*Connect* views. Views are being developed to address specific needs of consumers and providers taking into account specific practice areas, conditions, and treatment regimes. The priority views identified to date are the primary (or "critical") view and the health profile view.

Secondary users can also access data from event summaries across consumers, i.e., relating to populations, through Health*Connect* reports that will be extracted from the Health*Connect* databases in line with predefined requirements and a strict approval process.

A federation of Health*Connect* Records Systems (HRS) will perform the core function of Health*Connect*, the processing of Health*Connect* event summaries, and query transactions that maintain the primary Health-*Connect* repository. To exchange information with Health*Connect* users, each HRS interacts with Health*Connect*-enabled user applications via a common Health*Connect* message handling and transport system. The operating environment of Health*Connect* is illustrated in Figure 10-4.[31]

A provider will use a clinical information system to interact with Health-*Connect* (provided that the clinical information system is Health*Connect* enabled) or, where necessary, may use a Web browser to interact with Health*Connect* via a provider access portal running a provider front-end application.

Consumers will typically use a Web browser to access Health*Connect* via a consumer access portal running a consumer front-end application. It is expected that consumers may eventually be able to acquire Health*Connect*-enabled consumer health information systems that will allow them to interact with Health*Connect*.

Lifespan Considerations

One of the goals for Health*Connect* is to make information available throughout the lifespan of an individual. To enable this, the structure and content of Health*Connect* information is defined by Health*Connect* metadata, which will be used to format and exchange EHR information. All versions of Health*Connect* metadata that are actually promulgated and used for the formation and storage of Health*Connect* information must be retained indefinitely to allow future interpretation of the information. Event summaries will be defined by national terminology and data standards.

Accomplishments and Current Challenges

Accomplishments

The ongoing evaluation of the Health*Connect* trials and the Medi*Connect* field test has recorded a number of achievements since its inception in 2000.

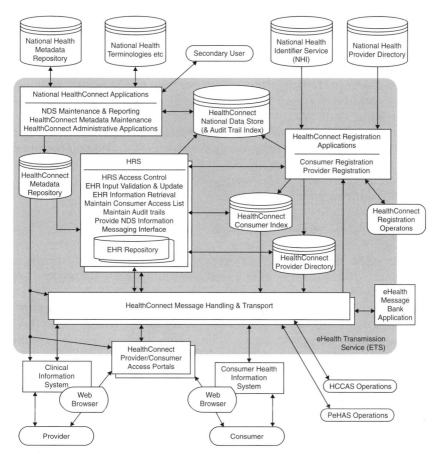

FIGURE 10-4. HealthConnect systems overview. (*Source:* Health*Connect* Business Architecture. Version 1.9. Commonwealth of Australia.)

These have been in the areas of architecture designs, policy development, key document development, the trial implementation of Health*Connect*, and the field test of Medi*Connect*.

Developed architecture designs. Achievements in the area of design include release of the Health*Connect* Business Architecture versions 1 and 1.9 with version 2 due to be released in 2005. The Health*Connect* Systems Architecture was also released in 2003. Development of all four design documents involved broad stakeholder consultation and input.

Developed critical policies. Core Health*Connect* policy components are well developed in a number of areas including privacy, consent, security and access control, registration, and identification arrangements.

Produced key documents. A number of critical documents have been developed to guide the implementation of Health*Connect*. These include the Health*Connect* Interim Research Report, Benefits Realization Framework, Implementation Approach, and Evaluation Strategy.

Implemented trials. Another significant achievement for the project has been the establishment of the Health*Connect* trial sites and the Medi*Connect* field test. Health*Connect* trials have been operating successfully in Tasmania and the Northern Territory since 2002, with two further trials now operational in Queensland.

Executed MediConnect field test. The Medi*Connect* field test was one of the largest e-health trials ever conducted in Australia. A decision was taken to incorporate Medi*Connect* into Health*Connect* because it is expected that a holistic record that includes medicine information will be more useful than the medicine information alone.

Challenges

The key challenges fall into four domains: Establishing a critical mass of users, managing technical issues, communicating with consumers and providers, and developing privacy and consent models.

Establishing critical user mass. The two main groups of participants that need to be considered are consumers and healthcare providers. Unless both of these groups are fully engaged and committed, planning or implementation efforts will face difficulties. One challenge is the need to establish a critical mass of participants. Critical mass is the point at which there are sufficient consumers and providers participating in an implementation site so that providers and consumers can begin to realize the benefits of participation.

For providers, an important element of this process is obtaining a high proportion of consumers participating in the program, because they will be likely to integrate the new workflow into their business practice and be encouraged to embrace the EHR. The same concept applies to consumers who seek a broad range of providers who view and enter information into Health*Connect*.

Managing technical issues. The Health*Connect* trials and the Medi*Connect* field test have shown that the interfaces between providers' clinical information systems (such as Medical Director which is used widely by GPs) and the Health*Connect* system need to be seamless, so that providers are not required to rekey information. Ideally, the information that populates Health*Connect* should be automatically extracted from the practice record.

The Health*Connect* system, including security mechanisms, needs to be technically robust and efficient, so that slow downs or interruptions to provider operations are minimized. The provider interface needs to be efficient and not time consuming, in order to encourage providers usage. Some providers have only a limited understanding of the hardware and software they use and need additional support. Providers and consumers must understand that data are secure as a basis for encouraging usage.

Communicating with consumers and providers. A key challenge arising from the Health*Connect* trials and Medi*Connect* field test is that communications material needs to be simple and easy to understand. It is important to avoid "information overload," which can overwhelm many consumers and providers. To minimize confusion, communications material should note where further information can be found without providing too much information at the outset.

One technique that can be used to assist the communications process is to market the program through local community groups. This helped build awareness of the system among various communities, and it will encourage people to register for, and participate in, the implementation. This technique has been used in several sites and has met with considerable success.

Developing the privacy and consent models. The development of an appropriate privacy and consent model is clearly critical to successfully engaging both providers and consumers in the project. The Health*Connect* trials and the Medi*Connect* field test have shown that consumers appreciate having a range of consent options available to them. However, they do not necessarily want to be immediately presented with many (often complicated) options at registration; rather, consumers need to be made aware of the availability of their options, and educated about how they can obtain further information should they wish to adjust the way their personal health information is kept secure.

United Kingdom

Overview of Universal Financing and Public–Private Delivery System

The UK has a centralized statutory universal healthcare financing system, a niche market for private insurers, and a mixed public–private delivery system; its national health policy includes rationing care through governmental control of funding for the public delivery system. The UK may be unique among countries with a statutory universal health system in that its National Health Service (NHS), established in 1948, underwent significant restructuring based on two independent reform strategies; however, the first was never fully implemented, and the second, initiated in 1998, was developed to usher in a comprehensive updating of the entire manner in which the NHS functions, with the intention of modernizing the NHS.[32]

Although universal financing represents the UK financial model, it has yet to be fully actualized. For this goal to be realized, the existing funding mechanism would need to be reassessed and aligned to include: 1) Paying

NHS trusts and other providers adequately for services delivered, while at the same time, managing demand and risk; 2) supporting the introduction of patient choice by ensuring that diverse providers can be funded according to where patients choose to be treated; 3) rewarding efficiency and quality in providing services; 4) matching capacity to demand; and 5) refocusing discussion from disputes over price to the volume and mix of services that meet population need and the pathway of care for patients.[33]

Healthcare Resource Groups (HRGs), referred to as Diagnostic Related Groups (DRGs) in other countries, will be introduced to Primary Care Trusts, in which the GP acts as a gatekeeper, will be at the heart of this model. Indeed, the model of a case mix adjustment payment method is the result of the UK's observation of global healthcare trends being deployed across other nations.

The NHS plan (a plan for investment, a plan for reform) sets out some very ambitious challenges for the NHS. It creates a historic commitment to sustain increases in funding coupled with reform and modernization and will transform the NHS into a health system fit for the 21st century.

The Formation of the NHS National Care Record Service Program in England

The Department of Health (DoH) created the structure for the EHR program and its National Program for Information Technology (NPfIT), now an executive agency of the DoH and renamed the NHS Connecting for Health (CfH) from April 2005. The current EHR project for England, the National Care Record Service (NCRS) program began implementation via a nationwide procurement process throughout 2003, resulting in the award of contracts in December 2003 to one National Application Service Provider (NASP) and five Local Service Providers (LSPs) (Figure 10-5). Consistent with the modernization of the NHS, the government has allocated funding for the NCRS program specifically for NHS trusts that serve the public sector. Although many components have been funded, the local trusts will retain responsibility for allocating funds to support a number of related, concurrent projects that support of the NCRS (e.g., infrastructure is a local responsibility as is legacy management). It is important to note that this procurement process represents both a public sector as well as a healthcare initiative.

Engagement of the healthcare community, especially healthcare professionals (HCPs), is key to the program's success. In preparation for the procurement process, special attention was given to defining key requirements of the NCRS program. As a result, documentation of requirements was termed as the first output-based specification (OBS1) and participation of pertinent members of the broader healthcare community was included.

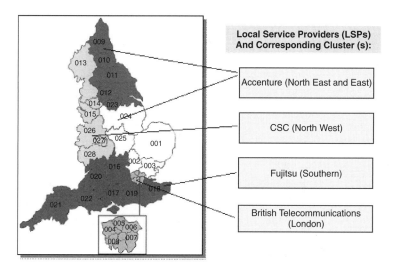

Local Service Providers (LSPs) And Corresponding Cluster (s):

Accenture (North East and East)

CSC (North West)

Fujitsu (Southern)

British Telecommunications (London)

FIGURE 10-5. The service providers and clusters for England. (*Source:* NHS National Programme for IT. © NHS Information Authority; 2004.)

A second iteration of the output-based specification (OBS2) was issued to tenders who qualified for the next stage in the procurement process. In advance of issuing OBS2, information was again solicited from a variety of healthcare sources such as the DoH, NHS organizations, the Royal Colleges, individual HCPs, and the local trusts. An interesting observation is that the requirements were not only related to required clinical functionality and technical requirement but also to the national guidelines and legal requirements.

As a government initiative, the NCRS program process was a tender process that began with an initial qualification of approximately 100 potential participants of which 22 were identified as candidates for LSPs and eight were identified as candidates for the National Service Provider. With the breadth of the requirements defined in the output-based specification, it was clear that no single vendor or firm could represent all the required expertise and capacity to deliver the program. As a result, the potential candidates formed a consortium to deliver the NCRS program.

The NHS CfH delivering the NPfIT continues to be a vital organization for monitoring progress across all five clusters, and for providing guidance for policy development for the NCRS program. Awarded contracts for each of the LSPs include a 7-year contract through 2010 because the structure of the program was designed to bring all trusts into a final stage of the NCRS program by that year. The funding over the life of the NCRS program has been budgeted for the 7-year process by the DoH.

With a workforce of more than 1.3 million, the NHS is one of the world's largest employers. The NHS CfH undertaking is the largest and most ambitious public sector IT procurement project to date with an original budget of £6.2 billion over 10 years. The rest of the world watches its progress with interest, as this kind of record sharing technology, although familiar in Web-based commerce, is very unusual in a large-scale health environment.

Investment, Model, and Strategy

The National Model and IT

The universal financing model continues to be widely supported as a key component of the UK's national agenda for healthcare reform—especially as it relates to benefiting citizens of the UK. With this in mind, EHRs emphasize patients' needs, their journey through healthcare services in the UK, and how IT will enhance healthcare and patient services via IT's four pillars of modernization: 1) improved access, i.e., reducing waiting lists of patients who are seeking services; 2) enhanced quality, i.e., ensuring that measures are in place for improvements in patient safety, quality of care, and patients' experience, etc.; 3) public and private care option choices for each patient; and 4) addressing health inequality, i.e., ensuring all citizens have access to quality health services.

From a strategic level, the entire government initiative for modernization is consistent with improving what is termed as the "Patient Journey." This patient-centric view focuses on how best to serve the population of England (50 million in 2003), while allowing patients to have a record that can be seamlessly accessed by all appropriate authorized healthcare professionals as they provide integrated patient care across service areas.

National Program for Information Technology

Some of the primary elements of the NHS CfH's National Program for Information Technology include, but are not limited to (Figure 10-6): 1) Choose and Book (previously known as the Electronic Booking Service); 2) an electronic NCRS program; 3) electronic transmission of prescriptions (ETP); and 4) a new national network for the NHS (N3) infrastructure to support the program (including the Spine, the national data repository).

Choose and Book

This element of the EHR is meant to facilitate the coordination of patient activities across care providers and enhance the level of convenience to the patient by offering a choice of when and where to be treated. It also allows for a more efficient administrative function and processing of requests to share medical information with other care providers when moving a patient across a variety of healthcare services.

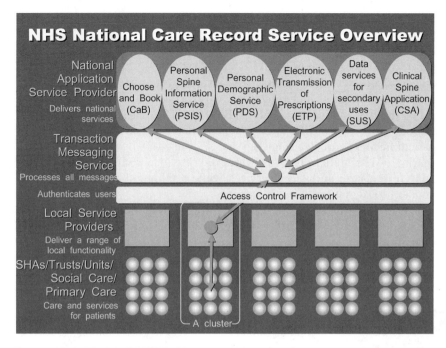

FIGURE 10-6. The NHS NCRS. (*Source:* NHS National Programme for IT. © NHS Information Authority; 2004.)

In its initial phase (during summer 2004), some Primary Care Trusts had their GPs, clinicians, and HCPs create an appointment for patients at the point of referral. In turn, patients completed the process initiated with their GPs by contacting the national call center and requesting their place and time of preference to receive their next care service.

During this first phase of the Choose and Book initiative, the two selected pilot sites used the functionality to book patients into the corresponding hospital trust to ensure patients received referral services. This constitutes a primary to secondary care referral model. In future releases of the Choose and Book initiative, there will be other types of functionality to allow for the scheduling of referred appointments in the following three configurations: 1) primary to primary, 2) secondary to tertiary, and, 3) follow-up bookings.

National Care Record Service

The NCRS is composed of the functionality and technology that support both administrative and clinical applications across the continuum of care. Currently, each NHS organization is like a separate franchise company with its own systems, methods of working, and information governance. The NHS

NCRS in England will link these disparate groups together to use IT to facilitate sharing of vital healthcare information on patients. This supports the NHS objective of improved and patient-centered care and choice. Figure 10-7 describes how the NCRS will dramatically improve care-related communications within and across a variety of organizations and geographical boundaries including home care, primary, and secondary care.

For the first time in England, NCRS will unify these sources by providing one portal for HCPs and, in time, other care services to access key patient history through a single service (Figure 10-8). It will enable national sharing of vital patient records from disparate local sources, such as hospitals, GP registers, and social services, while retaining the integrity of independent local systems.

The NASP will be responsible for applications common to all users nationally whereas the LSPs will accomplish the following: 1) Provide IT systems and services in the five regional clusters in England; 2) ensure that the national applications can be delivered locally; and 3) ensure that both national standards and local needs are met.

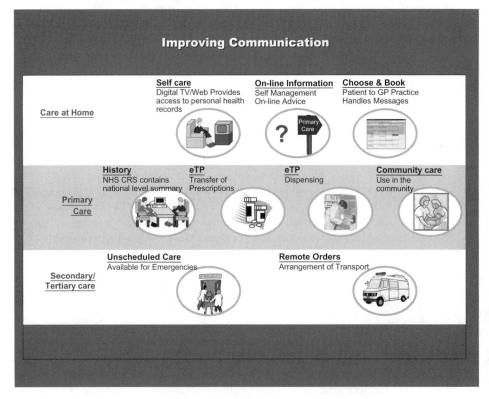

FIGURE 10-7. NCRS improvement in care-related communications. (*Source:* Department of Health. © NHS Information Authority; 2003.)

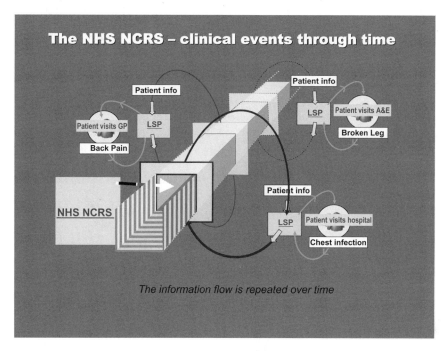

The NHS NCRS – clinical events through time

FIGURE 10-8. NCRS clinical events. (*Source:* NHS National Programme for IT. © NHS Information Authority; 2004.)

Electronic Transmission of Prescriptions

This initiative focuses on modernization of the primary care segment of patient care, with the purpose of: 1) providing benefits to patients that result in fewer trips to their GP to collect recurring prescriptions, and 2) enhancing patient safety by preventing efforts related to illegible or incomplete prescriptions. Patients will also be able to nominate their preferred pharmacy and collect their medications.

The ETP program will deliver a service that will allow prescriptions generated by GPs (and other primary care prescribers) to be transferred electronically among prescriber, dispenser, and reimbursement agency. Patient medication records held within the NCRS will be populated by information from local prescribing and dispensing systems connected to the ETP service, integrating ETP with the NCRS.

Pilots have also been conducted to transmit prescriptions between GPs, community pharmacies, and the Prescription Pricing Authority.

New National Network for the NHS

The New National Network for the NHS (N3) will provide IT infrastructure, network services, and broadband connectivity to meet NHS needs now and into the future. It will link all NHS organizations in England, enabling data to be exchanged reliably and securely. N3 will provide continuity of service from the existing NHSnet and satisfy the current and future wide-area networking requirements of the NHS.

The N3 Service Provider (N3SP) acts as an integrator, responsible for integrating an end-to-end service from a number of subcontractors procured by them. The N3SP is responsible for bringing together the separate elements into a complete and seamless network. They will also provide the national services needed to manage the network smoothly, for example, fault reporting and customer relationship management. It is estimated that delivering N3 services in this way can save the NHS an estimated £900 million over 7 years, relative to current NHSnet contracts.

Implementation

NHS's timeline for implementing specific levels of functionality has been identified over the course of this program. Beginning with contracts that were awarded to the LSPs in December 2003, each patient in England is expected to have a single, integrated, electronic care record that can be accessible anywhere and at anytime by any authorized provider of healthcare services by 2010.

Regional clusters were formed after consultation with Strategic Health Authorities (SHAs) on how best to deliver the local IT solutions as part of NPfIT. England was then divided into five geographic regions—each cluster comprising five, six, or seven SHAs—who agreed to work together to take forward the procurement and implementation of National Programme services at the local level. Table 10-1 identifies how each cluster contains a number of SHAs in which trusts exist in several configurations, specifically, Hospital Trusts, Mental Health Trusts (sometimes combined with Social Services), Primary Care Trusts, and Ambulance Trusts.[34]

TABLE 10-1. Trust distribution by clusters in the UK

Cluster in England	SHAs	Population (Millions)	Hospital Trusts	Mental Health Trusts	Primary Care Trusts	Ambulance Trusts
London cluster	5	7.172	32	10	31	1
Eastern cluster	5	9.461	34	12	70	7
North East cluster	5	7.58	28	14	50	5
North West and West Midlands cluster	6	11.982	52	17	73	14
Southern cluster	7	12.838	44	19	81	12

Source: Care Record Service Program. ©NHS Information Authority; 2003.
Note: Community hospitals can be included with the structure of a Primary Care Trust so the actual number of hospitals is higher than those labeled Hospital Trusts.

During the procurement process, the approach for selecting suppliers to become the National Service Provider and LSPs was conducted as a single procurement. Most importantly, all the trusts sought an LSP that could deliver in the areas of change management, benefits realization, solution (capable of delivering on nationally identified requirements by functional area), training, deployment services, and partnership model with the LSP.

Change management is most significant because the entire program relating to the IT initiative has been prefaced as a "change program" that uses IT as its enabler. The strong and consistent message about change and the efforts to support a change-management framework within the NHS is the strength of this program. In this way, it is positioned to complement the approach that is most consistent with clinicians as well as with all associated healthcare professionals.

Another pivotal component to the success is the request for partnership within the scope of the NCRS program. It is clear to all who are observing this program manifest that it constitutes a scale and complexity that is singular. Clearly, it is critical that the selected NASP and LSPs forge a framework with partnerships, not only at the local trust level, but also extending through various other organizations that support the national program (e.g., SHAs, Care Communities, NPfIT, DoH, and Social Services).

The intention of the NCRS program was to identify those bundles of functionality that, over the course of the 7 years (through 2010), would provide specific functionality to be delivered at key points. The functionality releases correspond to targeted dates by which the NCRS program provides significant contributions to support the corresponding changes concurrently in progress, and at the same time, keeping the focus on quality, outcomes, improved access to care, and access to a consolidated view of patient records across care delivery areas.

Table 10-2 provides a concise overview of identified requirements needed to support the NCRS program and the fact that the central funding for an EHR solution would be confined to bundles 1 through 12 whereas bundles 14 through 21 would be available—but at the expense of the local trusts. A bundle was defined in the procurement process as a batch of defined functionality that enables components of the EHR. Since the procurement process began, PACS bundle 13 has been redefined as a core offering, and central funding for the acquisition of the PACS solution available by cluster was granted in November 2004.[35]

Expanded functionality is available across a number of calendar-based releases of functionality. A detailed mapping of functionality, defined in the NCRS program requirements, corresponds to each bundle for each point in the release schedule. It is anticipated that each trust will adopt a predefined series of bundles identified with program requirements at a given point in time. When this occurs, each trust will implement subsequent bundles in a specified sequence in order to achieve compliance standards established in the national program.

Table 10-2. Care Record Service Program: Functional requirements represented by bundle mapping

Funding: Centrally Funded			
Bundle 1	Bundle 2	Bundle 3	Bundle 4
Connectivity, messaging, and access to PSIS and Spine Directory and eBooking Messaging	ICRS setup and basic patient administration	Assessment and clinical documentation (including social care)	Clinical support requesting and order communication, Decision support and ePrescribing
Bundle 5	Bundle 6	Bundle 7	Bundle 8
Scheduling	Integrated care pathways and care planning	Maternity	Information for secondary purposes
Bundle 9	Bundle 10	Bundle 11	Bundle 12
Emergency/unscheduled care	Surgical interventions	Alternative options for GPs	Prevention, screening, surveillance (some elements are identified as additional)
Bundle 13			
PACS and medical imaging (in Nov. 2004 Bundle 13 was changed from trust funding to central funding)			
Funding: Trust Funded			
Bundle 14	Bundle 15	Bundle 16	Bundle 17
Pathology	Financial payments	Health	Document management (excluding tracking)
Bundle 18	Bundle 19	Bundle 20	Bundle 21
Dental	Ambulance	Radiology Information Systems (RIS)	Pharmacy stock control

Source: Department of Health, United Kingdom.

Accomplishments and Current Challenges

Accomplishments

Major accomplishments have included managing a rapid procurement process, implementing a change management program, establishing and promoting standards, and establishing a unique patient identifier.

Managed a rapid procurement process. The procurement process was completed within calendar year 2003. This is quite an accomplishment, not only because of the scope of the project, but also because it incorporates both a combined public sector as well as a broader healthcare initiative.

Implemented change management. The NCRS program has been framed within the context of a change management initiative in which an IT component enables achieving the national agenda for modernization of the NHS.

Established and promoted standards. Policy development guidelines are in place to promote and support, whenever possible, standards as they apply and relate to various aspects of the NCRS program.

Established a unique national patient identifier. As a cornerstone to any EHR project, the designation of a unique patient identifier is key to managing the record. Therefore, an NHS number is assigned to every citizen, with the intention of providing a uniquely singular identifier for every citizen so that when they are treated across various service areas, multiple records can be avoided.

Current Challenges

The challenges of the NCRS program include managing HCPs' expectations, responding to local fiscal pressures at the trust level for IT investment, managing the scale of program, handling the number of concurrent national healthcare changes, responding to the talent pool shortage, working within labor laws, responding to the pace of change, integrating care services, managing vendor market contraction, and handling geographic influences.

Managing HCPs' expectations. HCPs (including consultants, GPs, allied health professionals, etc.) are concerned about the implications of NCRS and how it may directly impact their ability to deliver patient care in a secure manner. HCPs' expectations are one of the critical elements to securing not only agreement to proceed in a patient care environment, but more importantly, to adopting the NCRS program to achieve the desired outcome of a shared EPR for all citizens.

Numerous vehicles have been used to ensure HCPs' participation in the NCRS program at the trust level. Communication vehicles are in use to inform HCPs of NCRS activities, such as forums for best practice, solution discussions and demonstrations, and trust's program governance committees. HCPs' champions have been sought out and this approach will continue to be advanced and supported to ensure a maximum amount of involvement and input.

Responding to local fiscal pressures at the trust level for IT investment. There are many fiscal pressures for investment at the local trust level. Invariably a great number of trusts are challenged to spend at significant investment levels for the numerous interrelated projects that will ultimately deliver an EHR. Some of the most significant financial pressures can be found within the mental health and primary care trusts. The NCRS program has received investment from the DoH, although not all costs related to the deployment of this program are directly funded. Trusts now must also allocate the appropriate level of funding as they plan for their deployment slots.

Responding to program issues. The sheer scale of the NCRS program and the various component pieces of solutions that can be deployed at a given point in time provide a great challenge in coordination of multiple, time-sensitive initiatives that must meet government compliance targets. Other related challenges are extent of coordination of activities, dependencies, multiple governance bodies, and impact on all healthcare professionals that are continuing to discharge their daily duties while working on a historic program.

Negotiating many concurrent national healthcare changes. Within a given trust, staff and the organization as a whole are challenged because they are involved with a multiple number of major projects at the same time including the Agenda for Change, Modernization Agenda, and the NCRS program.

Obtaining the talent to support the NCRS program. There are natural market pressures that have emerged given the internal demand for staffing for the NCRS program as well as the demand from the supplier market. The pressure on the talent pool relates to more than the sheer quantity of required staff; it also applies to types of skills to assign to various projects that are in progress.

In addition, some trusts that have attained success with previous initiatives rely on a core employee team that is strategically placed in work groups or on a given project. Given the multiple projects that are being undertaken in some trusts, employers often are unable to effectively leverage key individuals who have previously contributed to successful projects.

Working within labor law constraints. Given the extensiveness of the NCRS program and additional concurrent NHS initiatives, achieving the aggressive timetables for deploying trusts can be supported and implemented given the stringent labor laws in the country. Expecting participating NHS employees to work beyond a sanctioned workweek would not be consistent with current labor practices. Although trusts have hired additional staff to support the program, the demand for human resources continues to be greater than trusts can supply.

Managing the pace of change in a public sector environment. The rate of deployment of the NCRS program for the entire NHS is being conducted at a rapid pace. Such comprehensive change has no precedence in the public healthcare arena in the UK. Concurrent to the NCRS program are also initiatives including the Agenda for Change, a national payroll and human resources initiative, and the Modernization Agenda.

Establishing fully integrated care services. The council and borough level of government funds only some segments of the healthcare delivery model such as Social Services. At the same time, this care community interacts with other healthcare professionals across trusts and other government agencies; it also operates with Information, Communication, and Technology, which lie outside of the NCRS program. Therefore, when providing care to certain populations, it will be difficult to provide an integrated level of care across multiple agencies and all responsible parties.

Responding to vendor market contraction. Because a number of healthcare information systems' vendors will have products that are phased out in lieu of the NCRS program, the healthcare vendor marketplace is experiencing a rapid compression. Existing systems will be required to meet national standards including messaging to the National Data Repository. As a result, there is concern that compliance cannot be achieved to transmit required data to the Spine.

Managing geographical influences. Whereas four of the five clusters comprise large geographic areas, patients in London can easily receive services from multiple trusts locally. An interesting and relevant concept, The Care Community, has been advanced since the inception of the London program in 2004. The concept of Care Community transcends the organizational and fiscal boundaries at the trust level. It contains those trusts that serve a given population within London, with the intention of promoting, planning, and making decisions that coordinate activities related to the deployment of the NCRS program across trusts, and which are within that Care Community.

An excellent reference document is the Electronic Record Development and Implementation Programme, Lessons Learned, Benefits Topic, April 2003.[36]

Review of Major Lessons Learned from Three Leading Countries

Introduction

Peter Schloeffel, Chief Executive Officer, Ocean Informatics Pty. Ltd., Australia, has observed: "There is a long way to go but there are encouraging signs that stakeholders are beginning to recognize that the very future of health systems depends on more efficient and effective information management. The EHR is arguably the most important foundation component in this pursuit."[37]

Canada, Australia, and the UK are three countries with national EHR programs that have advanced full EHR programs to the stage of cross regional or provincial implementations. Through the review of the independent assessments of these programs and through collaboration by the coauthors, representing in country EHR executives and implementation vendor partners, we are able to begin drawing useful lessons. Based on these actual program experiences, our observations are intended to inform EHR program planners in other countries currently working on large-scale EHR initiatives.

Major Lessons

Based on our research and observations, eight issues address the major lessons learned to date on the journey to implement EHRs on a national scale. They include the following: Sustaining national funding and leadership, building and maintaining medical consumer and physician acceptance, developing broad stakeholder support, adoption of critical data standards, building an initial critical mass of users, achieving legal and regulatory agreement on privacy and consent issues, and creating customizable technical solutions.

Lesson #1. Recognize that national EHR programs are industry-wide transformations developing within the relatively immature healthcare IT environments. A key success factor is a critical mass and core leadership representing various levels in the healthcare industry to not only sponsor but also actively promote fundamental change industry wide.

When considering national efforts in EHRs, we believe an industry-wide perspective must be adopted within each country. Within an individual enterprise, the leadership structure is generally well defined and roles and responsibilities are largely understood. In an industry transformation, the situation is far more ambiguous and leaders emerge from different places. No one enterprise has control in an industry-wide transformation and it is a much more turbulent environment. For example, in Canada, during the start up of *Infoway*, knowledgeable, actively committed leaders could be identified at the Deputy Minister level, the Assistant Deputy Minister level, and CIO level within governments across the country. In addition, early leaders could be found across the healthcare delivery organizations, the associations, etc. Without that critical mass of committed and outspoken leaders, *Infoway* would not be progressing.

In industry transformations, a critical mass of committed and visible leaders who are ready, willing, and able to promote and actively work toward a new vision is one of the keys to success. The EHR programs of Canada, Australia, and England are different from other countries because, to varying degrees, the countries have critical mass and core leadership in place to drive an industry transformation.

Lesson #2. Building and maintaining genuine physician and clinician involvement in the political and implementation process is absolutely essential to program success.

Every business transformation requires the participation of the end user. They bring the subject matter expertise and requirements for IT enabling the enterprise. They will bring the insights on how the business process needs to be changed to optimally use these new systems. Finally, they need to be the key champions of change.

Lesson #3. Developing support from all stakeholders in the healthcare enterprise, i.e., national, regional, or provincial governments, institutional and private providers are a recognized success component. The active engagement and management of the vendor community is critical to the success of a national initiative, a factor that is overlooked in some countries.

Undertaking an initiative as complex as a regional or national EHR will touch many stakeholders. First, one has to understand how to segment the stakeholders and involve them in the right ways and at the right levels. Low influence/low impact stakeholders should at least be engaged from a communications perspective. Low influence/high impact stakeholders should be informed for understanding. High influence/low impact stakeholders should be engaged for response and input. And finally, high influence/high impact stakeholders have to commit to be involved, and be engaged for their expertise and decision-making authority. Once the stakeholders are segmented, an engagement plan should be developed. This plan covers who, when, and how to engage.

We suggest that both Canada and England have taken a very active role in developing a vendor management strategy taking into consideration the role of the private sector, opportunities to invest along with public entities, and building support for industry standards. By comparison, the issue of working with vendors has been raised in Australia but no comprehensive vendor management strategy has been developed to date.

Lesson #4. Adoption and adherence to data exchange standards must be achieved early in the program planning process so that interoperative systems can be embedded into the overall system technical architecture.

Jeff Goldsmith, David Blumenthal, and Wes Rishel offer this perspective: "The United States lags well behind other countries, notably Great Britain, Australia, and New Zealand, in the adoption of computerized clinical systems, especially in the outpatient area. All of these countries have a greater ability to standardize clinical data systems, because they have national health services or a single payer, and they have used their financial and administrative muscle to facilitate widespread use of some information technologies."[38]

Peter Schloeffel ably defined the issue when he stated, "Lack of interoperability between EHR systems has been a major barrier to EHR deployment but the emergence of the open EHR model, the HL7 Clinical Document Architecture, and archetypes has provided a significant stimulus to the development of interoperability and other necessary EHR standards within major international standards organizations."[39] *Infoway's* approach in Canada shows the importance of standards that are endorsed on a pan-Canadian basis. *Infoway* has put in place a set of committees to collaborate on the complete standards development lifecycle, especially on business requirements with the users of the system using the standards. The objective is to develop standards that are adopted on a pan-Canadian basis. A core project team works on the standard (i.e., business analysts, clinicians, standards experts). The work is vetted by a cross-functional team of experts made up of clinicians, representatives of the various jurisdictions and governmental organizations, which must adopt the standard, and vendors. The work is endorsed by an advisory committee that looks across all the standards work *Infoway* sponsors. Ultimately, the work is approved by a steering committee.

Lesson #5. Developing initial momentum among stakeholders is essential for building a critical mass of medical consumer and healthcare provider users of the system.

Each country or health delivery region/organization must do its own analysis to determine what is best and most appropriate. First, it must establish the drivers and objectives of an investment. Second, analysis of the gaps in IT solutions to meet those must be determined. For example, if patient safety is a primary concern, it might invest in a system to manage patient medication history, physician order entry of medications, and decision support logic to check for adverse drug events. If efficiency and elimination of duplicate testing are objectives, it might invest in the electronic reporting and access to laboratory test results. Given this, the country or organization must also look at critical success factors related to those investments. For example, relevant to the two examples just given, if physicians in ambulatory practice do not have basic network access and computer systems in their office, then those capabilities will be impossible to deliver.

Lesson #6. Achievement of national legal and regulatory agreement on privacy and consent issues of electronic records is an essential enabling component of national programs.

Many believe that an electronic system of health records can be made more secure and private than the existing world of paper. That capability is enabled by privacy-enhancing technologies that are commercially available today. But those technologies can only be applied when there is clear understanding of the system requirements. Those requirements must be driven by policy and legislation, and, conversely, those requirements must be informed by what is doable and practical from an IT perspective. Debate in various countries continues on issues such as masking data for patient confidentiality and unique person identifiers to link the various systems that are sources of clinical data. There are no easy answers to these questions. Privacy concerns are critical, because these must be balanced in applying privacy-enhancing technologies impacting cost, system performance and scalability, system and data integrity, and system maintenance and administration.

Lesson #7. Substantial efforts must be applied to stakeholder communication to ensure successful participation and continued financial support for the program.

Publicly funded national programs are subject to significant public scrutiny and operate in highly political environments, often dealing with many jurisdictional stakeholders. It is critical to consistently demonstrate and communicate concrete progress and highlight the successes of jurisdictional and other key partners. Working with champions—successful EHR implementers, users or other supporters—by providing them with tools and information to share with their own communities has proven useful in building momentum and support.

Each country or health delivery region/organization should develop a communication and knowledge sharing approach adapted to the needs of different stakeholder groups. This can range from a corporate Web site and newsletter for broad groups to a password-protected site, online forum, and workshops for groups who need to be engaged more closely. The most influential stakeholders should be treated with particular care. For example, Canada's *Infoway* has created a Partnerships and Alliances group with regional representatives responsible for negotiations and regular, personal contact with key government and healthcare provider association stakeholders.

An overarching corporate communications plan should be developed and endorsed by the board of directors and management team. The plan's guiding principles and key messages should be reflected in the various communications strategies developed for specific programs and projects. The corporate plan should include a comprehensive issues management strategy to deal with privacy issues, risk of technology failure, and other sensitive matters.

Internal communications and knowledge sharing should not be neglected. Communicating business strategies, new developments, and lessons learned across the organization can help teams become more effective. Providing internal teams with key messages and question and answer documents can help ensure accurate and consistent messages.

Lesson #8. IT investment and deployment strategies and programs must be customizable. Each healthcare sector and the various healthcare delivery regions/organizations may be at a different point in their use of IT. Thus, the EHR investment programs must recognize those differences.

In most countries, IT has been deployed with great disparity across healthcare delivery settings. Acute care settings have for many years deployed clinical information systems, whereas primary care and ambulatory clinic settings have no semblance of IT. In countries such as Canada where health care is a provincial/territorial responsibility, there is significant contrast between the stated importance of healthcare IT and the corresponding investment allocation. As a state/province/territory/nation embarks on an EHR initiative, it must analyze the current use of IT, and then develop the desired future state. The future state systems deployment models and investment programs should respect the healthcare delivery organizational model(s) and processes; policy and legislation (particularly privacy); patterns of use by patients as well as referral patterns of providers (which ultimately affects data flow); custodianship of systems and data; an incremental approach to systems design and deployment (often constrained by the availability of financial and human capital, change management, and adoption); systems deployment, maintenance, and operations cost (leveraging economies of scale); and the performance and scalability of the solution.

Conclusion

In the article "Accelerating US EHR Adoption: How to Get There from Here," Blackford Middleton and coauthors have stated, "There is growing support for the widespread adoption of EHR as a fundamental strategy to improve US healthcare delivery, efficiency, quality, and safety. Despite considerable evidence to support adoption of EHR, progress has been slow to date. We suggest that the current HIT marketplace has difficulty due to several factors, including misalignment of financial incentives, absence of a clear business case for EHR adoption and for interoperability between EHR implementations, and incomplete specification and adoption of relevant standards."[40]

Appendix

United Kingdom Selected Program Bibliography

1. A First Class Service: Quality Care in the NHS. Department of Health; 1998.
2. Gillies AC. Computers and the NHS: an analysis of their contribution to the past present and future delivery of the national health service. J Inform Technol 1998;13(8).
3. Computers in the Consultation. The UK Experience Hayes, G SCAMC 1993:103–106. Accessed November 30, 2005.
4. Delivering 21st Century IT Support for the NHS. Department of Health; 2002.
5. Department of Health: The New NHS—Modern, Dependable, HMSO, Cmnd 3807; 1997.
6. Shaw NT, Gillies AC. Going Paperless. Abingdon: Radcliffe Medical Press; 2001.
7. Good Practice Guidelines for General Practice Electronic Patient Records. Version 3. General Practitioners Committee (GPC), Department of Health and Royal College of General Practitioners; 2003.
8. Roberts J. Health information systems—the same the world over? International Hospital Federation (50th Anniversary Issue); 1997.
9. Improvement, Expansion and Reform: The Next Three Years, Priorities and Planning Framework 2003–2006. Department of Health; 2002.
10. Roberts J, Szczepura A, Bickerstaffe D, Fagan R. Informatics—an enabler of health and social care interworking. HC2003 Proceedings, March 2003.
11. Information for Health—An Information Strategy for the Modern NHS 1998–2005, NHS Executive; 1998. Accessed November 30, 2005.
12. Information for Social Care—A Framework for Improving Quality in Social Care Through Better Use of Information and Information Technology. Department of Health; 2001.

13. Investing in General Practice: The New General Medical Services Contract. Department of Health; 2003.

14. Wanless D. Long Term Review of Health Trends. HM-Treasury; 2002.

15. National Programme for IT. www.dh.gov.uk/npfit.

16. Shekelle P. New contract for general practitioners. Br Med J 2003;326(7387):457. Accessed November 30, 2005.

17. Rogers RT. New initiatives in England to improve clinical practice through information. Infocus Proc 2000.

18. NHS plan: a plan for investment, a plan for reform. Department of Health; 2000.

19. NHS plan: building the information core. 2000.

20. NHS plan for England Department of Health. 2000.

21. Protti D. Proposal to use a balanced scorecard to evaluate information for health: an information strategy for the modern NHS (1998–2005). Comput Biol Med 2002;32(3):221–236.

22. Radical steps in health informatics: a think tank consultation, British Computer Society Health Informatics Committee (2002, 2003, 2004). www.bcshic.org. Accessed November 30, 2005.

23. Report on the Review of Patient-Identifiable Information. Caldicott Committee, Department of Health; 1997. Accessed November 30, 2005.

24. Gillies AC. Risk management issues associated with the introduction of EHRs in primary care. ePHI, 1,1 (2001).

25. Wanless D. Securing good health for the whole population: population health trends. 2003.

26. Wanless D. Securing our future health: taking a long-term view. 2002.

27. Shifting the Balance of Power: The Next Steps. Department of Health; 2002.

28. Shifting the Balance of Power. Department of Health; 2001.

29. The Health of the Nation. Department of Health; 1992.

30. Roberts JM, Hayes G. Validating national informatics policy—the importance of operational consensus to influence positive developments. IMIA MedInfo 2004 Proceedings. IOS Press; September 2004.

References

1. Ball M. International Approaches to the Electronic Health Record. CHIK Services Pty. Ltd. and Healthlink Inc.; January 2003.

2. Schloeffel P. Ocean Informatics Pty. Ltd., St. Peters; 2004.

3. Canada Health Act, 1984, c. 6, s. 1. http://laws.justice.gc.ca/en/C-6/index.html. Accessed June 23, 2005.

4. Noseworthy TW. In: Wieners W, ed. Global Health Care Markets: A Comprehensive Guide to Regions, Trends, and Opportunities Shaping the International Health Arena. San Francisco: Jossey-Bass, A Wiley Company; 2000:367–381.

5. Fyke KJ. Fyke Commission. Caring for Medicare: Sustaining a Quality System. Saskatchewan: Commission on Medicare; April 30, 2001.

6. Building Momentum: 2003/04 Business Plan. Montreal: Canada Health Infoway, Inc.; 2003.

7. Final Report: Building on Values—The Future of Health Care in Canada. Quebec City: Commission on the Future of Health Care in Canada; November 2002.

8. Electronic Health Record Blueprint Solution Architecture. Version 1.0. Canada Health Infoway, Inc.; July 31, 2003.

9. Personal Information Protection and Electronic Document Act (PIPEDA). Office of the Privacy Commissioner of Canada; April 13, 2000.
10. Privacy Impact Assessment Policy, May 2, 2002. http://www.tbs-sct.gc.ca/pubs_pol/ciopubs/pia-pefr/paip-pefr_e.asp. Accessed June 23, 2005.
11. http:// www.abs.gov.au. Accessed June 23, 2005.
12. Australia's Health 2004. Canberra: Australian Institute of Health and Welfare; 2004.
13. Australian Health and Ageing System: The Concise Factbook. Canberra: Commonwealth of Australia; August 2004.
14. Health and Aged Care in Australia. Canberra: Commonwealth of Australia; 1999.
15. Health and Aged Care in Australia. Canberra: Commonwealth of Australia; 1999.
16. Australian Government Department of Health and Ageing. http://www.health.gov.au/internet/wcms/publishing.nsf/Content/health-pbs-general-aboutus.htm-copy2. Accessed June 23, 2005.
17. Health Financing Series. Health Financing in Australia: The Objectives and Players. Vol 1. Canberra: Commonwealth of Australia; 1999.
18. Health Financing Series. Health Financing in Australia: The Objectives and Players. Vol 1. Canberra: Commonwealth of Australia; 1999.
19. Australian Institute of Health and Welfare. Australia's Health 2004. Canberra; 2004.
20. National Health Information Management and Information & Communication Technology Strategy. National Health Information Group and the Australian Health Information Council; April 2004.
21. A Health Information Network for Australia. Canberra: Commonwealth of Australia; July 2000.
22. HealthConnect trial documents can be accessed at http://www.healthconnect.gov.au/trials/index.htm. Accessed June 23, 2005.
23. Further information on NeHTA can be found at http://www.ahic.org.au/nehta/index.html. Accessed June 23, 2005.
24. HealthConnect Interim Research Report. Canberra: Commonwealth of Australia; August 2003.
25. HealthConnect Interim Research Report. Canberra: Commonwealth of Australia; August 2003.
26. HealthConnect Benefits Realization Framework. Version 1.0. Canberra: Commonwealth of Australia; October 2004.
27. Implementation Approach, Final Version. Canberra: Commonwealth of Australia; December 2004.
28. The HealthConnect Indicative Benefits Report. Canberra: Commonwealth of Australia; February 2004.
29. HealthConnect Business Architecture. Version 1.9. Canberra: Commonwealth of Australia; November 2004.
30. HealthConnect Business Architecture. Version 1.9. Canberra: Commonwealth of Australia; November 2004.
31. HealthConnect Business Architecture. Version 1.9. Canberra: Commonwealth of Australia; November 2004.
32. Duffy DA. United Kingdom. In: Wieners W, ed. Global Health Care Markets: A Comprehensive Guide to Regions, Trends, and Opportunities Shaping the

International Health Arena. San Francisco: Jossey-Bass, A Wiley Company; 2000:173–180.

33. Reforming NHS Financial Flows: Introducing Payment by Results. United Kingdom: Department of Health; October 2002.

34. Trust Distribution by Clusters in England, Care Record Service Program, Department of Health. United Kingdom: NHS Information Authority; 2003.

35. Care Record Service Program: Functional Requirements Represented by Bundle Mapping, Department of Health. United Kingdom: NHS Information Authority.

36. Electronic Record Development and Implementation Programme, Lessons Learned, Benefits Topic, Final Version. Birmingham: NHS Information Authority, NHSIA; April 11, 2003, p 1–20.

37. Schloeffel P. Informatics Pty. Ltd., St. Peters; 2004.

38. Goldsmith J, Blumenthal D, Rishel W. Federal health information policy: a case of arrested development. Health Affairs 2003;22(455).

39. Schloeffel P. Ocean Informatics Pty. Ltd., St. Peters; 2004.

40. Middleton B, Hammond W, Brennan P, Cooper G. Accelerating US EHR adoption: how to get there from here. J Am Med Inform Assoc 2005;12(1):13–19.

Section 3
Technology Infrastructure

11
Databases in Health Care

ALAN COLTRI

The heart of a modern information environment is the set of databases where data are stored and where data relationships are established. Databases in health care have generally followed the same evolutionary pattern as the use of databases in other industries. What marks health care as different is the enormous complexity of health data and the healthcare business model. The complexity of clinical data is driven by the highly detailed and different data needs of diverse care environments: inpatient, outpatient, specialist, intensive care, surgery, etc. With all the different activities in different areas, the modern hospital is in some ways more like a city than a corporation. All this complexity must be woven together. Government and consumers are demanding that order be brought about through the rationalization of healthcare information systems and processes.[1] Yet such rationalization must confront tensions that will change the way the next generation of healthcare information systems is constructed.

Conflicting Demands

This section is organized on the basis of some of these forces:

- Tension between the consolidation and independence of databases
- Desire for cross-institution, patient-based, data access
- Demands for more sophisticated data management
- Increasing expectations of users and regulators
- Horizontal versus vertical functional organization of data
- Transactions that help the user, push versus pull

This chapter was written from the perspective of a builder and integrator of healthcare information systems. Over the last 15 years, the author has been engaged in designing and supporting the clinical information systems of Johns Hopkins Medicine. He began as a project leader, selecting an early "provider order entry" system, then moved on to the installation of the first Health Level-7 (HL7) interfaces. These interfaces have delivered 1.5 billion

HL7 messages to dozens of vendor and homegrown systems. The author also spearheaded the consolidation of several legacy systems into Johns Hopkins' first "electronic patient record." Now Chief Systems Architect for Johns Hopkins Medicine, he is daily involved in the selection of information systems for various parts of the enterprise and in their integration into a coherent whole. This role has given him the opportunity to examine systems from the largest healthcare information system vendors down to the two-person "garage" operation, and from complete "Hospital Information Systems" down to systems designed to support a single sub-sub-specialty.

Tension Between Consolidation and Independence of Databases

The range of data held within the databases of a healthcare setting is both vast and constantly expanding. Classically, healthcare data were held in silos defined by function, such as laboratory management, pharmacy management, radiology management and imaging, third party insurance and billing, materials management, and patient admission/registration. In each case, the resulting database and associated applications needed to handle substantial data complexity, but most of the complexity was only relevant to the system operators, not their customers. A small subset of the total data was sufficient to link the functional silo with the rest of the organization. For example, a laboratory management system may keep track of the machine, reagents, and operator responsible for each analysis, whereas the orderer of the test only wants to know the end result. From a purely pragmatic perspective, this division into functional silos permitted the problem of designing and building database systems to be tackled in manageable units.

It is obvious that these silos have considerable data in common, such as the patient's identity, the care providers, and the service locations. Subsets of data must be shared as part of "cross-silo" transactions: an order communication system may generate an order for a laboratory test, the laboratory will perform and result the test, and a billing system will charge for it. Today's systems are generally constructed to be capable of independent operation (a necessary attribute for commercial offerings) with HL7 messages asynchronously transporting common information between the various silos where it is redundantly stored.

There are a number of responses to this problem of redundant storage. The first is the single-database model: "If we just used one database for everything," then things (coordination, operations, reporting) would become much simpler. Indeed, very powerful systems such as the Brigham Integrated Computing System (BICS) of Brigham and Women's Hospital, and very popular commercial systems, such as MEDITECH, have been built on this premise.

There are challenges with this solution. The single database must handle all the complexity found in all business functions. The database becomes very large and complex in an attempt to deal with the internal processes of each of its functional areas. Dealing with this level of complexity presents a huge challenge to system developers. Inevitably with these single-database systems, the depth of detail (functional features) within each domain has fallen behind the functionality available from the competing, domain focused, vendors.

The need to change design as business needs and technology change places another limit on the single-database solution. As systems evolve to include hundreds of tables and millions of lines of code, the design becomes stressed. Hundreds or even thousands of intricate functional relationships find their way into the systems, each solving some specific problem or satisfying some very specific need. The existence of these linkages and their proper operation must be preserved from software version to version. This preservation need creates a situation in which it is difficult to "restructure" existing functionality in any fundamental way. In the single-database solution, these restructurings can become traumatic.

In a federated database model, data continue to reside in multiple, domain-oriented, databases. But unlike in the traditional "silo" databases, the federated databases are logically interconnected and accessible, in combination, from multiple applications. In this case, integration is achieved, not by copying data between silos via HL7 message interfaces, but by using applications that directly access the data storage of multiple silos. Another integration architecture, evolving via the Internet, is called the Service Oriented Architecture (SOA). Generically an SOA is a form of distributed computing in which work is broken up into relatively independent, but communicating pieces. In this architecture, the various domain-oriented silos would "publish" services (useful chunks of business functionality) for other applications to incorporate and use.[2] Most SOAs are based on the World Wide Web and its standards are set by the World Wide Web consortium.

The vendor's business case for a single- or silo-based solution is clear. It is less clear that applications can be sold when built on other architectural models, because they require close cooperation among vendors, or embody "plug and play" levels of compatibility with as yet nonexistent standards (which is the current state of SOA in health care). The performance of the existing database engines in flexibly combining and manipulating data is greatest within the bounds of the single-database engine. Technology for ultra-large, distributed databases will enable alternative design strategies.

Desire for Cross-Institution Aggregation

That a patient may be receiving services from multiple healthcare businesses is well recognized but rarely addressed through real data sharing on a clinical level. The pressures for data sharing are driven both by a belief that better health care can be provided by clinicians who see more complete medical histories of their patients, and by the belief that health care can be delivered more efficiently when the medical history is fully available. This section is concerned with database issues in making this data sharing possible.

What was said in the previous edition of this book remains true: "We should begin by identifying a form of common patient identification, together with a record of what systems and databases have information about a patient. Initial transfer of information should then take place in a predominantly textural fashion while the necessary standards and data item definitions are developed to permit utilization of structured data and implementation of the proposed architecture."[3]

From consensus and from responses to the Office of the National Coordinator for Healthcare Information Technology,[4] it seems clear that data storage will remain the responsibility of the healthcare provider who collected (or produced) the information, and that the data will need to be made available to others when needed.

The ability to transfer data will depend on standards discussed in Chapter 12. The adoption of standards is especially slow when they must be defined with sufficient precision to provide a "plug and play" capability. Adoption of standards, in turn, will drive a series of revisions to currently deployed products. There will be many instances in which simple mapping of data elements will be unable to bridge the gap between applications, and instances in which the original data collection application will not be adequate for the job, having been designed with different core business logic, or using an incompatible terminology system.

Ever-increasing Demands for Data Management

The amount of data that is processed within the healthcare setting is constantly expanding. Consider the history of fetal ultrasound. Initially, doctors recorded short text of their interpretation of what they heard in auscultating the pregnant abdomen. With the fetal ultrasound, physicians recorded longer text of what they saw. Later, they pasted still pictures from the recording into the chart, which led to measurements made and stored (i.e., more text). Today, it is quite feasible to make digital video recordings of entire procedures. Storage, then, progressed from requiring 1 KB to requiring 100 MB, 5 order of magnitude. Multiply this by the number of observational and imaging technologies increasingly available—and including genomic data—and the complexity of an electronic health record (EHR) becomes truly daunting, in an environment that produces millions of documents per year, in dozens of specialty areas, and where the documents must remain readable for decades. The content used to compose the document is likely to be stored in multiple databases. But once the data are combined into a document, the document then must itself be managed as a coherent unit. The boundaries of the medical record are expanding rapidly.

The deceptively simple mechanisms of the Web for addressing, hyper linking, and markup have allowed an enormous system of interlinked information to evolve without detailed planning of the content links. But there are important differences between the Web and patient care. In general, the information on the Web is made available to anyone who wants it (not true in patient care); it is transmitted with display-oriented markup (HTML) but not with content-oriented markup (which is needed in the classical transaction-based model of clinical care); and is found by fuzzy searches and ad hoc selection (which provide a rich selection of things you might want, but not a definitive list of anything). This last item is the most striking difference—clinical systems are expected to be complete. A list of progress notes for an inpatient encounter is expected to include all the notes, in sequence. Anything less makes the system untrustworthy.

Expectations of Users and Regulators (and Patients)

Core expectations concern confidentiality, patients' access to their records, and the providers' need for rapid, targeted access to complete data. Databases will need to tailor what they provide based on both the role of the requester and the requester's current context.

Databases as the repositories of the data, and applications as channels for the appropriate distribution of data, both have major roles in meeting these expectations. There will be expanded needs for automated auditing of system access, expanded use of encrypted transmission and storage of data, increasingly powerful and flexible authentication, and authorization systems.

Horizontal Versus Vertical Organization of Data and Function

We now see specialty systems for Gastroenterology, Pulmonology, Cardiology, Oncology, Obstetrics, Emergency Medicine, and many specialties and care settings, beyond the old, enterprise-wide, but functionally specific systems, such as laboratory and pharmacy. To the users of these new systems they are wonderful—tailored to their specific practice needs and providing full services: Scheduling, registration, data collection, machine/modality interfaces, automated documentation and billing, referring physician communications, etc.

But, what happens at the intersection between these vertical systems and the horizontal systems of the enterprise? For example, when the person using the Emergency Department System wants to order a laboratory test or a medication, is the order management system involved? Or does the

Emergency Department System have its own application for generating orders? Does the Emergency Department System have the same knowledge of patient allergies as other systems? Does it independently perform drug allergy checking, which in other contexts would be provided by the order communication system?

The tension between central services (horizontals) and specialty "all-in-one" systems is increasing. Some new model is required that allows the specialty user to see a system designed for them—full functionality, easy navigation; exactly what they need. At the same time, this new model needs to treat the underlying services as consistent enterprise-wide functions: If someone is ordering a medication, it should be checked against the known patient history no matter what specialty application the user is operating from. If someone is placing an order, it should be known to the order management systems so that all orders are available in common context and can be checked for duplication and conflict.

SOA may provide some help in this new model. Flexible aggregations of user interface components may help as well.

Transactions that Help the User, Pull Versus Push

The huge increase in scope of data collected as part of a medical record has not been accompanied by increases in the amount of time clinicians have available to review the record. In the early days, before the 1980s, systems were designed around performing (or recording) transactions, exhibiting their billing-system ancestry. Even as the application suites expanded to include clinical transactions (patient orders, medication administration, flow sheets), the primary mode of nontransactional use of the electronic record was browsing. Applications presented the user with an interface that allowed them to wander about in the record assimilating information. Such a user interface is a "pull" system—the user initiates the search, and draws the data to themselves. To make pulling easier or more effective, applications have attempted to anticipate what the user will want to see and to present it. These attempts usually presume that the user will engage the computer periodically, providing the system with the opportunity to show some selected data to the user.

There are occasions when important data become available while the person who needs to know is not engaged with the computer (or is engaged looking at something else). In these cases, the information system may be designed to force or "push" the data upon the user. What kind of "push" best gets the user's attention? The initially simple approach of "highlight the data new to the current user" requires the user to be engaged with a computer system. If they are offline, will the system generate a "page," or an e-mail, or a phone call, or all of these?

The solution to these design questions will place enormous demands on the databases, for they will not only need to expose a transaction history, and parrot back documents, but will also need to store and process sufficient contextual data to guide the data presentation. This contextual data might need to include "who has seen each element of data previously," "how long ago," "which result types are most relevant for which diagnoses," "what data are most used by which medical specialty," "what result ranges are normal— for this specific patient at this time and under these circumstances."

Beyond this intelligent presentation lies the issue of decision support and automated alerts. To what degree should the computers be attempting to detect patterns or events, and who should they tell about them? And, what data are needed to make these decisions?

Historical Perspective

Throughout the history of computing there has been a powerful connection between the way data were stored and the types of applications that could be built using the data. A look back at this connection between data storage technology and the ability to construct data-oriented applications may give some insight on how database technology and usage will evolve in health care.

File Systems and the Emergence of Database Engines

Before 1960, data management meant record processing. In the simplest sense, data existed in a list (of library book check outs, of bank deposits, of social security enrollees) and programs would run through the list, "processing" the data. The processing might include filtering (only acting on certain records), sorting (rearranging the sequence of records), calculation, or copying selected records. Complex tasks could be performed in a series of processing steps, with each step in its turn acting upon one or more lists. In application systems that were built this way, the meaning of the data in the records is dependent entirely on the processing applications. These multipass, sequential operations were consistent with the storage mechanisms of the day, which featured tape as the primary medium, not disk drives, and were referred to as Sequential Access Method (SAM) applications.

As systems evolved, disk drives became widely available, and with them came the ability to access data randomly based on indexes called ISAM (Indexed Sequential Access Method) and later VSAM (Virtual Storage Access Method, 1974). If the "index" of a record was known, the file need not be read sequentially from the beginning. One could skip ahead to the disk location where the desired record would be found. In consumer electronics, a similar evolution occurred during the conversion from the use of tapes and vinyl records (which are both sequential access devices) to CDs, which are indexed sequential devices. It was not practical to play the songs on a cassette or vinyl record in any order except the one in which they were recorded.

With this ability to reach into a list (a dataset) and pluck out an individual record came a new set of capabilities. Each record had a key. If one knew the key, one could get the record without reading the entire dataset from the beginning. So we made the keys meaningful, for instance a medical record number plus an encounter date.

In all these cases, the actual content of the record was defined implicitly by the applications that wrote the records. A program reading the record would have no knowledge that positions 10 through 20 of the record contained a person's last name and positions 21 through 24 contained their birth year. In fact, there would be no enforcement, within the storage system, of columns 21–24 even needing to be numeric. Enforcement of the data locations and data types occurred at the application level, often through the use of common "record maps" imported into each module of application code. Many a mess has occurred when one of the programs operating upon a dataset has had a different opinion about the positions of the fields, or the type of data to be recorded.

Because the arrangement of the contents of a record was simply a gentleman's agreement among the application programs, complex forms evolved, limited only by the imagination of programmers, in which different types of records could be packaged in a single dataset. An early medical record might have as the first two fields of a dataset a patient identifier and a record type. The value of the record type (demographics, encounter, laboratory result, etc.) would be used to determine the layout of the remainder of the record. The record has a simple hierarchical data structure.

The relationship between storage architecture and performance was dramatic. On-computer Random Access Memory (RAM) was expensive, so most data were held on disk. Keeping the system efficient meant minimizing the number of times the head of a disk drive needed to move to access a patient's data. If all accesses were clustered together on the disk, and could be read at one pass, performance would be acceptable. This simple fact led file-based hierarchical systems to organize the physical storage of their data to correspond with the access pattern that was anticipated to be the most likely.

Perhaps the best known example of a hierarchical-storage system is MUMPS (MGH Utility Multi-Programming System), also known as M, which was developed in the 1960s, and although now an aging technology, continues to be widely used in health care, particularly in the federal sector.[5,6]

MUMPS is a high-level procedural programming language with distant roots in the language JOSS, and was designed for interactive computing applications with emphasis on text-string processing, and on building and managing highly dynamic hierarchical databases. The MUMPS data storage mechanism is the "global"—a persistent, sparse, dynamic, multidimensional array with string subscripts and string data values. All manipulations of globals are performed by MUMPS application code, with no implicit separation between the application and database layers.

Applications of the 1980s (typically mainframe, Unix, or VAX) evolved as complex sets of operating system files, with all data management being handled by custom-written application code. Changes to an application and its related datasets involved substantial analysis and code changes because of the low-level access programming. Issues such as concurrent access, and transaction integrity were also handled by application code, and functions such as reporting and query operations also required that individuals write applications, or use file-oriented utilities.

Into this scene of datasets and programmers, the database engines appeared, which changed the landscape by providing an application layer (the database engine) which was responsible for core data management functionality. This functionality could then be used by application programmers to produce far more robust and complex applications.

Emergence of Relational Databases

In the 1970s, theoreticians developed the concepts underlying the now ubiquitous relational database. These were famously summarized in several articles by E.F. Codd for *Computer World* in 1985, where he stated a set of 12 rules for the behavior of relational databases.[7]

Essentially, Codd's rules for relational databases define a method of organizing data based on the attributes and relationships found within the data itself; a mathematically precise query and data manipulation language that expressed all allowable operations; and a guaranteed set of underlying services that assured data integrity. These elements are deeply connected. Despite the limitations of the "real database products," these rules have formed the core of database thinking and development for many years.

In the relational model, all data are stored in tables, two-dimensional structures with rows and columns. The definition of the tables, and relationships among tables, is intended to reflect the real world from which the data are obtained, at a level of complexity appropriate to the purpose of the database. Consider a simple data element, "last name." A database whose purpose can be achieved by recording only the current "last name" of a person will likely have a table where a row represents an instance of a "person" with each of the attributes of a person, across people, forming a column (in this case, a column, "last name," in the table "person"). If the database needs to record changes in "last name" over time, it would need additional tables and fields to handle these facts. Similarly, databases that must record multiple name aliases for a person will need yet another structure.

It is the structure of the database, the set of tables and columns created for a specific application, that defines the data and data relationships that can be recorded. The definition of tables, columns, and relationships is called the database schema. And what can be recorded is, almost always, a simplified model of the data existing in the real world. "Schema change," during a database upgrade, means that the structure of the database, the arrangement of its tables and their fields, is being changed in order to allow it to record some new information, or some additional complexity, which was not previously encompassed by the database's structure.

Relational Appeal

The appeal of the relational database model, and the database engines based on it, stems from a synergistic combination of capabilities that are explored in the following sections.

Structured Query Language

An ANSI (American National Standards Institute) standard, Structured Query Language (SQL), is essentially a language for accessing and modifying data that are organized according to the relational model. The language uses the core concepts of the relational model in its operations. All operations within the SQL are used to select and act upon sets of records. It may be that the "set" has been so narrowly identified that it only contains one row, or maybe no rows at all, but it is still a set. The entire language is actually a collection of mathematically precise "set" operators, such as union, intersection, subset. Whereas the language is used to specify the set of records and the action desired by the user, it provides no (standard) mechanism for the user to tell the database how to accomplish its objective. The optimization process of translating the request into a specific series of actions is left entirely to the database engine.

Transaction Integrity

Database engines (applications such as Oracle, DB2, SQL Server), which provide database functionality, evolved into powerful pieces of software whose jobs were to protect and preserve data. To this end, they provided many services, related to their primary function of data storage, which were completely invisible to casual users. These services allowed programmers to use the database with the assurance that "things will (automatically) work the way they are supposed to." Core among these functional attributes are the ACID properties.[8] This term refers to four properties of transaction behavior in databases and are summarized below.

Atomicity—the "all or none" rule. A transaction that involves changes to multiple pieces of data will either successfully change all the items, or will fail, and not change any of them. This prevents the partial-change problem—for example, saving an "order" without saving all the "line items" of the order.

Consistency—the data integrity rule. The properties and relationships of the data in the tables and columns of the database cannot ever be left in an illegal state. For example, if a database is defined such that a particular value (think of a medical record number) must be unique within a table, then no combination of operations can ever leave the database in a state in which the value is not unique.

Isolation—the independence rule. This rule states that each transaction is executed as if it were completely independent of all other transactions. In multiuser systems, it is always possible for different users simultaneously to request conflicting changes. Isolation essentially "serializes" the requests—one transaction will execute first and complete its changes with complete consistency, then the other will attempt to execute. If for some reason this serialization cannot be accomplished, it is considered a serious database error called a "deadlock."

Durability—once a transaction has been processed the changes are permanent within the database.

With a relational database, the programmer can easily achieve high-integrity transactions with very little direct effort. Storing a complex data object becomes relatively simple. For example, a data object that includes rows in four tables, and where each of the tables has two indexes, requires a "writing" data in 12 logical locations (four tables and the corresponding eight indexes). Doing this with file system storage, presuming ACID properties, would take great skill and a great deal of work. Within a database engine, this collection of actions is simply declared to be a logical transaction—and the ACID properties will automatically be enforced by the database engine.

System Administration

In addition to transactional attributes, the relational databases also provide a number of system-level data management features such as backup and recovery machinery, transaction journals that allow "point-in-time" recovery, data replication, user authentication, data access authorization, performance monitoring, system auditing, and system health monitoring.

These database administration functions are, for the most part, hardware platform and operating system independent. They represent another area in which the delivery of high-end system services allow applications to be developed with very powerful data management capabilities at virtually no cost in custom development.

Schema Modeling

One of the extraordinary attributes of relational databases is that one can intelligently discuss the "correctness" of a data structure or schema. During relational database design, one can transform the knowledge of a domain expert into a data structure and argue that the structure is "correct"—that all the objects and their relationships are defined, and organized in a way that satisfies the objectives of relational modeling, and which represents a functionally correct model of a real world data domain. This type of modeling is generally called Entity-Relationship (ER) Modeling and was originally proposed by Peter Pin-Shan Chen in 1976. This was truly the new world—structures that were objectively "correct," and whose definition was safely ensconced within the database itself as a byproduct of the act of creating the structures.[9]

In the database, the schema is itself stored as data. Sometimes called "meta-data," or data about the data, it is usually stored in a special set of tables, called catalog tables, which store the definitions of all the tables, the columns in the tables, the attributes of the columns, and the relationships between the tables. Unfortunately, the structure of these catalog tables varies among the various database engines, requiring specific knowledge to use the meta-data. A common method of accessing the meta-data eventually was developed and will be described next.

Tools

Construction of a database application requires many functions to be performed, and tools have grown up around them. These tools are generally not proprietary to any one database vendor, and encompass a broad range of tool types, including programming language connectors, data modeling tools, reporting tools, and query interfaces. These tools all benefit from the expression of the structure of the database as just another set of data. This "self-documentation" provided by the meta-data allows the tools to tailor their behavior uniquely to each database instance.

Programming interfaces and database catalogs were nonstandard. In the early days, each database vendor supplied software modules called "drivers" which provided an access path between various programming languages and the database. Similarly, the database catalog tables were not standard in their structures. These two proprietary factors forced developers to construct applications with a specific target database in mind.

The programming interface and database catalog problem was effectively solved by Microsoft with the development of an Open Data Base Connectivity (ODBC) driver. ODBC was initially released in 1992 and was based on a Call Level Interface specification developed by the SQL Access Group. A major revision occurred in 1994.[10] ODBC drivers are now available in many forms and from many vendors, and essentially allow applications to be written to a vendor-neutral database interface. This approach was also adopted by Sun for the Java community, which built upon the ODBC standard, and produced the Java Data Base Connectivity (JDBC) standard.[11] In both cases, these standards also translate the proprietary catalog structures of the various vendors into a vendor-neutral catalog representation. Although ODBC/JDBC standardize some aspects of database access, a factor in their success was their accommodation of proprietary constructs through the use of the pass-through mechanism. Although the basics of SQL are well established, and common among most implementations, proprietary extensions are still part of the landscape.

Limitations

The relational database approach is not just about a language (SQL) or a modeling method (ER Modeling) or a set of behavioral rules (Codd's 12 rules). Rather, it is the combination of all three that is so compelling. Developers now had a logical way to think about the organization of data, and if they followed the rules for organizing data, they could use a powerful language for reading and writing the data, no matter how complex it became. The engines that provided all these facilities also assured the integrity of transactions with guaranteed ACID properties. The net result was a change in the thought process of an industry and the dawning of the relational age.

Although elegant and powerful, some fundamental capabilities, which were often needed by real world systems, were missing:

- Sequential processing: Relational databases operate upon "sets" of records. Sometimes the set may be ordered (for example, alphabetical by patient last name). But there is no notion of the "third" record in a set, or of related concepts such as "add the value from each record to the value of the record before it." This type of function must be performed by procedural logic—not SQL.
- Hierarchy: Relational database tables can be constructed to store data of fixed hierarchies (states have many counties, and counties have many townships). One may operate on these fixed hierarchies with relational operators. But it is difficult without nonstandard SQL extensions to handle an open-ended hierarchy, such as "list all the descendants of John Smith."
- Conditional logic: SQL cannot easily perform simple logical choices: "Build a list of people with their home address unless they are current inpatients in which case use their unit location instead."

The three issues above revolve around the need to include logic in the database, with standard procedural processing constructs such as "loops," and "ifs." Standardization has been less successful here, with database vendors offering proprietary languages that are tightly coupled to their databases, such as Transact SQL used by Sybase and Microsoft.[12,13]

Logic in the Database

Databases have long ago shed their role as exclusively data persistence devices. They enforce simple business logic via their definition of table relationships, and data types. They can enforce simple data access rules by their definition of user roles, and role-based table access rights. These control methods are based on symmetries in the database relationships: "Everyone in the 'manager role' can update the table 'budget estimate' "; but, trying to enforce, "Everyone in the 'manager role' except Jeff," breaks the symmetry and becomes suddenly difficult, and requires different approaches. Two forms of database logic have been widely adopted and are described below.

Database Triggers

Database triggers extend the capability of a database engine by automatically detecting changes to the data within its tables, and reacting to these changes. Typically, each table in a database is allowed to have triggers for the "create, update, and delete" functions on the table's records. For example, a "create row" trigger could be placed on a "patient demographics" table—each time a new "patient demographic" record is created, the trigger will fire (execute) and do something. What the trigger does is entirely up to the database designer. A typical action might be to write a database row to an event logging table with some relevant information about the event that occurred: "At 11:55 p.m., a new patient record for Josiah Hawthorne was created by Maggie Smith at the Blueberry Clinic." The crucial attribute of the trigger as a design technique is that it operates entirely within the database engine and executes whenever specific data changes occur. No application programs are involved. If 10 or even 100 applications are written that create rows in our "patient demographics" table, they will all have their activity logged in exactly the same way—because the applications are not doing the logging themselves—it is occurring as an integral part of the database's activity.

Stored Procedures

Stored procedures extend the capabilities of the database engine by allowing database actions to be bundled and executed in a repeatable and controlled manner. Unlike individual SQL statements, stored procedures add capabilities for individual, sequential, row processing and have basic looping and conditional programming capabilities ("next," "if-then," and "while"). Stored procedures bring programming into the database engine, opening up a whole world of possibilities for the database designer. The use of these procedures can be controlled by the database security system where the ability of users to "execute" the stored procedure can be granted.

Whereas stored procedures are generally written in the proprietary procedural languages of databases (Transact-SQL and PL/SQL), several major database vendors, including Sybase, Oracle, and IBM, now provide the ability to write database procedures in non-database-oriented languages, such as Java, as well.

A typical use of the stored procedure is to place all data-modification processes inside stored procedures. Users may be allowed to read from a table, but never to create, update, or delete records. These data modification operations are far too dangerous in the hands of users: "Delete from patient_demographics where medical_record_number = 12345678" may be reasonable for a user who needs to delete a single row, but from the perspective of the database engine, this user must have "delete" authority on the rows in the "patient_demographic" table (and that permission applies to all of the rows). So the statement, "Delete from patient_demographics," which requires the same user security rights, can have the catastrophic effect of emptying the table of all data.

The stored procedure protects us from this danger. Users may be granted execution rights on a "delete_patient_demographics" stored procedure. The stored procedure may be written to require the user to supply a single patient's medical record number guaranteeing that it will delete only one patient row. This combination strategy of providing "read" access to all tables, and "create," "update," "delete" only through "execution" of stored procedures, is very common among client server clinical applications from the 1980s and 1990s.

The evolution of our ideas regarding information privacy has created problems for this design strategy. Note that the user has "read" access directly on the tables—they can see everything. If they access the data exclusively through an application, then the application may limit their visibility to what they really ought to see. But, if they can use their credentials (user name and password) to access the database directly (through any one of hundreds of SQL query and reporting tools) then they can see everything, extract it, copy it, etc. Furthermore, because few databases are ever set up to audit "read" accesses, the user can probably do this without detection. One common solution for systems that were designed this way is to provide two sets of credentials for each user. One set, which is known to the user, is used to gain access to the clinical application. The second set, known to the application but not the user, is then used to connect the application to the database on the user's behalf. The end result is that the user cannot exploit direct access to the database.

More Limitations of the Relational Model

Several other limitations, more specific to health care, remain to be described.

Increasing Complexity of Data Models

Because relational databases rely on data modeling in two dimensions (tables and the relationships between them), real world domains with complex data relationships can require many tables and relationships in order to be accurately recorded in a relational database. In the case of some real world domains, which have intrinsic hierarchy, or unlimited nesting, relational modeling may be extremely difficult. Working with the data model using standard tools such as report writers becomes increasingly complex.

Data models incorporating hundreds of tables are commonplace and frequently models exceed a thousand tables. This complexity changes the dynamics of application development. A state is reached in which virtually no individual can be trusted to know the entire data structure. Extensive documentation of the models becomes an absolute necessity. Query and report writing become tasks for specialists, working against the original promise of SQL to make querying available to a wide range of users.

Need to Manage Complex Objects as Units

One cause for large data models is the wealth of detail needed to store a logical data object. Consider for a moment a clinical report, which includes a minimally useful set of data elements: A patient, an encounter, a location, a patient history narrative, a list of procedures performed, a list of diagnoses, a list of allergies, a list of medications administered during the procedure, and a list of the staff participating in the procedure. Recording this "simple" clinical report in relational structures involves many tables. In order for the coherence of the report to be maintained, changes to the data in all the tables must be managed as a unit according to the ACID properties of transactions.

But can the data in the various tables be managed independently? Clearly, there could be a patient "diagnoses" table that could be updated outside the context of an individual report, but there is also the concept of "diagnoses" as they were known at the time of the report and were applicable to the clinical report. Changing the data that underlie the report essentially changes the report itself. So the diagnoses at the time of, and related to, the clinical report are different data elements than those in the "general" diagnoses table. Data elements become logically bound in well-defined collections: "This is the set of values that were in the collection at the time it was signed by the responsible clinician." The collection is commonly known as a document.

Relational databases have no intrinsic notion of documents—of collections of rows from many tables that form a complex object. It is true that one can store large text objects, but to the relational engine, those have no internal structure.

These strange creatures—documents—may also have strange editing rules. They can be composed and edited by various staff members (including transcriptionists), but must eventually be signed by the clinician responsible for the care described in the document. After the clinician signs, even they cannot edit the document again. It can be amended (changed), however, with special permission and a recorded rationale, and including various visual highlights to emphasize its changed state. So it seems that documents need to have versions. Relational databases do not work easily with versions either. Would version two of our mythical document store a complete second set of rows in all the tables, or try to just store the ones that changed? The mechanical details become complex, because the concept of data collections is absent.

This notion of collections that must be managed as units will return shortly, in our discussion of XML.

Medical Data Typing

Databases and programming languages, healthcare considerations aside, are often described in terms of the strength of their data typing. Strength means the precise and enforced use of data types, for example, integers, character strings, or dates. In a relational database, it is simply not possible to store a character string in a field defined to hold integers. Strong data typing avoids many problems in building computer systems. Programs do not need to be written to protect themselves against unexpected data types. In the relational world, a value that came out of an "integer" column is absolutely going to be an integer (or a null).

Unfortunately, for those of us who design clinical systems, the reality of data typing in medicine is more murky, because reality gets in the way. A laboratory instrument, for instance, may have a lower detection limit of 10. When a specimen is measured as below that level, the value is neither 10, nor any specific number under 10, but "below 10." An instrument may report values in ranges "10–20," or an attribute may be reported according to nonparametric scales, such as "cloudy, hazy, clear." These problems create major dilemmas for the designer. They want to keep all the laboratory results in one table with "analyte name, value, units," but although values are numeric 99% of the time, the field cannot be "typed" as numeric, if it is also to hold the non-numeric exceptions. But if it is not typed as a numeric, then many of the standard SQL operators cannot be used. For example, the values cannot be sorted properly (numeric and alpha sorts are very different) nor can they be used in numeric operations and filters such as "multiply by 10," or "get the values over 100." One solution is to store two columns for the same data, one expecting integer data and the other text.

Interfacing and Databases

During the decade from 1987–1997, HL7 messaging moved from the draft version 2 through its establishment as an ANSI standard. Our own use of HL7 interfaces at Johns Hopkins began in 1990 with eight systems. Successful interfacing requires that the databases at both ends of the interface transaction must have some similarity in their structures. For example, perhaps one system distinguishes between a patient's home address, and current temporary address (which can be an issue when patients and their families travel to tertiary care centers from long distances and stay for a while). If there is an attempt to interface this system with one that has a simpler world view—that patients have one address—this attempt will inevitably encounter problems. If the simpler system maps its single address to the patient's permanent address, then someone using the simple system may try to contact the patient by calling their home a thousand miles away, when the patient is in a hotel across the street. Conversely, if they map the temporary address to their single address, then the opposite effect will occur. They will be able to reach the patient while the patient is in town, but months later, they may be sending the patient's bills to the hotel across the street, not to the patient's actual home.

Similarly, a simple data element such as patient name can cause problems. Many legacy systems have fixed maximum field lengths for their data elements. Many also combine several name elements into single fields. So one can find that they are attempting to synchronize names over a set of variations such as these:

- System A—very modern and complete. Has fields, without maximum lengths, for all six HL7 defined name parts (first, middle, last, prefix, professional suffix, given suffix).
- System B—a relatively new system with all six HL7 name parts, but with each one having a maximum length.
- System C—somewhat older, with only two name fields, one for last name and one for everything else ("Coltri" and "Mr. Alan James III MD").

For many common names, these systems can exchange data without difficulty. But at the edges of their capabilities, the exchanges break down. System A is capable of sending name parts that exceed System B's ability to store them (think of fully spelled out Welsh and Hindi names). System C must use algorithms to untangle its "everything else" field into the explicit parts of the other systems—is "Senior" a name or the first individual of a name? Is "Major" a name or a rank?

Accuracy in interfacing requires that the systems at both ends of the exchange, and the messages passing between them, are all able to handle a logical data structure, and are making consistent use of data domains for all the individual fields.

The HL7 standard does identify coded fields where tables are used to define the allowable values, and it does allow multiple representations of data elements, each marked with the coding scheme used. However, these adaptations simply acknowledge the existence of the problem, and provide mechanisms for coping with it in specific implementations.

This section, however, is not a critique of HL7, but rather of database designs. Data storage designs are tailored to the needs of the application being written. There is not any standard for the "storage format" of medical records data. HL7 tries to encompass all reasonable message exchanges, and allows enormous optionality and content nesting within messages.

HL7 version 3 attempts to solve many of the problems of data exchange, but faces an uphill battle against the large installed base of version 2.1–2.4 implementations. Complex healthcare environments often have hundreds of existing HL7 interfaces, involving dozens of vendor products, each of which has been carefully woven into a fabric of data exchanges unique to the specific environment. Even if HL7 version 3 allows perfect expression of content within the message, the endpoint problem will still exist. The databases must both store the logical relationships of records and field data including all constraints of data typing and data domains.

Database Auditing

In the "database trigger" example described earlier, a database trigger was used to create a log record of a data change. This type of design is common, with application designers using the capabilities of the database to perform the logging function. But it is worth noting that databases often have additional built-in auditing capabilities. These may take the form of a set of database tables which, once created, are not entirely under the control even of the system administrator, and which have some (almost) irrevocable behavior. Once the audit subsystem is created, the system administrator identifies the events they want to audit. Common choices might include every attempt to connect to the database, every creation or deletion of a user account, or every SQL statement that updates specified tables. The system may even support an investigation mode where it records every SQL statement issued by a particular user connection.

We have not seen these "built-in" auditing capabilities exploited in the vendor products we have used. They may have been present, and certainly are more likely to be used as security concerns increase. Remember though, that these systems focus on "what events are happening on which connections," and "which user account initiated the connection." In the modern world, there are often processes between the user and the database that mask this trail of accountability. Although the database itself may not be used for this type of auditing, many applications include auditing within the application software. This approach has the merit of recording "audit" events that are easily understood in terms of the "functions" of the application, not in terms of the storage mechanics of the database.

Alternative Forms of Storage

XML for Storage

In recent years, XML (Extensible Markup Language) has been given as the answer to most questions about the future of information processing. This is an unfortunate overstatement. XML is a wonderful concept, a way of creating languages that allow data of almost any degree of complexity to be recorded and communicated precisely. However, it is up to the resulting XML-based languages to solve our technical communication challenges. Some excellent examples of the use of XML in the sciences include MathML (Mathematical Markup Language),[14] CDA (HL7 Clinical Document Architecture),[15] and MAGE-ML (MicroArray and Gene Expression Markup Language).[16]

In the simplest possible terms, XML is a tag-based, hierarchical way of writing documents that are both machine and human readable. "Tag-based" means that the data structure and data values are identified using a system of beginning and ending markers that look much like HTML tags; for example, a "last name" data element might look like:

⟨lastname⟩Smith⟨/lastname⟩

"Hierarchical" means that the elements of an XML document may be nested; one element may include another. For example:

⟨patient name⟩
    ⟨first name⟩John⟨/first name⟩
    ⟨last name⟩Smith⟨/last name⟩
⟨/patient name⟩

Any collection of data can be expressed in XML, whether we think of the collection as a document or not. However, XML's basic unit of organization is the document, and all XML data exist within the context of a document. It is the definition of the tags and the definition of allowable nesting that create XML-based languages for various purposes.

Remembering the earlier discussion of relational database limitations one can see that XML solves two of the big problems of SQL—hierarchy, and complex collections. Unlike the SQL database, which is a continuous fabric of interrelated data, XML is intrinsically oriented toward a document or complex collection view.

There are two levels of standards compliance in the XML world. The first, "well formed," is enormously flexible, but not very precise. It requires that documents follow basic structural rules, but does not require any rigorous definition of meaning. The second level, "valid," follows the same structural rules, with the additional requirement that the content of each document conforms to a detailed specification. These specifications can be written in either a document type definition (DTD) or XML schema. The document definitions rigorously define the set of "tags" that may be used in the document, and the allowable hierarchy of tags. For example, a document definition for a book may specify an allowable set of tags that include ⟨chapter⟩, ⟨section⟩, and ⟨paragraph⟩, and may define hierarchy rules such that chapters may contain sections and sections may contain paragraphs (but paragraphs may not contain chapters). Documents that conform to a DTD may be tested for obedience to all the rules of the DTD. If a document obeys all the rules of the DTD, it is a "valid" instance of the document type. Historically, the DTD represents an earlier technology generation, and was inherited from XML's conceptual ancestor SGML (Standardized Generalized Markup Language). When XML is used for well-defined purposes, such as a book chapter or an electronic transaction, the semantics of valid XML provide the definition needed for precise communication.[17]

Once XML is used for storage, it can be used to find documents with some particular content to perform a query. The query language, XQuery, allows one to specify a search based on structural locations within a document, and the values found at the location. This is similar to SQL, which allows queries based on tables and fields. However, relational databases include well-defined mechanisms for indexing data, and automatically include the use of query optimization techniques for performance. XML storage implementations have been lacking these functions, and the process of query execution is usually one of inefficiently "opening" and examining each document individually to determine if the document meets the query criteria.

Combination Systems—XML Stored in the Relational Database

The power of the Relational Database Engines and their market dominance have placed them in a position to try to absorb the upstart XML. To this end, a wide variety of hybrid designs have evolved.[18] In the simplest form, the relational database is used to list, catalog, and index the XML documents that are being stored. This approach utilizes all the data management strengths of SQL. Documents can be organized by author, date, type, subject matter, etc. The documents themselves can be stored as entire objects in the large data object fields of a database. Consider the HL7 CDA. It defines an XML document that has a well-defined and consistent "header" (who, what, when, where) and a potentially very complex "body" of clinical data. What could be easier than to use the "header" data to catalog the document in a relational database, and then store the entire document in its XML form? In reality, it is the entire document that is usually wanted for clinical use—for it is a logically complete object, whereas the "header data" is most useful in locating the documents desired.

Queries against XML documents handled in this way can benefit from the combination of language strengths. The data held in the relational database can be used to drastically reduce the number of candidate documents, whereas XQuery can then take the search inside this much reduced set for individual document evaluation.

An alternative approach, most suitable for relatively simple valid XML documents, is to completely decompose or "shred" the document into relational tables down to its individual data elements.[19] The transformation is most useful if there is an XML schema definition for the documents that defines their structural possibilities and can be used to aid the mapping of data into relational structures. Structures that are simple in either one of these forms can be horribly complex in the other—it all depends on the natural organization of the data.

Database vendors have produced various language extensions to support these hybrid approaches and the technology has now evolved to the point where standards such as ISO/ANSI SQL/XML are beginning to be used.[18,20]

XML as Transport—Not as Storage

In addition to its success as a document format, XML has had great impact as a technology-neutral transport format. SOAP, the Simple Object Access Protocol, uses XML for transport. SAML, the Security Assertion Markup Language, is an XML language for transporting security information. Many other examples exist.

Movement of data from one system to another can be thought of as the delivery of a series of documents, each attesting to some set of facts. The structure of HL7 messages is entirely hierarchical, and the nesting of structures is entirely consistent with XML's requirements. It is easy to conceive of HL7 messages being transformed to, and transported as XML, and that has in fact been done with standard DTDs available from www.hl7.org for versions 2.3.1 and 2.4. Version 3.0 messages are natively XML.

XML and Security

In the earlier discussions of security, some limitations of the relational model were highlighted. These primarily surrounded the use of table-oriented security controls for trying to manage access to complex objects spanning many tables. Versioning of complex objects was noted as being difficult to accomplish. Because XML treats complex objects naturally, the access control system can be much simpler, operating directly at the document level. This ease extends beyond access control to any security feature in which a complex object is the natural unit of operation. Versioning is simple, adding non-repudiation checksums to documents is simple, and providing document level encryption keys is simple.[21]

The development of XML was initially associated with the desire to separate the content and presentation of documents. It was believed that the receiver of a document should be allowed to determine how to display it. Or perhaps the document, as a unit, would not be displayed, but instead have some portion of its contents extracted and used in some way. There are obviously situations in which this is appropriate and good, but are clinical documents one of them? For example, if one sends a blood sample for a series of hematology tests, one gets back a report of all the results from the specimen (with units and reference ranges). Do we really want someone to "restyle" the data omitting the reference ranges? Or to combine the data, with data from other specimens that were collected under very different circumstances? Are data ever "the same" after they are restyled? As we talk about building regional medical records by extracting and displaying data from a variety of systems, we will need to be very careful not to inadvertently alter the meaning of the data by allowing too much flexibility in their presentation.

XML and Archiving

How to deal with archiving of complex medical records and their documents as they change in format over time is a policy and legal matter that goes well beyond a discussion of databases. But from the technology perspective, we need to be careful about embedding our data in databases with proprietary schemas, which require live applications to interpret. In 10 years' time, we may no longer use or own the application; the vendor may no longer even exist.

XML archiving provides a possible avenue of approach to this problem. If we can define the elements of the record we need to preserve, and package them as a series of XML documents, we would then have an easily archived, platform and technology neutral representation of the record.

EAV Databases

EAV is a term meaning "entity, attribute, value" and describes a way of storing data as entities whose properties are defined by attribute–value pairs. For example, in the "name" examples used earlier, one could define an "entity" of "HL7 name" with six attributes (prefix, first name, middle name, last name, given suffix, professional suffix) (Table 11-1).

Because of the dominance of relational databases, their excellent transactional abilities, and their high performance, EAV designs frequently use a relational database engine in their implementation, essentially embedding the entity-attribute-value triad as the columns of a single "long, narrow" table. Sometimes several tables are used, allowing for "value" columns in

TABLE 11-1. Example of an EAV database

Entity	Attribute	Value
HL7 name	Name-prefix	Mr.
HL7 name	First name	Joseph
HL7 name	Middle name	Albert
HL7 name	Last name	Smith
HL7 name	Given suffix	Jr.
HL7 name	Professional suffix	MD

the different tables to be defined with strong data types (integers in one table, strings in another, etc.).

The power of an EAV database and its associated applications lies in the fact that no new data structures need to be created, or new applications written, when the database is extended to new uses. The "new use" is expressed as new "meta-data" describing the new entities. The new "meta-data" defines how the entity is to be stored in the preexisting EAV "long, narrow" tables, and further defines how data entry and display applications are to operate on the data. In medical use, this type of structure is ideal for applications in which "users" are defining many similar data collections, such as flow sheets. In a reporting application that we produced at Johns Hopkins, one set of EAV tables, meta-data tables, and applications is currently driving several hundred flow sheet-like data collection forms. A benefit not to be overlooked is the reduction in testing demands. Once the base functionality of the system has been tested thoroughly, no additional testing of application code is needed as new EAV entities are defined. It is true that the meta-data of each new entity must be verified, but because no new programs have been written, the system will behave predictably.

EAV suffers from a few problems, largely related to the abstraction it places between the "real world" and the SQL database. Because the data structure is abstract, and not the direct mapping of real world entities to tables and attributes to columns, some of the normal relational database strengths are missing. Ad hoc queries are very difficult to construct, and standard report writers, which expect "real world meaningful" tables and columns, are virtually useless. In general, these limitations are mitigated by providing transformation software that can create traditional relational tables using the meta-data definition of the entities, and then move data from the long, narrow tables of the EAV model to the traditional relational tables for use by query and reporting tools.[22,23]

N-tier Architectures

Direct interaction between the user and the data storage is not usually a good idea. Data storage and modification are the end result of business processes that may be quite complex. The user should be performing processes, which in turn perform the associated data management. This led to the phrase "three-tier" architecture, in which there is a client application (user interaction and display), a business logic tier (processes), and a persistence tier (data storage and retrieval).

As applications became more complex, involving services on multiple machines, the notion of "tiers" began to break down leading to the term "N-tier" systems—meaning that the system contained many interacting layers with a division of functional responsibilities.

Architectures, which centralize database access services, often use a technique called connection pooling. For instance, if 100 people are using a database through a Web Application Server, it is highly unlikely that the user has their own personal "connection" through to the database. (If you were to ask the database "who is connected," it would not list out these 100 people—in contrast to an old two-tier client server application which would have listed them all.) Instead, the Web Application Server will have a few connections, managed as a pool (a group of interchangeable resources), and will route requests from all the users down these few pipes. In a connection pooling, additional connections are created as needed, based on aggregate workload. There are two basic facts to remember about this architecture: First, it is much more efficient than individual user connections; and second, the database engine can no longer know to whom it is speaking by knowing which account created the connection. This implies that the database engine itself can no longer provide the auditing capability on database actions. Auditing requires the assistance of the software layer that is using the connection pool to inform it of which requests to attribute to which users.

This simple example of the role of the "business layer" in managing a connection pool and auditing actions (or assisting the database in auditing), is only the beginning of the functionality it may provide. For example, a "lab order" business logic might ultimately store its data in an "order table," but it may also do many other things as well—send out an HL7 order message, log the placement of the order in a log event recording subsystem, and validate the legitimacy of the order (who placed it, from where, for what). The users of the business logic unit do not know (and should not care) about these process details, nor should they know if these process details change.

Service Oriented Architectures

SOA can serve as the extension of the "business tier" of the N-tier architecture above, in the sense that services may be provided from one or many sites (anywhere on the Web), they may be discovered by inquiry into standardized registry services, and they provide implementation neutral, standards-based programming interfaces.

Virtually all of the data exchanges involved in the use of SOA—in the discovery of services, the definition of services, and the use of services—are expressed in various XML languages. The vision is that services dynamically assemble into complex applications. The trivial example is often given of a "restaurant locator" service, which gives individuals a listing of restaurants near wherever they happen to be, followed by a "menu" service which would display menus and prices, and a "reservation" service.

Can healthcare functions be divided into such modular "services"? One possibility is the replacement for many of our current message-based interfaces with on-demand services. Today, when a new clinical specialty system needs to be integrated and needs to know (as virtually all do) who the registered patients are (so that service can be provided, and the proper patient account can be billed), the only real alternative is to send that application an HL7 admissions/registrations message stream. The application then processes vast amounts of data trying to keep track of every patient who might require service, when it really only needs to know about a few patients whom it ultimately does serve. How much nicer it would be if a simple lookup service could be invoked to import a patient's demographic and visit information when it is needed.

Another possibility lies in the pursuit of the national and regional medical records. It seems likely that there will not be a physical aggregation of records, and that the data will largely remain in the hands of its producers. What needs to be sought then is a method of "finding" and "querying for" the parts of the distributed record.

Predictions

The complexity of modern systems virtually demands that a powerful and flexible business logic/service tier exists, and that it is positioned largely outside the database. This implies that the more rigid control systems (authentication, authorization, triggers) built into the fabric of the database engines will see less use. Two-tier client servers will disappear for medium-to large-size systems.

Databases store information at a very granular level, but the next round of development will focus on data collections—documents with internal structured data, and complex document forms including images and annotation. Regional data sharing will begin with the sharing of very small, high-value, subsets of the patient record. These will be delivered on an SOA architecture. Clinical applications will evolve to become more "active" in their interaction with clinicians, with far more emphasis on pushing critical data forward, not waiting for it to be browsed.

Databases and data structures will continue to be the core engines underlying EHRs.

References

1. Information for Health: A Strategy for Building the National Health Information Infrastructure, Report and Recommendations from the National Committee on Vital and Health Statistics, Washington, DC. November 15, 2001. Available at: http://aspe.hhs.gov/sp/nhii/Documents/NHIIReport2001/default.htm.
2. Web Services and Service-Oriented Architectures. Available at: www.service-architecture.com.
3. Ball MJ, Collen MF. Aspects of the computer-based patient record. New York: Springer-Verlag; 1992.
4. Office of the National Coordinator for Health Information Technology. Summary of Nationwide Health Information Network (NHIN) Request for

Information (RFI) Responses. Washington, DC: DHHS; June 2005. http://www.os.dhhs.gov/healthit/rfisummaryreport.pdf. Accessed June 9, 2005.

5. MUMPS. Wikipedia. http://en.wikipedia.org/wiki/MUMPS. Accessed June 29, 2005.

6. Brown SH, Lincoln MJ, Groen PJ, Kolodner RM. VistA—U.S. Department of Veterans Affairs national-scale HIS. Int J Med Inform 2003;69:135–156.

7. Codd E. Is your DBMS really relational? Computer World 10/14/1985, 10/21/1985.

8. Gray J, Reuter A. Transaction processing: concepts and techniques. San Mateo, CA: Morgan Kaufmann Publishers; 1993.

9. Chen PP. The entity-relationship model—toward a unified view of data. ACM Trans Database Syst 1976;1(1):9–36.

10. Richter J. ODBC 2.0 further establishes cross-product data sharing standard. Byte November 1994.

11. JDBC Overview. Available at: http://java.sun.com/products/jdbc/overview.html.

12. Kline KE, Gould L, Zanevsky A, NetLibrary Inc. Transact-SQL programming. Sebastopol, CA: O'Reilly & Associates; 1999.

13. Feuerstein S, NetLibrary Inc. Advanced Oracle PL/SQL programming with packages. 1st ed. Sebastopol, CA: O'Reilly & Associates; 1996.

14. W3C Math Home. Available at: http://www.w3.org/Math/.

15. HL7. Available at: www.hl7.org.

16. MicroArray and Gene Expression—MAGE. Available at: http://www.mged.org/Workgroups/MAGE/mage.html.

17. XML Schema Part 0: Primer Second Edition. Available at: http://www.w3.org/TR/xmlschema-0/.

18. Dayen I. Storing XML in relational databases. Available at: http://www.xml.com/pub/a/2001/06/20/databases.html?page=1.

19. Udell J. The future of XML documents and relational databases. Available at: http://www.infoworld.com/article/03/07/25/29FEdocs_1.html.

20. Information technology—database languages—SQL. Part 14. XML-related specifications (SQL/XML). Available at: http://www.incits.org/tc_home/h2sd4.htm.

21. Simon E, Madsen P, Adams C. An introduction to XML digital signatures. Available at: http://www.xml.com/pub/a/2001/08/08/xmldsig.html.

22. Nadkarni PM, Brandt C. Data extraction and ad hoc query of an entity-attribute-value database. J Am Med Inform Assoc 1998;5(6):511–527.

23. Chen RS, Nadkarni P, Marenco L, Levin F, Erdos J, Miller PL. Exploring performance issues for a clinical database organized using an entity-attribute-value representation. J Am Med Inform Assoc 2000;7(5):475–487.

12
Standards

Linda F. Fischetti, Peter Schloeffel, Jeffrey S. Blair, and Michael L. Henderson

The first edition of *Aspects of the Computer-based Patient Record* observed that "Numerous sources of machine-ready medical information already exist. However, the information is located on separate machines within hospitals, medical practice offices, pharmacies, commercial laboratories, and nursing homes. . . . The only solution to this fragmentation and redundancy is standards."[1] Later, it stated that "Health data standards are now developing, but not as rapidly as the situation demands. . . . The lack of data standards remains a major barrier to achieving many significant milestones in health care and broad deployment of CPRs [computer-based patient records] and CPR systems."[1] Regrettably, these assessments are still largely true.

Most electronic health records (EHRs) now in use are tightly bound to the physical implementation models of the particular system developers who provide them, that is, to a proprietary EHR system (EHR-S) that has its own display tools and applications. Standards support interoperability and portability, breaking these bonds. The use of increasingly standardized language to discuss EHR scope and function, EHR infrastructure, information and communication models, methods for interfacing, clinical content, and the standards that enable EHRs will free EHRs and the information they contain from constraints. It will also enable EHR-Ss to provide the tools to more effectively and efficiently move information into, out of, and across the EHRs. Thus, freeing the EHR from the EHR-S allows the creation of lifelong, shareable EHRs.

The creation of longitudinal, interoperable records is today the goal in the United States (US) and the focus of nationally sponsored activities in England, Canada, Australia, Denmark, and Brazil. These governmental initiatives are accelerating progress in health informatics standards, adopting and building on the work of standards development organizations (SDOs) over the past decade.

Standards Development Organizations

In the international arena, three SDOs cover the main broad areas of health informatics. Two are based in Europe: Technical Committee 215 (TC 215) of the International Organization for Standardization (ISO)[2] with 38 member countries (the US is represented here by a single delegation chosen by a national Technical Advisory Group) and Technical Committee 251 of the European Committee for Standardization, or CEN (Comité Européen de Normalisation)[3] with 28 member countries. The third is Health Level 7 (HL7),[4] a US-based SDO with 25 countries as international affiliates.

Increasingly HL7 has been responding to government requests for targeted work in specific areas and signing Memorandums of Understanding for cooperative work with other SDOs, such as the Object Management Group (OMG) and the American Society for Testing and Materials (ASTM). These efforts involving both international and US-based SDOs are an important step toward accelerating and coordinating standards development to reduce redundancy and prevent gaps in standards coverage.

Specific areas are addressed by other SDOs, for example, imaging by Digital Imaging and Communications in Medicine (DICOM), medical devices by the Institute for Electrical and Electronic Engineers (IEEE), and e-prescribing by the National Council of Prescription Drug Programs (NCPDP). In the US, many other organizations are involved in health informatics, but the main broad-based health informatics SDO is Technical Committee E31 in the ASTM, now collaborating with HL7.

Breaking the Nexus Between the EHR and the EHR-S

There is an important distinction between the EHR and the EHR-S. Whereas the EHR is a repository or store of a patient's health and medical information, the addition of the term "system" reflects the tools and applications that facilitate the use of the data from the EHR by the end user. The EHR-S thus becomes a more comprehensive application consistent with what many mean by the term EHR. In 1991, the Institute of Medicine provided the definition of the CPR system; this continues to be the benchmark for the use of the word "system."[5,6]

Those wishing to further their knowledge of the terms used to describe EHRs should consult ISO/TR 20514 EHR Scope, Definition, and Context.[6] This technical report provides additional definitions for shareable EHR, Core EHR, Extended EHR, and others.

This new target of interoperable longitudinal information that can be shared across multiple EHRs and presented to clinicians via whatever

EHR-S the clinician is using is dependent on universal standardization. To date, standards for development of EHR communication, terminology, and others have allowed for individual interpretation and uniqueness of implementation. As a result, implemented EHRs tend to be insular, unable to communicate with or understand data from other EHRs. This leads to presenting "foreign" data in such a way that is human readable but not computable within the "host" EHR's clinical reminders and decision support systems. Standardization of terminology and information models within the database used for storage (the EHR) can make the information available for display to the clinicians independent of the display tool (the EHR-S) in use. Without standardization, the healthcare industry has naturally migrated to the more common physical information model which includes technological constraints to enable the building of a particular implementation (e.g., an EHR-S built for a particular hardware and software platform).[6]

One international standards activity that is gaining domestic interest as key to EHR interoperability is the concept of standardized information models. If the EHR is based on a standardized logical information model, then it can be completely independent of any particular EHR-S. International SDOs are focused on logical information models that specify the structures and relationships between information but are independent of any particular technology or implementation environment.

Interoperability, although initially seen as a threat by commercial EHR-S vendors, may in fact offer them a significant opportunity. Freeing the EHR from the EHR-S will not in any way limit the ability of vendors to value-add and differentiate in their EHR-Ss. The ability to share EHR information beyond a single healthcare organization (or even between different applications within an organization) will open up the EHR-Ss market which to date has had minimal penetration in any healthcare sector.

Classifications of Standards

For purposes of this chapter, standards are divided into two classifications: EHR standards and EHR-enabling standards. The first includes standards directly related to the EHR, including interoperability, infrastructure, information and communication, interface, clinical content and datasets, functionality, framework, and special interest standards. The second classification consists of the large group of related health informatics standards needed to support an integrated clinical information system where the EHR-S may be viewed as the central component. These enabling standards include most of the current areas of health informatics standardization activity, such as health concept representation (HCR) (terminology), demographics (identification), messaging, decision support, and privacy and security.

EHR-S Standards

We focus on a number of concerns: *Focus* and *functionality* define what the standards need to accomplish. Standards are needed for the *domain*, for *interoperability*, and for *infrastructure*. These, in turn, are supported by *information and communication models*, standards for *interfaces* (*messaging and common services*), standards for *clinical content and datasets*, standards for the *framework* (*meta-standards*), and standards for *special interests*. The following sections are based on these concerns.

Scope

In 2001, ISO/TC 215 established an EHR ad hoc Task Group to identify gaps and requirements for international standards for EHRs. The final report of this group in 2002[7] made ten recommendations. The first three advised ISO/TC 215 to:

- Develop a comprehensive consensus definition of the EHR.
- Define EHR standards as part of a family of standards based on a "system-of-systems" approach that collectively represent the major services in a distributed health computing environment.
- Restrict the scope of EHR standards to a conception of the EHR that is concerned with a single subject of care, has as its primary purpose the support of present and future health care, and is principally concerned with clinical information.

The first of these recommendations was implemented in the ISO Technical Report, Electronic Health Record: Definition, Scope, and Context.[6] The second and third recommendations implicitly define the scope of EHR standards activity, at least for ISO. As defined in the report, there are two distinct views on the scope of the EHR and of EHR-Ss.[6] The first view, the "Core EHR," is consistent with those recommendations: It includes clinical information and the care of individual patients and excludes other components of a comprehensive clinical information system such as demographics, security, terminology, and decision support. The "Extended EHR" view includes not only the related EHR "building block" services such as terminology and security, but also nonclinical functions such as patient administration, scheduling, billing, and resource allocation.

Functionality: The HL7 EHR-S Functional Model

The EHR has no functionality per se because it is "a repository of information" that is processed by an EHR-S. Functionality standards are therefore relevant to EHR-Ss but not to the EHR. There have been a number of EHR-S functionality standards in the past (often wrongly denoted as

EHR functionality standards), but the most important and recent is the HL7 EHR System Functional Model.

Scope

In July 2004, HL7 released its EHR System Functional Model as a Draft Standard for Trial Use (DSTU).[8]* Prepared by HL7's EHR Technical Committee, the draft standard thus became available for public comment before being reballoted as a fully normative standard. Consistent with HL7 practice, if the trial period did not result in subsequent ballots, the draft status would expire at the end of a 2-year period of 2004 to 2006.

The DSTU defines a standardized model of the functions that may be present in EHR-Ss, clearly distinguishing them from the EHR as a singular entity. The model is agnostic as to specific clinical disciplines or settings. It does not, for example, list specific functions potentially useful for research. Rather, its support for researchers consists of ensuring that the functions for an EHR-S support the clinical documentation processes and ensures that the data are captured in a way that follows the required protocols for privacy, confidentiality, and security. In like manner, the model does not specify implementation: The EHR-S may be either a system-of-systems or a single system providing the functions required by the users. The model makes no statement about the technology used or about the content of the EHR; it does not dictate how EHR-Ss are developed or implemented now or in the future. The DSTU is not a specification that addresses messaging, implementation, conformance, or the EHR as a singular entity. It is neither a conformance testing metric nor "an exercise in creating a definition for an EHR or EHR-S."[8]

Composition and Use

The model presented in the DSTU consists of a functional outline that can be used to create functional profiles that are specific to clinical users or clinical settings. These profiles overlay the outlined functions, and assign priorities for the functions in the profile. Although the outline is not intended as a list of all functions to be found in a specific EHR-S, it should include all reasonably anticipated EHR-S functions. The profiles can be used to constrain functions to an intended use. Thus, customizing the model involves the creation of profiles defined by users. For example, clinicians develop "use profiles" to provide care to their patient population, and vendors develop "product profiles."

The functional outline for the EHR-S is divided into three sections: Direct Care, Supportive, and Information Infrastructure functions as shown in Figure 12-1. These three sections include 13 subsections and more than

---

* Information in this section is extracted from two documents published by HL7; see Reference 8.

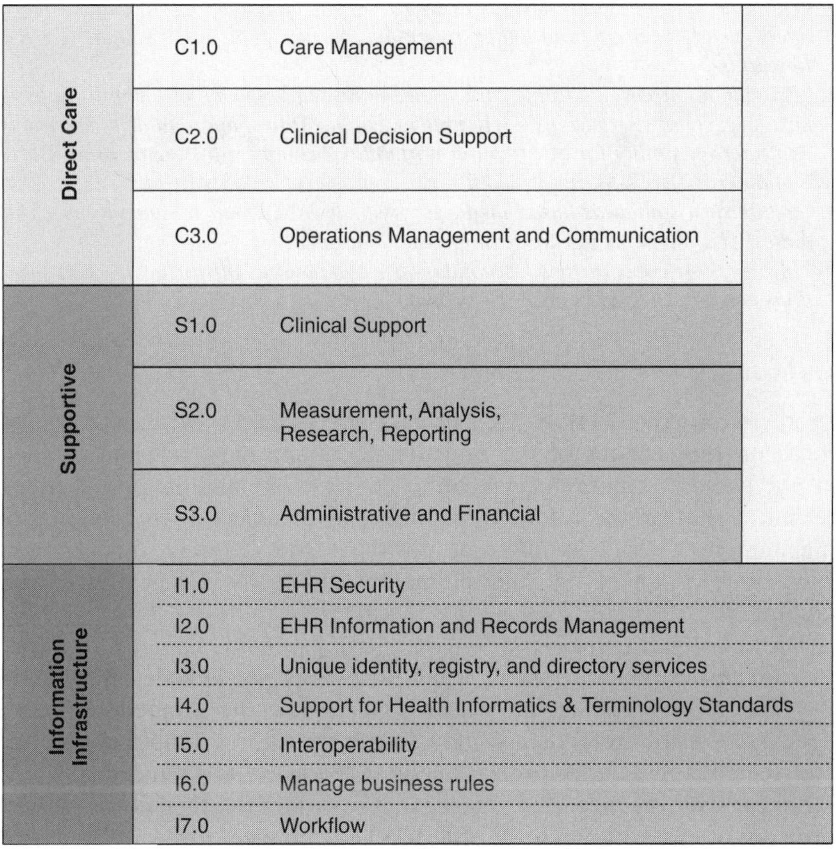

Direct Care	C1.0	Care Management	
	C2.0	Clinical Decision Support	
	C3.0	Operations Management and Communication	
Supportive	S1.0	Clinical Support	
	S2.0	Measurement, Analysis, Research, Reporting	
	S3.0	Administrative and Financial	
Information Infrastructure	I1.0	EHR Security	
	I2.0	EHR Information and Records Management	
	I3.0	Unique identity, registry, and directory services	
	I4.0	Support for Health Informatics & Terminology Standards	
	I5.0	Interoperability	
	I6.0	Manage business rules	
	I7.0	Workflow	

FIGURE 12-1. The framework for the EHR Functional Specification DSTU (*Source:* Dickinson et al.[8])

125 individual functions, each with a Function Name, Function Statement (normative), and associated information such as description, rationale for inclusion, and citation (reference information). The functions for Clinical Decision Support functions interact with the Direct Care and Supportive functions.

Simply put, the intent of the model is to provide users with a superset of functions from which they can select a subset to illustrate what they need within their particular EHR-S. Functions describe the behavior of a system in user-oriented language that key stakeholders can understand. These standard EHR-S functions can be used to:

- *Facilitate describing end user defined benefits such as patient safety, quality outcomes, and cost efficiencies in terms of standard EHR-S functions*

- *"Promote a common understanding of EHR functions upon which devel-opers, vendors, users, and other interested parties plan and evaluate EHR-S functions.*
- *"Provide the necessary framework to drive the requirements and applications of next level standards, such as EHR content, coding, information models, constructs, and interoperability for information portability between sub-systems of an EHR-S and across EHR-Ss.*
- *"Establish a standards-based method by which each realm (country) can apply these EHR functions to care settings, uses, and priorities.*
- *"Inform those concerned with secondary use and national infrastructure what func-tions can be expected in an EHR system."*[8]

DSTU Review

In reviewing the EHR-S DSTU package, users in each organization focus on the sections of the Functional Outline most relevant to their everyday work. Clinicians focus on the Direct Care and Support sections, technical staff on the Information Infrastructure section. Three scenarios highlight how users in different positions and different organizations can study, comment on, and ultimately utilize the DSTU Functional Outline.[8,Appendix B]

The first scenario involves a 50-person group practice planning to replace its clinical information system which that does not include an EHR in 2 years. In this setting, physicians first review the Ambulatory Care documents in the reference section to see what the example use setting and scenario and its prioritization of individual EHR functions would mean for their practice. Their subsequent review of the Functional Outline provides them with input to the DSTU comment process regarding several terminology issues; it also produces a list of functions they can use in discussions with vendors about their next information technology (IT) system.

The second scenario depicts a large hospital with a two-year-old IT system that does not include clinical decision support, performance moni-toring, or public health reporting. The chief information and chief medical officers organize teams to review the model, beginning with the Acute Care profile documents in the reference section, to see how the EHR-S might be used within a hospital. The teams then focus on the Functional Outline, and a small group of providers and IT staff meet to discuss their conclusions. As part of the DSTU comment process, they suggest revisions to some func-tions, some sections of the Informative text, and the reference materials. They plan to use the list of functions in discussions with vendors about adding functions to their existing system.

The third scenario describes a large health IT company. Their product line includes dedicated EHR-Ss and integrated systems with an EHR that provide some decision support for medication ordering. In anticipation of the Medicare Reform law, which provides financial incentives for providers who use IT to track patients, the company wants to add performance monitoring/reporting functionality to its products. The head of the clinical division asks her staff to review the model. Based on the care setting examples in the reference section, they identify a small number of functions to be added to their products. When their review finds that a supportive function they already provide is not included, they plan to discuss its inclusion with HL7 during the DSTU period. They plan to use the EHR-S model in discussing upgrades or new purchases with clients.

Domain Standards

Development of standard formats for exchanging medical event and domain data began in the 1970s, when interactive computer systems started to gain acceptance in clinics and hospitals. Development of domain messaging standards was well underway by the 1980s. With the assistance of Dr. Clement McDonald and others, ASTM developed the 1238 standard for laboratory results and order exchange. In 1985, a joint effort between the American College of Radiology and the National Electrical Manufacturers Association produced connectivity and transmission standards for imaging objects. Known as DICOM (Digital Imaging and Communications in Medicine), this standard is now in its third version (version 3.0).[9] More information on DICOM is available at http://medical.nema.org (see Chapter 16).

By themselves, however, domain messaging standards could only provide limited amounts of the information needed to enable clinicians to make well-formed decisions at the point of care. Integrated views of broad portions of the patient record required the development of standards that supported exchange of both data and meaning across disparate domains.

Interoperability

At its most basic level, interoperability allows two or more systems to exchange information so that it is readable by a human receiver. This level is achievable through the use of non-information-model-based messaging standards such as HL7 version 2.x (V2.x). However, a higher level is required to underpin intelligent decision support, care planning, and other value-added applications. This is called semantic or knowledge-level interoperability, whereby information shared and exchanged between systems is "understood" by the system at the level of formally defined domain concepts, i.e., information is automatically computer-processable by the receiving system.

Semantic interoperability is not an all-or-nothing concept. The degree of semantic interoperability depends on the level of agreement on terminology and the content of data models (such as archetypes and templates) used by the sender and receiver of information. When not all of the standardized components are available to both sender and receiver, transformations between sender and receiver reference models and mappings between different archetypes and terminologies can assist to some degree. However, the complexity and information loss often inherent in these processes may limit their practical use.

The HL7 messaging standards have to date represented the mainstream of the effort to provide cross-domain information interoperability. Beginning in 1988, the HL7 SDO has issued a series of V2.x standards that define relatively simple formats for serializing data about persons and events in treatment and administrative domains. These standards are still being maintained and are sufficiently widely implemented among disparate systems to satisfy the expectation that an HL7 V2.x interface can be crafted to pass data in recognized formats between most pairs of systems in the enterprise.

However, three concerns grew from the early work of HL7 standards developers. First, it had been decided very early to use delimited formats, rather than tagged formats, for the HL7 message structures. These delimited formats, in which the contents of elements are implicitly understood by position rather than explicitly indicated by element tags, are often referred to today as "railroad tracks," from the use of the vertical-bar character as the primary element delimiter. Delimited message formats introduced relatively difficult parsing issues that were not widely mitigated until the introduction of enterprise middleware and of XML encodings in the late 1990s.

Second, HL7—whose name was derived from the concept of the HL7 messages resting atop the seventh (application) layer of the Open Systems for Interoperability (OSI) model—was silent with respect to normative guidance about lower-layer communications protocols and message specifications. By contrast, the DICOM standard provided explicit structures for connection maintenance and for conformance assertions; early DICOM versions even mandated certain kinds of hardware connections.

Third, HL7 was not the result of formal development processes as they are understood today. HL7 was (and, in V2.x, largely remains) a consensus standard in which the commonality of message and vocabulary elements is derived from message definitions rather than inherent in any sort of standard-wide model. Thus, HL7 interfaces, although facilitating large-scale data interchange, faced issues of constraint deficiency and of divergence of meaning which limited semantic interoperability.

To fill this need, HL7 instituted a version 3 (V3) development effort at whose center—built over a decade-plus time span—is the Reference Information Model (RIM). The HL7 RIM is its primary repository for message element definitions and taxonomies in V3. By offering rich expressivity and ensuring agreement on meaning and expression of the elements of messages, the HL7 RIM makes it possible to deliver a real-time information snapshot to the clinician or administrator working with a patient.

Infrastructure Standards

In order to be able to share and exchange information held in EHRs and between EHR-Ss, agreement on a number of different types of standards is required. These standards include:

- EHR Reference Model—the semantics of EHR generic information structures
- Service interface models—the semantics of interfaces between the EHR and other services in a comprehensive EHR-S such as demographics, terminology, and security
- Knowledge concept models—information models, data models, archetypes, and templates that define the structure of clinical and other domain-specific concepts and constraints on them
- Terminologies/vocabularies—the language of health
- Data types—the semantics of data values assigned to a given data element
- Identification—one or more attributes that uniquely identify the EHR subjects of care, healthcare providers, and origin of the information

The main standard in this group is the ISO EHR Definition, Scope, and Context.[6] Although a technical report rather than a normative standard, this is fundamentally important in that it effectively sets the boundaries of the EHR and of EHR standards. Moreover, some countries may decide to develop normative national versions of all or parts of this technical report to give legal weight to its definitions. This may be important as part of the legal framework underpinning national and regional EHR initiatives in both the public and private sectors. Australia is planning to base a normative standard on the ISO technical report.

Data type standards are relevant to messaging as well as EHRs, but are included here because they are not easily classified elsewhere. Standardized data types are essential for interoperability in both EHR and messaging systems. Together with terminologies and vocabularies, they are the lowest level entities requiring agreement to enable interoperability of communicated health data.

At present, there are two main health-specific data type standards internationally. The first is the HL7 V3 data types standard.[10] The second is the CEN data types standard used in Europe[11] and based on the HL7 standard. Much work has been done between HL7 and CEN to harmonize these two standards, and there are now only a few small differences between the two. A project within ISO/TC 215 is producing an international standard that will have a fully harmonized subset of the HL7 and CEN standards.[12]

Information and Communication Models

Requirements for Models

The only comprehensive requirements standard for EHR models available to date is the ISO Requirements for an Electronic Health Record Architecture.[13] This is a Technical Specification rather than a full normative standard because there is as yet little practical implementation experience of applying this standard against specific EHR model standards or implementations of these standards. The ISO/TS 18308[13] requirements are presented under a framework that includes EHR structure (record and data organization, type and form of data, and supporting HCR); clinical and record processes; communication; privacy and security; medicolegal; ethical; consumer/cultural; and evolution requirements.

"A compliance mapping" is essentially a document listing the compliance of a particular model against each of the requirements in the ISO/TS 18308. To date, compliance mappings have been done for the *open*EHR Reference Model[14] and the CEN 13606-1 Reference Model.[15] Ideally, there should be requirements standards and information model standards for each of the EHR enabling standards areas (demographics, terminology/HCR, security, etc.). This has not yet been achieved within any SDO.

CEN EN13606-1 EHR Reference Architecture

The original CEN ENV13606** EHR interoperability standard was a four-part standard that was published in 1999/2000. ENV13606 had limited uptake, attributed mainly to difficulties with implementation inherent in its single-level modeling approach. In November 2001, a decision was taken by CEN to revise ENV13606 and to adopt the *open*EHR archetype methodology[16] as a key to improving interoperability and overcoming the earlier implementation difficulties.

When completed, the revised EN13606 will contain five parts. Part 1 of the standard is the EHR Reference Architecture (i.e., logical RIM). CEN prEN 13606-1 was successfully balloted into ISO in early 2005 and will form the basis for the development of the international (ISO) EHR interoperability standard. It is also expected that Parts 2–5 of EN13606 (discussed individually under their relevant sections below) will be progressively introduced into ISO/TC 215.

** "ENV" denotes a "Pre-standard" (now renamed a "Technical Specification" to comply with ISO terminology) whereas "EN" denotes a full de jure European standard. All CEN standards are ENVs for a period of 3 years, which enables implementation experience and feedback before becoming a full standard. At the end of the 3-year period, a pre-standard can be converted without change to full EN status, or it can be revised to become an EN, or it can be scrapped. "PREN" denotes a draft of a full European standard.

HL7 Clinical Document Architecture

Traditionally focused on health messaging standards, HL7 modified its mission statement in 2000 to include the EHR. The first EHR-related HL7 standard development was for the Clinical Document Architecture (CDA). The CDA is not a full EHR specification, but it forms an important subcomponent of the EHR and is broadly compatible with the equivalent EHR subcomponents in CEN 13606-1 and *open*EHR.

The CDA was not initiated as an EHR project but rather as a means of identifying and tracking the numerous clinical documents that are created and transmitted every day in the US as part of the transcription process. CDA release 1.0 was completed in 2003.[17,18] An XML specification with no formal data model, it standardized the headers of clinical documents, in order to safely communicate and identify unstructured clinical documents. There have been a number of successful implementation projects of release 1 in the US and other countries. However, it was recognized within HL7 that substantial value could be added to the CDA by including further structures within the clinical document.

Release 2 of CDA was completed in 2005. It contains two further levels of structure in addition to the document header: Sections, which contain semantics for clinical headings reflecting the workflow and consultation/reasoning process; and Entries, which contain the semantics for clinical statements and detailed structures for data. Release 2 also has its own UML model and a formal mapping to the HL7 RIM. The CEN EN13606-1 Reference Model has been harmonized to CDA release 2.

EHR Persistent Data Storage Standards

There are at present no model-based standards for persistent EHR data storage. Despite the absence of any standards in this area, there is increasing recognition that high-level interoperability may be dependent on data stored in standardized format to facilitate sharing. The EN13606-1 Reference Model comes closest but has several limitations. Designed as a standard for EHR extracts, not as a standard for persistent EHRs, it does not define the semantics of the EHR as a whole. Moreover, it may offer too much optionality for storage. For example, its Entry class is appropriate for communication of EHR extracts but is too generic for persistent EHRs (e.g., it does not contain classes for Observation, Evaluation, and Instruction and does not support lists, trees, and tables). It also has incomplete version control as it does not support change sets (contributions).

The *open*EHR specification contains all of the necessary semantics for EHR storage as well as exchange and is likely to form the basis for the European, Australian, and perhaps international standard.

Interface Standards: Messaging and Common Services

Messaging

Messaging standards such as HL7, DICOM, and the United Nations Electronic Data Interchange standard, UN/Edifact, have crucial roles for interoperability between medical devices, other health IT systems, and components of EHR-Ss (e.g., laboratory, radiology, pharmacy) and EHR-Ss or between two nonstandardized EHR-Ss (i.e., EHR-Ss not sharing the same information model). Messaging standards will always be necessary for laboratory, imaging, and pharmacy orders and results because laboratory and similar systems do not contain/operate on patient-centered EHRs (this is neither their primary purpose nor operationally efficient).[8]

The Venn diagram seen in Figure 12-2 illustrates that health service messaging has a much larger domain than the EHR. Patient administration, billing, and materials management are examples of areas within the scope of messaging but generally considered to be outside the scope of the EHR. Currently, messaging interfaces are point-to-point interfaces that require developers from each system to pre-agree on coding conventions and program their systems to send and receive based on the pre-agreements. Current messaging standards lack the specificity to prevent customization based on the developer level point-to-point agreements. This makes it difficult to interface with multiple partners because of variability of conventions that must be accommodated with each new partner.

Laboratory tests, radiology, and pharmacy are examples of areas where both messaging and the EHR have a role in communication. As stated above, messaging is necessary in these areas when placing orders and receiving results but the results could then be communicated to another standards-based EHR-S more easily and efficiently using EHR extracts rather than messages.

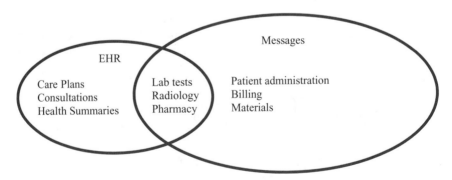

Figure 12-2. Venn diagram of health service messaging.

Common Services

Service interface standards are required to ensure that the various components of an integrated clinical information system (e.g., demographics, terminology, access control/security) can interoperate with the core EHR service. A number of open specifications for health service interfaces have been developed by the OMG. HL7 is currently developing a Clinical Terminology Service (CTS) and may build other service specifications in the future. CEN/TC 251 is currently revising its prestandard ENV12967, "Health Informatics Service Architecture" (HISA).[19]

CEN EN 12967 HISA. The CEN HISA*** is a three-part standard. HISA defines a high-level architecture which is applicable to the whole health informatics space. It "sits above" and is compatible with standards such as EN13606 and the HL7 RIM.

The revised standard uses the methodology of the ISO RM-ODP (Reference Model for Open Distributed Processing) standard[20] which defines a service-based architecture for distributed systems and five viewpoints within this architecture: Enterprise, Information, Computational, Engineering, and Technology.

HISA uses the first three of these viewpoints:

- Part 1—Enterprise (business) viewpoint: Aims to describe the business context in which the system will reside, by identifying the user activities being supported, the objectives and limits of the system, and the expected benefits.
- Part 2—Information viewpoint: Describes the information being managed by the system and their mutual relationships, both within the local business context and with respect to the relevance outside of the system (if any).
- Part 3—Computational (functional) viewpoint: Describes the functions of the system with respect to the services and interactions between the system and the rest of the "world."

The three-part HISA standard will provide a reference model for healthcare IT services, facilitating the building and purchasing of interoperable systems. Its focus is on intraorganization communication (which may be geographically dispersed), but it can also be used for interorganization communication.

OMG Health Domain Task Force (HDTF) Clinical Observation Access Service (COAS). The OMG HDTF (previously known as CORBAmed) (http://healthcare.omg.org) is another SDO that has produced interface standard specifications. Its EHR interface specification is known as the COAS.[21] This is a set of interfaces and data structures through which a server can supply clinical observations from an EHR.

*** See http://www.centc251.org/WGI/WGIdoclist.htm. Accessed December 12, 2005.

The OMG HDTF has also completed health interface specifications for other services such as demographics (PIDS—Person Identification Service), terminology (LQS—Lexicon Query Service), Security (RAD—Resource Access Decision), and Imaging (CIAS—Clinical Image Access Service).

Unfortunately, these services have not been widely implemented and some are now in need of revision. A new activity that has promise to facilitate future work on services interfaces is a memorandum of understanding between OMG and HL7 that was signed in 2004. This cooperative activity will make the HL7 RIM available to OMG and make the OMG technologies available to HL7 development groups.

Clinical Content and Dataset Standards

Meta-data Standards

Archetypes as meta-data specifications. A new class of EHR standards, meta-data specifications, may be viewed as the previously "missing link" between the reference model and terminology in the quest for semantic interoperability in health information management. The key artifact in this group of standards is archetypes.[16,22–27] A descriptive definition of an archetype is "a model of a clinical or other domain-specific concept which defines the structure and business rules of the concept" whereas a more technical definition is "a computable expression of a domain-level concept in the form of structured constraint statements, based on some reference information model."[6] Archetypes may define simple concepts such as "blood pressure" or "address," or more complex compound concepts such as "family history" or "microbiology results." Archetypes have so far been built for a number of different reference models including *open*EHR, CEN EN13606-1, HL7 CDA, and the HL7 V3 Refined Message Information Models (R-MIMs), which constrain the classes and relationships required to express a specific closely related set of actions within a single domain under the HL7 RIM. CEN EN 13606 part 2 will incorporate Archetype Interchange Specification while part 3 will cover and Reference Archetypes and Term Lists.

HL7 templates specification. HL7 templates have a very similar meaning to CEN/*open*EHR archetypes, but their development is currently at an earlier stage than archetypes and there are as yet no balloted standards or software tools to build HL7 templates. CEN and *open*EHR also use the term "template" but with a somewhat different meaning which has unfortunately caused some confusion in the standards and health informatics communities. In CEN and *open*EHR, templates are structured collections of archetypes used to narrow the choices of archetypes for local or specific purposes such as a screen data entry form.

EHR Data Content Specifications

In the past, some SDOs have attempted to define the EHR through the exhaustive and prescriptive specification of data content. This is a daunting task given the huge number of clinical concepts [more than 300,000 in the Systematized Nomenclature of Medicine Clinical Terms (SNOMED-CT) alone]. If such a specification could be achieved, it would be rapidly out of date and would drastically restrict flexibility and usability of EHR-Ss. A far more achievable and flexible goal is the definition and specification of a limited set of key clinical concepts (a few thousand), together with appropriate terminologies, placed into standardized knowledge models (called archetypes or templates). Clearly, there is a need for standardized minimum datasets for disease and other clinical registries. There is also utility in developing a standardized core dataset for the EHR that can be extracted and exchanged in a standard manner. The ASTM Continuity of Care Record (CCR) is one important project in this area.

Continuity of Care Record. The CCR[28] is a standard specification jointly developed by ASTM, Healthcare Information Management Systems Society (HIMSS), and several medical groups including the Massachusetts Medical Society, American Academy of Family Physicians, American Academy of Pediatrics, and the American Medical Association (AMA). This standard has already been balloted; the implementation guide was balloted in March 2005. The CCR is "a core dataset of the most relevant and timely facts about a patient. . . . It includes a summary of the patient's health status (e.g., problems, medications, allergies) and basic information about insurance, advance directives, care documentation, and care plan recommendations." The CCR has accelerated its timeline to implementation because of a memorandum of understanding between ASTM and HL7 to achieve an HL7 CDA V2 transport mechanism for this important dataset.[8]

Framework (Meta) Standards

This group consists of high-level standards, in support of what the RM/ODP terms the Enterprise view. These meta standards include the ISO Health Indicators Conceptual Framework, the ISO Health Informatics Profiling Framework, and the ISO Emergency Data Sets Framework (EDSF). An EHR Enterprise Architecture standard covering the scope, policies, and high-level (conceptual/enterprise) architecture for the data management and knowledge management components of the EHR would be another example of an EHR meta standard.

Although these standards tend to be non-normative technical reports, they can serve a useful and important function in the broader EHR standards context. For example, the EDSF[29] [ISO/DTR 22219 2004] presents an approach for the classification of health informatics datasets. More specifically, it aims to provide a standard method for defining and classifying datasets within the domain of emergency care. It establishes a common vocabulary and perspective in the form of a framework for describing the complex domain of emergency medical care and its supporting datasets. Thus, the EDSF is a guide for how to build a good quality emergency dataset. This is a common feature of most framework "standards" in health informatics and is frequently used in the field of HCR (i.e., how to build a good quality terminology or classification).

Special Interest Standards

The development of EHR standards for particular technologies, health sectors, and/or stakeholders should be undertaken only where absolutely necessary to avoid the problem of incompatibility between "special purpose" and "generic" EHR standards. There should be no reason, for example, to develop an EHR architecture standard for a personal health record (PHR) that differs from that of a generic EHR architecture standard. Although a consumer/patient with a PHR and a physician using a hospital electronic medical record clearly have different requirements for data input and presentation, the needs of both end users can be accommodated by a single standardized generic EHR architecture. This will have the major benefit of enabling sharing of information (i.e., interoperability) between the PHR and the electronic medical record versions of the EHR, if and when appropriate, and with appropriate privacy and security measures in place.

Special interest EHR standards arise when there is no relevant generic standard or when the requirements of a technology, health sector, or stakeholder group cannot be met by a more generic standard. Development of the current set of EHR standards for Health Cards within ISO/TC 215 responds to both conditions:

- The need to standardize specific aspects of Health Card use that are unique to the Health Card technology
- The lack of an adequate generic standard for this EHR architecture that the Health Card standardization group can adopt

Thus, it may be necessary eventually to modify this aspect of the Health Card standards to comply with the architecture of a more generic EHR standard when it becomes available.

The ISO 21549 Patient Healthcard Data standard[30] is an eight-part suite consisting of (1) general structure; (2) common objects; (3) limited clinical data; (4) extended clinical data; (5) identification data; (6) administrative data; (7) electronic prescription; and (8) links. The first three parts have been completed and are now full international standards; the other five parts are at various stages of progress.

EHR Enabling Standards

Demographics Standards

There are as yet few health-specific demographic standards at the international or even the national level. Although generic demographic standards are available, the health industry has special needs because people (patients) are the core business of health care. In most other industries, such as banking, insurance, manufacturing, and telecommunications, people are ancillary to the workflow.

Subject of Care (Patient) Identification

Australia was one of the first countries to issue a national standard for patient identification. Its identification standard, AS5017, "provides a framework for improving the positive identification of clients in health care organizations. . . . It defines demographic and other identifying data elements suited to capture and use for client identification in health care settings, provides guidance on their application, and provides an overview of data matching strategies. It also makes recommendations about the nature and form of health care identifiers."[31]

The Australian standard does not assume or depend on the availability of a Unique Patient Identifier (UPI), although it recognizes that such identifiers can significantly improve positive identification and matching. In many countries, including the US, considerable political sensitivity surrounds the introduction of UPIs. Only a few countries have yet implemented national UPIs, for example, the United Kingdom and New Zealand.

An ISO standard for "Identification of Subjects of Health Care" (ISO/DTS 22220) is currently under development, using the Australian standard as its starting point.

The OMG PIDS[32] is a health-specific model-based demographic service interface specification and as such is different from but complementary to identification standards such as AS5017.

Provider Identification (Clinicians, Organizations, Locations)

Australia has been one of the first countries to issue a provider identification standard. It is similar in structure to the Australian Client Identification standard and can be used to identify individual providers (physicians, allied health professionals, etc.) and organization providers (hospitals, ambulatory clinics, laboratories, pharmacies, etc.) including location details. However, the standard ". . . includes only the minimum dataset required for unambiguous identification. It is recognized that specific applications such as provider directories or service locators will require additional data to fulfill their purposes. The Standard provides a generic set of identifying information which is application independent."[33]

ISO/TC 215 has commenced the development of an international provider identification standard, using inputs such as the Canadian and Australian provider ID standards as inputs.

Country Identification

With increasing globalization and international travel, together with the emergence of national and potentially transnational shared EHR initiatives, there is a need to be able to uniquely identify countries as well as providers and patients. An ever-increasing number of people in a variety of categories (e.g., business, tourism, military, refugees) will require emergency and short-term healthcare services outside of their own country and will benefit from the timely availability of information from their home-country EHR.

ISO/TC 215 has developed a country identification standard[34] which gives guidance to healthcare providers on the appropriate use for healthcare purposes of the two main generic international country identifier standards.

HCR Standards

A broad field, HCR includes terminologies, vocabularies/nomenclatures, classifications, and ontologies. It may also include nontextual modes of concept representation such as pictures, symbols, icons, and graphs.

The majority of formal SDO consensus standards in the field of HCR are meta-standards, i.e., frameworks and standards about how to build good quality terminologies, etc. There are very few formal standards for structure and content of specific terminologies, vocabularies, and classifications, although there are a number that can be regarded as de facto standards.

HCR Meta-standards

The first ISO HCR meta-standard was "controlled health terminology— structure and high-level indicators"[35] (ISO/TS 17117). It consists of a set of definitions of terms frequently used in the field of terminology and quality indicators for controlled health terminologies. Its scope is the specification of ". . . the principal ideas which are necessary and sufficient to assign value to a controlled health terminology. It is applicable to all areas of healthcare about which information is kept or utilized."

In contrast, the second published ISO HCR meta-standard relates to a health subdiscipline, "integration of a reference terminology model for nursing"[36] (ISO 18104). Other ISO HCR meta-standards under development include "conceptual framework for patient findings and problems in terminologies" and "vocabulary for terminological systems." A less technical and very useful adaptation of ISO/TS 17115 for nonexperts with an interest in HCR is the Australian standard "the language of health concept representation."[37]

Archetypes and Micro-vocabularies

Terminology is perhaps the most problematic area within the field of EHR enabling standards. Many health terminologies have been developed or have grown from an original core in a rather haphazard way, hence the need for terminology meta-standards for the future development of better quality terminologies. Many large terminologies are "polluted" by a combinatorial explosion of precoordinated terms in addition to core atomic terms, making them difficult to use and sometimes problematic when terms are postcoordinated in EHR-Ss for decision support and other applications.

Another significant problem with current terminologies, particularly large reference terminologies, is that most are proprietary. To ensure at least de facto standard status, it is necessary for such proprietary terminologies to be available to healthcare providers everywhere, usually through a national license.

The advent of archetypes and micro-vocabularies means that significant interoperability of patient information can be achieved without having to wait for the "big terminology problem" to be solved. HL7 has already developed some 400 micro-vocabularies to populate HL7 messages from its Clinical Terminology Service. CEN is adopting the same strategy for naming nodes of archetypes and populating list variables within archetypes. These micro-vocabularies enable a significant degree of interoperability without any reliance on the availability of external terminologies. However, they can be bound to any available external terminology such as SNOMED or Logical Observation Identifier Name Codes (LOINC) at run-time. Comprehensive reference terminologies will still be required for large groups of terms such as diagnoses, laboratory tests, and anatomic terms.

Core and Related Terminologies

In 2000, in its advisory capacity to the Secretary of Health and Human Services (HHS), the National Committee on Vital and Health Statistics (NCVHS) called for "the adoption of uniform data standards for patient medical record information (PMRI) and the electronic exchange of such information." In subsequent recommendations, NCVHS specified message format standards and identified a core set of clinical data terminology standards that included SNOMED-CT, LOINC, RxNorm, and NDF-RT (details appear below). NCVHS stressed that a cohesive, internally consistent terminology resource requires integration of these core terminologies through the creation of relationships within the Unified Medical Language System maintained by the National Library of Medicine. The relationships should be maintained in concert with changes to the constituent terminologies.

In addition, NCVHS recommended that the federal government recognize a number of "important related terminologies" not included in the core set of PMRI standards. NCVHS asserted that because these terminologies will continue to be used, compatibility of the core set of PMRI terminologies with them would be key to enhancing the value and accelerating the adoption of the PMRI terminology standards. Thus, NCVHS recommended mapping to the important related terminologies in two groups prioritized as follows:

Priority 1: Terminologies previously designated as Health Insurance Portability and Accountability Act (HIPAA) medical code sets:
- CPT-4 (Current Procedural Terminology)
- CDT (Current Dental Terminology)
- Level II HCPCS (Healthcare Common Procedure Coding System)
- ICD-9-CM (International Classification of Diseases—Clinical Modification)
- NDC (National Drug Codes)

Priority 2: Terminologies in common use as enablers of important healthcare functions. These terminologies include but are not necessarily limited to:
- DSM-IV (diagnosis codes for mental disorders)
- Terminologies in private sector drug information databases (e.g., First-Databank NDDF Plus, Medi-Span, Micromedex, Multum Lexicon)
- ISBT 128 (coding system for describing blood products and tissues)
- Medcin (codes for structured entry of clinical notes)
- MedDRA (international code set for use by drug regulatory agencies)
- Nursing terminologies not otherwise included in SNOMED-CT

Consolidated Health Informatics Initiative

As part of the Consolidated Health Informatics (CHI) initiative, HHS and the Departments of Defense and Veterans Affairs joined with other federal agencies to identify appropriate, existing data standards and endorse them for use across the federal healthcare sector. In 2003, CHI identified its first set of five standards, including the following:

- HL7 messaging standards (see Interoperability section).
- National Council on Prescription Drug Programs (NCPDP) SCRIPT standards for communicating electronic prescribing information between prescribers and dispensers. The dispensers in this case are commercial and retail pharmacies. The NCPDP SCRIPT standards complement the NCPDP telecommunications standards which were previously selected as standards under HIPAA. The NCPDP telecommunication standards are the message format standards that transmit healthcare claims between commercial and retail pharmacies and payers/PBMs.
- Institute of Electrical and Electronics Engineers 1073 (IEEE 1073)[38] is a set of medical device communication standards also known as ISO 11073 standards. These standards communicate patient data from medical devices typically found in acute and chronic care environments (e.g., patient monitors, ventilators, and infusion pumps).

- DICOM (see Chapter 16)
- LOINC to standardize the electronic exchange of clinical laboratory results.[39]

In 2004, CHI identified 15 further standards. Federal agencies agreeing to these standards will use them as they develop and implement new IT systems. These standards are:

- HL7 vocabulary standards for demographic information, units of measure, immunizations, and clinical encounters, and HL7's CDA standard for text-based reports. (Five standards)
- SNOMED-CT[40] for laboratory result contents, nonlaboratory interventions and procedures, anatomy, diagnosis and problems, and nursing. A division of The College of American Pathology, SNOMED has been recognized by ANSI as an accredited SDO. The National Library of Medicine has made SNOMED-CT available for use in the US at no charge to users. (Five standards)
- LOINC to standardize the electronic exchange of laboratory test orders and drug label section headers. (One standard)
- HIPAA transactions and code sets for electronic exchange of health-related information to perform billing or administrative functions. These are the same standards now required under HIPAA for health plans, healthcare clearinghouses, and those healthcare providers who engage in certain electronic transactions. (One standard)
- A set of federal terminologies related to medications, including the Food and Drug Administration's (FDA's) names and codes for ingredients, manufactured dosage forms, drug products and medication packages, the National Library of Medicine's RxNORM[41] for describing clinical drugs, and the Veterans Administration's National Drug File Reference Terminology (NDF-RT) for specific drug classifications. (One standard)
- The Human Gene Nomenclature (HUGN)[42] for exchanging information regarding the role of genes in biomedical research in the federal health sector. (One standard)
- The Environmental Protection Agency's Substance Registry System for nonmedicinal chemicals of importance to health care.[43] (One standard)

Classifications

Generally used for statistical, reimbursement, and other secondary uses of EHR data, classifications are of less use for direct patient care. They are usually less granular than clinical terminologies and lack the rich semantic networks needed to underpin computerized decision support. There are hundreds of health classifications in use around the world, with the majority of them being used for subdomain classifications such as procedures or specialist disease coding, for example, for cancer.

The best known, oldest, and most widely used classification in health is the International Classification of Diseases (ICD-10). The origins of ICD go back as far as the eighteenth century and the statistical bills of mortality, but the first official version of ICD was issued in 1893. The current endorsed version of ICD is ICD-10,[44] but the US still uses a modification of the previous ICD-9 version[45] [ICD-9-CM 2005]. A modified version of ICD-10 for use in the US is currently in preparation.

The World Health Organization (WHO) Family of Classifications includes the ICD series and the International Classification of Functioning, Disability, & Health (ICF).[46] In 2003, the International Classification of Primary Care (ICPC)[47] was added to the WHO Family of Classifications.

Privacy and Security Standards

Most people consider their personal health information more sensitive than their banking, taxation, or social security information. Ultimately, the success of any EHR-S will depend on public trust, on patients and providers trusting in the system's ability to protect the privacy and security of personal health information. Open consensus standards, together with legislation where appropriate, are an essential underpinning for a health information privacy and security framework.

Privacy

The protection of privacy of health information in most countries has largely been through legislation and privacy codes developed by governments, rather than SDO-developed consensus standards. Many countries rely on generic privacy legislation to cover health as well as all other industries such as taxation, social security, finance, and telecommunications. However, the rapid growth in e-health clinical information systems over the past few years has fueled an increasing trend for governments to enact health-specific privacy legislation such as the HIPAA in the US. There are also increasing numbers of government-developed and monitored health information privacy codes, some of which carry significant penalties for privacy breaches in both the public and private sectors.

Where there are SDO-developed health information privacy standards, they tend to be broad privacy frameworks that complement the more detailed and prescriptive privacy codes and legislative acts. There are currently no international standards available for health information privacy.

One example of a national standard in this area is the Australian Standard "Personal Privacy Protection in Health Care Information Systems" published in 1995.[48] This has been well accepted in Australia and has been useful in framing both health information privacy legislation and privacy codes that have since been developed.

Security

It is often thought that the security requirements for standards and systems for health information should be no different from those for information in any other industry. This is unfortunately only partially true because the special privacy requirements for health information have implications for security systems as well, particularly in the area of access control to personal health information held in EHRs and other health repositories. The role-based access models and policies being developed for health are generally different and more complex than those of most other industries.

The first international health information security standard was the ISO Public Key Infrastructure standard published in 2002 as a Technical Specification and now being upgraded to a full ISO International Standard.[49] This was followed by "Guidelines on Data Protection to Facilitate Transborder Flow of Personal Health Information."[50] Other important health informatics security standards currently under development are "Health Informatics Privilege Management & Access Control,"[51] Health Informatics Functional & Structural Roles,"[52] and "Health Informatics Guidelines for Backup & Restore/Recovery."[53]

The only international service interface standard for security is the OMG "Resource Access Definition" specification.[54]

Clinical Decision Support Standards

To date, work on formal clinical decision support (CDS) standards has been limited. As of this writing, neither ISO/TC 215 nor CEN/TC 251 has any group working in this area. HL7 has a CDS Technical Committee and is one of the very few SDOs currently active in the CDS field. It has so far produced one CDS ANSI standard, for the Arden Syntax[55] for Medical Logic Systems.

A rule-based method for specifying decision support guidelines, Arden Syntax was first developed in 1989, making it one of the first CDS methods. HL7 is also working on standardizing other CDS methods such as GLIF (Guideline Interchange Format),[56] a computer-interpretable language for modeling and executing clinical guidelines, and GELLO,[57] an object-oriented query and expression language for CDS, derived from GLIF. ASTM has also produced an ANSI standard, the Guideline Elements Model (GEM), an XML-based guideline document model.[58] Details regarding specific CDS approaches are provided in Chapter 7.

Patient Safety and Quality of Care Standards

In the absence of definitive international standards for patient safety and quality of care, healthcare associations and agencies in the US have developed an array of measures, including quality indicators, datasets, guidelines, and barcodes.[59]

Quality Indicators

"Standards" in this domain comprise standard measuring tools and approaches. In what is called the ORYX initiative,[60] the Joint Commission on Accreditation of Health Care Organizations (JCAHO) developed a set of quality indicators for acute myocardial infarction, heart failure, community-acquired pneumonia, and pregnancy and related conditions.

The AMA developed clinical performance measurement tools.[61] Derived from evidence-based clinical guidelines, these tools can be used by physicians to gather data from their own practice, measure their own level of performance, and ultimately enhance the care of their patients. Measurement sets are available for many chronic diseases.

Datasets

The Health Plan Employer Data and Information Set (HEDIS)[62] developed by the National Committee for Quality Assurance (NCQA) includes quality performance measures for osteoporosis, urinary incontinence, colorectal cancer, appropriate use of antibiotics, and chemical dependency in its 2004 dataset.

Guidelines

Over the last few years, practice guidelines/parameters have been developed by national, regional, and local organizations, such as professional associations, government agencies, providers, consulting firms, and vendors. The Agency for Healthcare Research and Quality (AHRQ) maintains the National Guideline Clearinghouse (NCG).[63] Developed in partnership with the AMA and the American Association of Health Plans, the Clearinghouse is a publicly available database of evidence-based clinical practice guidelines and related documents.

Bar Codes

In 2003, the FDA proposed drug bar code regulations to help reduce medical errors related to prescriptions and medication administration. These regulations would standardize and require the use of bar codes on prescription drugs, over-the-counter drugs packaged for hospital use, and vaccines. The final rule covers blood and blood components.[64] ANSI has given the Health Industry Business Communications Council (HIBCC)[65] accreditation as the SDO for bar codes used for human drug products and blood.

Information Technology Standards Enablement

ASTM, HL7, DICOM, X12, and other standards organizations realized, in the mid-1990s, that they were in many cases running side by side and in some cases were exchanging similar kinds of data. The increasing number and broadening implementation of standards raised several concerns. Common data such as patient demographics were being defined in multiple standards, often with widely varying structures and constraints. Moreover, it was not always clear what standards were most appropriate for certain kinds of application data: For example, should X12 or HL7 be used for financial data? And except in the case of DICOM, little guidance was offered to implementers or software vendors who wished to issue fully constrained specifications or to make conformance assertions.

Fortunately, standards bodies usually recognized the need at least to be aware of one another's work. In the case of DICOM, imaging standards developers and implementers went a step further. They recognized that DICOM and HL7 existed side by side in many implementations. Lest interoperation cause harm or disruption, it was important that, for elements used throughout the healthcare delivery organization, common definitions (preferably) and mappings (if necessary) be available, and furthermore that a common transaction profile format be available and easily constrainable into a site or product specification.

Integrating the Healthcare Enterprise Initiative

With these requirements in mind, a group of IT professionals and clinicians from the Radiological Society of North America (RSNA) and HIMSS joined forces in 1998 in the Integrating the Healthcare Enterprise (IHE) Initiative.[66] IHE produced in 1999 the first of the Radiology Technical Framework (TF) documents. The IHE Radiology TF, which is revised annually, profiles workflows in the imaging domain and presents a common specification template for DICOM and HL7 standards. Importantly, IHE also provides mappings between the standards for such common elements as patient name.

IHE workflows have been demonstrated to a broad and enthusiastic audience at the annual HIMSS meetings every year since its inception. Starting in 2002, the IHE Radiology TF adopted standards beyond HL7 and DICOM. It now includes support for standards developed by the Internet Engineering Task Force (IETF), the International Telecommunication Union (ITU), the Network Time Protocol (NTP) project, ASTM, and the World Wide Web Consortium (W3C). Additionally, starting in 2003, IHE technical framework documents were developed or published in the Laboratory, IT Infrastructure, and Cardiology domains, and additional work was planned for the domains of Nuclear Medicine, Ambulatory Medicine, and Pharmacy.

EHR-Ss in the Near Future

Around the globe, national initiatives for EHR-S adoption and interoperability are forcing the standards community to deliver standards solution that are robust, scalable, and able to carry specific information across EHR-Ss without losing or changing the original information or its context. Achieving this demands continued cooperation and collaboration among, between, and even within standards organizations. Increased collaboration will benefit the production of uniform standards by allowing re-use of standards products that work well, thereby decreasing variation across standards organizations and their products. Increased cooperation will also help detect "black holes" in the standards landscape. In the near future, standards communities will be challenged to meet the need for:

- Standardized data models that are understandable by multiple systems
- Common services architecture as the framework for interoperability
- Common data elements, templates, and archetypes

Consumers will become increasingly involved as the EHR begins to populate the PHR. Some see a future in which all health data will be owned by individuals, as their personal finances are now kept in banks of their choosing. Others believe consumers will be specifically targeted for research clinical trials based on recent diagnoses entered electronically, or for reimbursement by drug companies and others willing to pay for access to a subset of patient data at the time a specific drug is ordered. Still more see the EHR-S used for population health surveillance and bioterrorism detection. The challenges and the opportunities are daunting.

The EHR-S industry is experiencing a period of unprecedented rapid growth and innovation. The dynamism of the commercial health IT sector is likely to affect the standards industry. Some standards now considered essential and mandatory may quickly be outmoded; others now on the fringe or not yet conceived could rapidly become accepted standards. The standards communities and standards organizations that support health care must be nimble, strategic, and open to the constantly changing demands coming to them from the healthcare industry.

References

1. Ball MJ, Collen MF, eds. Aspects of the Computer-based Patient Record. New York: Springer-Verlag; 2002:4,300.
2. ISO/TC 215. International Standards Organization, Health Informatics Technical Committee 215. 2004. Available at: www.iso.ch/iso/en/stdsdevelopment/tc/tclist/TechnicalCommitteeDetailPage.TechnicalCommitteeDetail?COMMID=4720. Accessed December 12, 2005.
3. CEN/TC 251. European Committee for Standardization, Health Informatics Technical Committee 251 (CEN/TC 251). 2005. Available at: www.centc251.org. Accessed December 12, 2005.

4. HL7. Health Level Seven Inc. 2005. Available at: www.hl7.org. Accessed December 17, 2005.
5. Institute of Medicine. Committee on Improving the Patient Record. The Computer Based Patient Record: An Essential Technology for Healthcare. Washington, DC: National Academy Press; 1991.
6. Health Informatics—Electronic Health Record: Definition, Scope and Context. ISO Technical Report. ISO/TR 20514. Geneva: ISO; 2005.
7. Schloeffel P, Jeselon P. Standards Requirements for the Electronic Health Record and Discharge/Referral Plans. ISO/TC 215 EHR Ad Hoc Group. Final Report; 26 July 2002.
8. Dickinson G, Fischetti L, Heard S, eds. HL7 Electronic Health Record System Functional Model Draft Standard for Trial Use. July 2004.
9. Digital Imaging and Communication in Medicine (DICOM), PS 3. Rosslyn, VA: National Electronic Manufacturer's Association; 2004.
10. Pratt D, Schadow G, ed. Version 3 Data Types [ballot draft]. Ann Arbor, MI: Health Level Seven; 2001.
11. Health Informatics. Data Types. Document number: BS DD CEN/TS 14796. British Standard; 2004.
12. CEN/TC 251. Health Informatics—Data Types. European Committee for Standardization, Health Informatics Technical Committee 251. TS 14796; 2004.
13. ISO/TC215. Health Informatics—Requirements for an Electronic Health Record Architecture. ISO/TS 18308. Geneva: ISO; 2004.
14. Beale T. Mapping of *open*EHR to ISO/WD 18308. Requirements for an EHR Reference Architecture. Version 1.4. March 2003.
15. Health Informatics—Electronic Health Record Communication. Part 1. Reference Architecture. CEN prEN13606-1. Brussels: CEN; 2004.
16. Beale T. Archetypes: Constraint-based Domain Models for Future-proof Information Systems. OOPSLA Workshop on Behavioural Semantics. 2002. http://www.openehr.org/downloads/archetypes/archetypes_new.pdf. Accessed December 12, 2005.
17. Dolin RH, Alschuler L, Beebe C, et al. The HL7 clinical document architecture. J Am Med Inform Assoc 2001;8(6):552–569.
18. Alschuler L, Dolin RH, Boyer S, Beebe C, eds. Clinical Document Architecture Framework Release 1.0. Ann Arbor, MI: Health Level Seven; 2000.
19. CEN/TC 251. Health Informatics—Health Informatics Systems Architecture. European Committee for Standardization, Health Informatics Technical Comittee 251. prEN 2005;12967:1–3.
20. JTC 1/SC 7. Information Technology: Open Distributed Processing—Reference Model: Overview. ISO/IEC 10746-1. Geneva: ISO; 1998.
21. OMG COAS. Clinical Observation Access Service (COAS) Specification. Object Management Group, Healthcare Domain Task Force. Version 1.0. April 2001. Available at: http://www.omg.org/technology/documents/formal/clinical_observation_access_service.htm. Accessed December 12, 2005.
22. Beale T, Heard S, eds. Archetype Definitions and Principles. Rev 0.6, March 2005. Available at: http://svn.openehr.org/specification/TRUNK/publishing/index.html. Accessed December 12, 2005.
23. Beale T, Heard S, eds. The Archetype Object Model. Rev 0.6, June 2005. Available at: http://svn.openehr.org/specification/TRUNK/publishing/index.htm. Accessed December 12, 2005.

24. Beale T, Heard S, eds. The *open*EHR Archetype System. Rev 0.3.1, December 2003. Available at: http://svn.openehr.org/specification/TRUNK/publishing/index.html. Accessed December 12, 2005.

25. Beale T, Heard S, eds. The Archetype Definition Language (ADL). Rev 1.3, June 2005. Available at: http://svn.openehr.org/specification/TRUNK/publishing/index.html. Accessed December 12, 2005.

26. Beale T, Heard S. A Shared Archetype and Template Language Part I. Rev 0.3, May 2003. http://svn.openehr.org/specification/TRUNK/architecture/am/language/language_design/archetype_language_1v0.3.doc. Accessed December 12, 2005.

27. Beale T., Heard S. A Shared Archetype and Template Language Part II. Rev 0.7, December 2005. http://svn.openehr.org/specification/TRUNK/architecture/am/language/language_design/archetype_language_2v0.7.doc. Accessed December 12, 2005.

28. ASTM E31.28. WK4363 Standard Specification for the Continuity of Care Record (CCR). West Conshohocken, PA: ASTM; 2005. Available at: www.astm.org. Accessed December 18, 2005.

29. ISO/TC215 WG1. Health Informatics—Emergency Data Sets Framework. ISO 22219. Geneva: ISO; 2004.

30. ISO/TC 215. Health Informatics—Patient Healthcard Data. ISO 21549:1–8. Geneva: ISO; 2005.

31. Standards Australia. Health Care Client Identification. AS5017.2002. Sydney: Standards Australia; 2002. Available at: http://www.standards.com.au/catalogue/script/details.asp?DocN=AS675618737075. Accessed December 12, 2005.

32. OMG PIDS. 2001. Person Identification Service (PIDS) Specification. Object Management Group, Healthcare Domain Task Force. Version 1.1. April 2001. Available at: http://www.omg.org/cgi-bin/doc?formal/2001-04-04. Accessed June 6, 2005.

33. AS4846. Health Care Provider Identification. Australian Standard. 2004. Available at: http://www.standards.com.au/catalogue/script/details.asp?DocN=AS0733758487AT. Accessed December 12, 2005.

34. ISO/TC 215. Health Informatics—Country Identifier Standards. ISO/TS 17120. Geneva: ISO; 2004.

35. ISO/TC 215. Health Informatics—Controlled Health Terminology. Structure and High-level Indicators. ISO/TS 17117. Geneva: ISO; 2002.

36. ISO/TC 215. Health Informatics—Integration of a Reference Terminology Model for Nursing. ISO 18104. Geneva: ISO; 2003.

37. AS 5021-2005. The Language of Health Concept Representation. Sydney: SAI Global; 2005. Available at: http://www.standards.com.au/catalogue/script/details.asp?DocN=AS0733767486AT. Accessed June 30, 2005.

38. IEEE 1073: Medical Device Communications. IEEE 1073, 2005. Available at: http://www.ieee1073.org/. Accessed December 12, 2005.

39. Logical Observation Identifiers Names and Codes (LOINC®). Indianapolis: Regenstrief Institute; 2004. Available at: http://www.regenstrief.org/loinc/. Accessed June 7, 2005.

40. SNOMED International. Welcome. Northfield, IL: Snomed International; 2005. Available at: http://www.snomed.org/. Accessed December 17, 2005.

41. RxNORM. Bethesda: National Library of Medicine; 2005. Available at: http://www.nlm.nih.gov/research/umls/rxnorm_main.html. Accessed December 17, 2005.

42. Wain HM, Bruford EA, Lovering RC, et al. Guidelines for human gene nomenclature. Genomics 2002;79(4):464–470. Available at: http://www.gene.ucl.ac.uk/nomenclature/guidelines.html. Accessed December 17, 2005.
43. Substance Registry System. Washington, DC: US EPA; 2004. Available at: http://www.epa.gov/srs/. Accessed December 17, 2005.
44. International Classification of Diseases (ICD). Geneva: World Health Organization; 2005. Available at: http://www.who.int/classifications/icd/en/. Accessed December 17, 2005.
45. International Classification of Diseases. 9th Revision. Clinical Modification (ICD-9-CM). Hyattsville, MD: National Center for Health Statistics; 2005. Available at: http://www.cdc.gov/nchs/about/otheract/icd9/abticd9.htm. Accessed December 12, 2005.
46. WHO. The World Health Family of Classifications. World Health Organization. 2005. Available at: http://www.who.int/classification/. Accessed December 12, 2005.
47. WONCA. International Classification of Primary Care. World Organization of Family Doctors. 2005. Available at: http://www.globalfamilydoctor.com/. Accessed December 12, 2005.
48. Personal Privacy Protection in Health Care Information Systems. Canberra: Australian Standard AS4400; 1995.
49. ISO/TC 205. Health Informatics—Public Key Infrastructure. Parts 1–3. ISO Technical Specification. ISO/TS 17090. Geneva: ISO; 2002.
50. ISO/TC 205. Guidelines on Data Protection to Facilitate Trans-border Flow of Personal Health Information. ISO International Standard. ISO 22857. Geneva: ISO; 2004.
51. ISO/TC 215. Health Informatics—Privilege Management and Access Control. ISO Draft Technical Specification. ISO/DTS 22600. Geneva: ISO; 2005.
52. ISO/TC 215. Health Informatics—Functional and Structural Roles. ISO/DTS 21298. Geneva: ISO; 2005.
53. ISO/TC 215. Health Informatics—Guidelines for Backup and Restore/Recovery. DTR 21547. Geneva: ISO; 2004.
54. Resource Access Decision Facility. Needham, MA: OMG; 2005. Available at: http://www.omg.org/technology/documents/formal/omg_security.htm#RAD. Accessed December 12, 2005.
55. HL7. Health Level Seven Arden Syntax for Medical Logic Systems. Version 2.1. ANSI/HL7 Arden V2.1-2002. New York: ANSI; 2002.
56. GLIF. Towards a Representation for Sharable Guidelines. Available at: http://www.glif.org/. Accessed December 12, 2005.
57. Sordo M, Boxwala AA, Ogunyemi O, Greenes RA. Description and status update on GELLO: a proposed standardized object-oriented expression language for clinical decision support. Medinfo 2004;11(pt 1):164–168.
58. ASTM E31.28. E2210-02 Standard Specification for Guideline Elements Model (GEM)-Document Model for Clinical Practice Guidelines. West Conshohocken, PA: ASTM; 2005. Available at: http://www.astm.org. Accessed December 17, 2005.
59. Blair J, Cohn S. Critical areas of standardization. In: Demetriades JE, Kolodner RM, Christopherson GA, eds. Toward HealthePeople. New York: Springer; 2005.

60. Facts about ORYX® for Hospitals, Core Measures and Hospital Core Measures. Oakbrook Terrace, IL: Joint Commission on Accreditation of Health Care Organizations; 2005. Available at: http://www.jcaho.org/accredited+organizations/hospitals/oryx/oryx+facts.htm. Accessed December 17, 2005.
61. Measurement Sets. Chicago: AMA; 2005. Available at: http://www.amaassn.org/ama/pub/category/4837.html. Accessed December 17, 2005.
62. NCQA. The Health Plan Employer Data and Information Set (HEDIS®). Available at: http://www.ncqa.org/Programs/HEDIS/. Accessed December 17, 2005.
63. National Guideline Clearinghouse. Available at: www.guideline.gov. Accessed December 17, 2005.
64. FDA. Bar Code Label Requirements for Human Drug Products and Biological Products; Final Rule. 21 CFR Parts 201, 606, et al. Federal Register: February 26, 2004; Vol 69 (Number 38), p 9120 ff.
65. HIBCC: Healthcare's B2B Standards Development Organization. Phoenix, AZ: HIBCC; 2005. Available at: http://www.hibcc.org/. Accessed December 17, 2005.
66. Integrating the Healthcare Enterprise. Available at: http://www.ihe.net/. Accessed December 17, 2005.

13
Privacy and Security

Darren Lacey

Fifty years from now our grandchildren may well wonder how something as fundamental as the Internet was built on such an insecure foundation. The networked information technology (IT) "revolution" progresses unabated, while evidence of its inherent insecurity continues to mount. Any server connected to the Internet is almost certain to be scanned and prodded within minutes of connection. New forms of malicious code—viruses, worms, and spyware—are introduced daily. Vulnerabilities in major applications and systems are exposed at nearly the same rate. We fear that the Internet could come undone at any time—possibly from intentional attack or from the sagging weight of a remarkably complex communications system.

Even so, up until now the Internet has proven surprisingly resilient: Perhaps because of its great size and redundancy as well as the necessarily piecemeal, yet generally effective, security measures put in place. Whatever security concerns they might have, every major industry—including health care—has nonetheless embraced computer technology and the Internet.[1] As other chapters in this volume amply illustrate, there is in medicine at least a new era dawning, one built on integrated delivery systems, electronic health records (EHRs), telemedicine, and improvements in diagnostics and decision support tools. IT has begun to transform medical care and public health in ways that are remarkable and likely permanent. All this transformation has taken place square in the middle of a supposedly insecure cyber-space.

As information systems became ubiquitous in the seventies and eighties, so grew a large and increasingly professional labor force and set of practices that together have formed what is now called informatics. The same thing is occurring today in the somewhat narrower field of information security. And just as informatics grew organically out of the business needs of myriad organizations, information security has emerged for generally mundane operational reasons rather than high-flown commitments to protecting national security or maintaining some overarching information "infrastructure." And it is in this context that we will discuss the role of security in informatics, and EHRs in particular, and emphasize its complex relationship with personal privacy concerns.

Privacy

Advances in technology are often followed by changes in the law, and few legal concepts have seen changes as dramatic as in personal privacy. The rapid increase of IT and the Internet has accelerated changes in many of our common conceptions of privacy. Just as older technologies such as photography and audio recording led to a contraction of the private space a hundred years ago, the more powerful and pervasive tools of cyber-space could diminish our privacy to the vanishing point.

Eventual Supreme Court Justice Louis P. Brandeis and a lawyer colleague Samuel Warren raised just these concerns in an 1890 article that also set forth one of the most comprehensive and provocative cases for privacy rights even to the present day.[2] Most of what has been written on privacy— before 1890 and since—has focused on the relationship of the individual and the state: Civil investigations, abortion laws, and criminal search and seizure are examples of incursions, whether justified or not, by the government in the personal space of its citizens. The genius of the Brandeis-Warren piece is that its arguments are equally appropriate in all settings where privacy might be infringed, whether by the government or a private third party, such as in media exposés, the selling of private data, or surveillance. It is the latter concerns of privacy, whereby individuals and organizations potentially violate the privacy rights of their neighbors, that interested Brandeis and Warren and that continue to interest us today. For it is here that we begin to understand the responsibilities that those of us outside the government owe to the privacy concerns of our customers, patients, and employees.

Throughout the eighteenth and nineteenth centuries, courts drew a clear distinction between public and private personae and attached rights of privacy accordingly. One's private actions—those inside the home or office—were considered sacrosanct, and the courts therefore disallowed reference to such actions in civil actions and greatly circumscribed what could be discussed even in criminal cases. Personal journals, notes, diaries, and even letters sent under presumed confidence were generally seen as beyond the scope of legal discovery or of publication by others. Whereas the private realm received almost categorical protection in law, what one did or said in public received almost none. The distinction between public and private lives began to dissolve with the rise of consumer markets, expansions of credit markets, and increasingly complex professional services in law, medicine, and accounting for example. Because so much everyday activity resisted easy reduction to public or private selves, the traditional understanding of privacy laws seemed likewise antiquated.[3]

Brandeis and Warren attacked traditional theories of privacy on two fronts. First, they suggested that one of its traditional justifications, "domestic setting," could not be sustained across the wide range of locations and circumstances in which private information could be recorded or disclosed. It struck them as peculiar to determine the privacy of an instance on how closely the setting resembles a home. The second pillar of privacy law was equally shaky. The authors disputed the common notion of the time that violations of privacy were either always the result of, or roughly equivalent to, trespass. At the time, publication of personal papers was prohibited mainly based on the notion of the "fruit of the poisoned tree," a bar on benefits derived from an original "bad act," in most cases a trespass on person or property. Brandeis and Warren pointed to many cases at the time in which courts would prevent publication of such papers even where there was no claim of trespass, thus suggesting that courts recognized in deed if not always in word how privacy protection had outgrown its foundations. They also contended that trespass theory, whatever relevance it might have had in the past, would almost certainly undermine many privacy claims in the future. They foresaw that with "recent inventions" such as photography and sound recording it would be possible to conduct surveillance without any breach of property rights at all. Brandeis and Warren argued persuasively that as the realm of the observable grows, the practical realm of privacy contracts, perhaps to the vanishing point. Under their theory, rather than asking how certain information was originally procured, the more fundamental inquiry should be on the information's content, that there may be something inherent to the word or deed that should trigger privacy protection. A great deal of private information is disclosed voluntarily to all manner of individuals and organizations: Banks, physicians, employers, government, among others. In no way are these disclosures "domestic occurrences," nor are they the result of "trespasses," yet their content may very well be private and deserving of protection under law. Should the mere fact that one discloses information to someone voluntarily, say a hospital or bank, negate all claims for privacy?

For all their objections to other understandings of privacy at the time, Brandeis and Warren were unable to propose a well-thought-out alternative. They presented an elegant turn of phrase by stating that privacy is, "the right not merely to prevent inaccurate portrayal of private life, but to prevent its being depicted at all." Yet even they understood that this somewhat radical formulation could not be sustained in practice, and immediately started to backtrack with respect to public figures, political issues, etc. The simple fact is that an open and free society must allow for the occasional—and usually more than occasional—airing of private information. Brandeis and Warren knew this and struggled unsuccessfully to introduce a test that would balance rights of privacy with other rights, such as press, speech, and a general need to use some private information in commerce and everyday life.

Recently, scholars have taken up the challenge of articulating a theoretical and legal justification for privacy. Jeffrey Rosen among others seeks to support privacy by appealing to contemporary sociological theories of identity.[4] In tribal or small agrarian societies, individuals have numerous opportunities to make themselves known, to demonstrate the many aspects of their character and personality. Today, however, our relative anonymity means that we usually have a more difficult time succeeding in "impression management." People rarely have time to gather more than a partial sense or understanding of the character of others. When the sum of knowledge regarding others is so limited, individuals are "in danger of being judged, fairly or unfairly, on the basis of isolated bits of personal information that are taken out of context."[3] Rosen argues that greater transparency, and consequently less privacy, distorts impressions by focusing on a small number of facts or incidents. It is not difficult to imagine how health and medical histories, for example, could unfairly and inaccurately prejudice against a prospective professional colleague or social contact.

Whatever the merits of Rosen's case for privacy, these issues are clearly difficult. There is a legal truism that hard cases make bad law, and privacy is rife with hard cases and contradictory results. Although much of the view that Brandeis and Warren first presented has carried over into present day privacy law, much has also been lost through the rise of technology and the administrative state. According to Rosen and others, the current state of privacy law is a dangerous muddle—not clear enough to predict results but on an inexorable path toward reducing the sum of our privacy rights. In the absence of clear direction from the courts, the federal and state legislative branches have become increasingly active in regulating privacy. The last 30 years has seen a patchwork of privacy laws and regulations covering the privacy rights of individuals and responsibilities of those collecting information. The first significant advances took place in the 1970s with the passage of the federal Fair Credit Reporting (finance) and Privacy (government data use) acts. These laws brought to fore standard ways of handling data, especially private data, and helped cement an emerging set of requirements, the Fair Information Practice Principles (FIPP). Computer technology was addressed in the Electronic Communications Privacy and Computer Security Acts during the 1980s. Around that time, Congress addressed privacy of library records, book purchasing, and video rentals, and issues regarding research and academic freedom. In the last decade, further laws were made regarding financial services (Gramm-Leach-Bliley), business records (California Senate Bill 1386 and the European Union Privacy Directive) and medical records [Health Insurance Portability and Accountability Act (HIPAA)]. These laws recognize in ways that common law does not that private information is often disclosed for any number of purposes and that the use of such information should be administered according to reasonable standards.

HIPAA and FIPP

Throughout this section and the remainder of the chapter, both security and privacy will be discussed in terms of the most important piece of legislation on the topic in the healthcare field (and perhaps in any field), the Health Insurance Portability and Accountability Act of 1996 (HIPAA, Public Law 104-191). HIPAA was enacted to simplify and standardize healthcare administration and in so doing to facilitate greater portability of health insurance coverage for people changing jobs or otherwise experiencing life changes.

HIPAA standards may achieve greater portability, but there have been questions from early on in its legislative process as to whether these standards would also threaten the privacy and confidentiality of patient records.[5] With all records in a standard and intelligible form, it would be possible for attackers, once having accessed patient information, to read and aggregate such data more easily. In a standardized environment, an attacker need only learn taxonomy and semantics once and then apply this knowledge each time he launches an attack, rather than have to learn a unique taxonomy for each system. Security professionals refer to attacks that can be multiplied with little additional effort as "scalable," and it is the emergence of scalable attacks that has concerned many in the healthcare field. In response, privacy and security standards were included in HIPAA, and the Secretary of the Department of Health and Human Services was required to develop standards for both. The document on standards of privacy, the "Privacy Rule," was finalized in 2002 and all "covered entities" (e.g., providers, insurers, health plans, and information clearinghouses) were to have reached compliance in 2003. The "Security Rule" was completed in 2003 with compliance by covered entities completed in April 2005. Already, HIPAA privacy and security requirements have changed the practice and business of medicine. HIPAA also seems to be increasing patient awareness of the value of personal medical information and creating new expectations regarding how such information should be collected, handled, and disseminated. The regulation of privacy in HIPAA has counterparts in other private sector industries, principally banking, yet in its detailed set of prescriptions it is unprecedented. It is something of an experiment to subject a major private sector industry to specific standards of care for the protection of the private information of its customers. The next few years will likely demonstrate how close regulation of an industry in this matter will work, and if successful, the model could be replicated across multiple industries.

Particularly in the Privacy Rule, HIPAA includes a number of unique regulatory statements, yet the overall structure is familiar to those in the privacy advocacy community. It is based on a vocabulary and taxonomy that has been in place for more than 30 years. Fair Information Practice

Principles (FIPP, not to be confused with Federal Information Processing Standards or FIPS) has provided business and government a model for assessing information handling and privacy. Widely known in government, it is understood in the commercial sector principally through its progeny (the Internet privacy standard P3P, for example). Every major effort to plan and adopt privacy owes at least part of its substance to FIPP, a relatively straightforward statement of privacy principles that are intended to underscore the main responsibilities of those collecting personal data.

Notice/Awareness

The first principle, both in terms of priority and importance, is notice. Individuals disclosing data [called here "Discloser(s)"; those receiving data are "Collector(s)"] should be made aware of a Collector's information practices before disclosing any personal information. Disclosers must receive notice before they can make informed decisions as to whether and to what extent to disclose personal information. According to FIPP, Disclosers should be provided notice of the following:

- Identity of the Collector
- Uses for the information collected
- Potential recipients of the information
- Nature of the information
- Whether providing information is voluntary
- Steps taken by Collector to ensure confidentiality, integrity, and quality of information

Under HIPAA, covered entities are required to provide to patients a "Notice of Privacy Practices" that closely follows the privacy requirements set forth in this principle. It is the primary privacy control measure for the main activities of healthcare entities: Patient treatment, payment, and operations. For other activities undertaken by healthcare entities, such as research, marketing, or fund-raising, notice is by itself insufficient—and covered entities must obtain Discloser consent.

Consent

Notice defines subject matter and participants. Consent takes the next step by providing the Discloser an opportunity to establish his preferences regarding use and disclosure of personal information, particularly secondary uses beyond those contemplated at time of disclosure. A patient, for example, discloses personal information when visiting a physician and the physician would provide notice of her (or her office, clinic, hospital, or payer) set of privacy practices. Using FIPP terminology, HIPAA regards treatment, payment, and operations as the *de facto* contemplated uses of information in the healthcare setting. If the collecting physician has another use in mind—for example, medical research, hospital fundraising, or disclosure to a public health clearinghouse—she must first receive from the disclosing patient consent ("authorization" in HIPAA parlance) for these intended uses. A good portion of the Privacy Rule involves determining when authorizations are required from patients and how these should be processed and maintained. Although it would perhaps be desirable to require authorization and hence consent by all patients for any intended use, healthcare providers have been quick to point out the costs involved. Where covered entities intend to use aggregations of patient data—a common occurrence in many hospitals or clinics—obtaining and processing patient authorizations presents significant administrative burdens.

Consent generally comes in two forms: Opt-in or opt-out. Authorization under HIPAA requires affirmative steps (signing a form) by the Discloser to allow certain uses of personal information, an opt-in. In an opt-in world, nothing is permitted—that is, the Collector may not collect or use personal information—until the Discloser does something to remove the prohibition. Opt-ins do not always require a signature or other documentary evidence. In many cases, a click box at a Web site may be deemed adequate to indicate an affirmative statement of choice.

Opt-out regimes require affirmative steps to prevent collection and/or use of personal information. This means that in an opt-out regime, everything—to be precise, every reasonable use or practice—is permitted until the Discloser acts to set limits or prohibitions. In some cases, opting out is easy—removing checks from check boxes on a Web page, for example—yet in others it requires some effort on behalf of the Discloser. Several years ago, financial institutions were required to send consent forms to their customers regarding disclosure of personal information between business affiliates. Consent notices were sent by mail to nearly all customers, and many customers received several notices from the same bank or financial services company. Yet, to effectively opt out (to disallow information from being shared with an affiliate), customers were required to perform a concerted action: Calling a phone number, returning the consent form by mail, or filling in a Web form. Predictably, few people took the trouble to opt out, and information sharing continued much as it had before this change in the law.

Access/Participation

Under this principle, a Discloser has the right to review his personal information being maintained by a Collector to ensure accuracy and completeness. One of the driving forces behind the HIPAA Privacy Rule has been a growing interest among patients in the transparency of patient records and the rights of patients to review their records.[6] Access can give the patient a sense of ownership of his/her medical record and be an effective check on integrity and accuracy. As an example of access rights, the standard Notice of Privacy Practices at Johns Hopkins includes the following language:

- *Right to inspect and copy*. With certain exceptions (such as psychotherapy notes, information collected for certain legal proceedings, and health information restricted by law), you have the right to inspect and/or receive a copy of your medical information.
  - We may require you to submit your request in writing. We may charge you a reasonable fee for copying your records.
  - We may deny access, under certain circumstances, such as if we believe it may endanger you or someone else. You may request that we designate a licensed healthcare professional to review the denial.
- *Right to request an amendment or addendum*. If you feel that medical information we have about you is incorrect or incomplete, you may ask us to amend the information or add an addendum (addition to the record). You have the right to request an amendment or addendum for as long as the information is kept by or for Johns Hopkins.
- We may require you to submit your request in writing and to explain why the amendment is needed. If we accept your request, we will tell you we agree and we will amend your records. We cannot take out what is in the record. We add the supplemental information. With your assistance, we will notify others who have the incorrect or incomplete health information. If we deny your request, we will give you a written explanation of why we did not make the amendment and explain your rights.[7]

These policies seek a balance between the rights of patients to see and amend information with the complexities of Johns Hopkins' operational environment. Interestingly, patients are not given the right even by request to delete information in a record even if that information is incorrect. To maintain the integrity of records and patient safety, records may only be marked and supplemented with corrections; not erased or deleted.

Integrity/Security

FIPP combines the idea of integrity (preserving accuracy of data) with security, an idea that, as we will see in this and the next section on Information Security, includes a great deal more.

Enforcement/Redress

The last element considers the real-world mechanisms for ensuring compliance with standards, enforcement, and recourse. Enforcement focuses on the Collector, usually involving an enforcement entity and a set of procedures that come into play when there is a question of compliance by a Collector or its affiliate. However, recourse concerns the rights of those potentially wronged as a result of noncompliance. These ideas are mutually reinforcing: The former addresses the overall compliance environment for an organization or sector, and the latter considers justice in the individual case. Both enforcement and redress rely on (1) self-regulation, (2) private remedies, and (3) government enforcement. For example, healthcare entities self-regulate enforcement through internal or external audits, certification procedures, and adoption of industry-wide standards of care. The federal government enforces HIPAA through the Office of Civil Rights at the United States (US) Department of Justice for HIPAA privacy and the Center for Medicaid and Medicare Services (CMS) for HIPAA security. State governments also have enforcement arms for privacy and security. Redress for privacy and security is self-regulated through institutional complaint processes or ombudsmen. Although individuals cannot sue under HIPAA, it will be interesting to see how private actions on related grounds, such as common law torts or state law, will be used as first a means of redress and then more broadly of enforcement of HIPAA requirements. As medical privacy law develops over the next few years, so will new theories underlying lawsuits and determinations of damages caused by privacy and security breaches.

Today HIPAA is a hodgepodge of approaches to data collection and data uses—treatment, billing, research, public relations, and fund-raising—and detailed standards for compliance in each have yet to be drawn. Compounding this uncertainty is the fact that most states have their own medical privacy laws that will likely give rise to conflicts and contradictions. The uncertainty of the law will keep lawyers and judges busy for a while, and it is likely that many of the same issues underscored by FIPP will return in many forms and guises.

Information Security

Information security draws from at least four distinct disciplines. The first and oldest is the history of cryptography that David Kahn documented in his classic book, *Code Breakers*.[8] The art of "secret writing" to protect communications reaches back thousands of years—the Caesar cipher, a common technique taught even today to beginning cryptography students, is named after the man who spread its use, Julius Caesar. Thomas Jefferson received a patent on a mechanical encryption tool, a wheel cipher that was used by the US Navy as late as World War I. The allied victory at the Battle of the Midway in World War II is at least partly attributable to the US successfully unlocking the "Purple" code, thought by its creators in Japan to be unbreakable. There is general recognition that code writing and breaking are the foundations of much of what has now become information security; the terminology and practice in both are strikingly similar. Evidence of this close relationship is found in the government itself. The National Security Agency has been designated as both the leading code breakers and code makers for the defense and intelligence communities since the fifties. To put it another way, the same organization that is in charge of uncovering the secrets of others ensures that our own national secrets remain secret. This illustrates a fundamental truth of information security: Security can only be effectively planned and implemented by those who can think like attackers.

For most of its history, the science of information security was largely concerned with creating, testing, and evaluating ciphers and encryption algorithms. Today, practically unbreakable encryption is widely available, and the discussion has generally shifted from the quality of algorithms to the quality of their implementation in real-world systems. It is now possible to build security into systems through careful engineering rather than by calling upon esoteric mathematics. Security is thus within the reach of any organization and industry, even those relatively underinvested in IT such as health care.

At about the same time that cryptography became widely available in the seventies, the US intelligence community began to work through another series of security models, one that is less recognized but ultimately more important for regulatory regimes such as HIPAA. Researchers in the intelligence community began to explore formal models for sharing information across organizational lines and to individuals with different purposes and levels of trust. Military intelligence protects information by matching the sensitivity of a specific datum to an individual or systems level of clearance (e.g., CONFIDENTIAL, TOP SECRET) in a formal process known as Multi-Level Security (MLS).[9] MLS was created to solve a problem that had been bothering intelligence professionals for many years. How can information from many sources and with many purposes be shared among individuals and organizations when the data "owner" cannot be aware of all potential recipients? By the height of the Cold War, the military/industrial intelligence community had simply grown too large to control information flow in an ad hoc manner. The security clearance and certification processes of individuals and systems were established to form baseline sets of controls for sharing information. There is some controversy on how well formal MLS models work in practice and even greater question whether they could work where there are looser organizational structures, such as in health care. MLS is conceptually useful because it self-consciously connects information security issues to their counterparts in physical, personnel, and systems. Because the HIPAA Security Rule was drafted largely by government security experts, it is easy to see the echoes of MLS throughout the regulation, and the HIPAA approach to information management retains much of the MLS flavor. This leads to the second discipline from which information security flows, information management. Information security is a subdiscipline in the field, one that overlaps with data privacy, quality assurance, networking, and a number of other subdisciplines. It is tempting to view information security as yet another subdiscipline of IT rather than information management. Yet, the latter is more germane to the broad sweep of HIPAA. It is why, for example, the Security Rule is as expansive in the administrative as technical components of information security. The focus of HIPAA is not information systems per se, particularly the IT systems, but rather on the value and attendant risk of the underlying information.

As Eric Raymond noted with respect to software applications, the value of information varies dramatically based on its form, content, and possible uses.[10] Information security professionals, especially in health care, are principally concerned not with how or how much collectors of information value it (high value is often assumed), but how potential attackers could find value in such information. It is not difficult to see how attackers could value financial information generated by banks because that is where the money is. Although it may be harder to place a value on medical information to the Dillingers of cyber-space, it is impossible to plan an effective security program without doing just that. Good information management asks whether a particular datum is first valuable to the organization. If not, then why is the datum being collected in the first place? Once having determined that certain information does indeed have internal use value, we ask whether it would be valuable to anyone else, specifically a thief, a blackmailer, or other bad actor. Out of these determinations we can arrive at a formal or informal data classification scheme that adjusts security on the basis of both internal value and the risks posed by its potential value to others. Information systems that handle such information can likewise be classified according to these calculations of value and risk, and thus we see the outlines if not the precise structure of MLS.

The third discipline and the one most familiar to many readers is computer security and its attendant component network security. It is the rise of the network, specifically the Internet, that has vaulted computer security from its place as a sleepy computer science subdiscipline of interest primarily to those in the defense and intelligence communities to its current central place in contemporary informatics. The increase of computer security is almost entirely a function of the increase of networked computing. If an attacker needs physical access to a specific machine to execute an attack, the universe of possible attackers—those with the motivation, technical skill, and means—is usually quite small. If, however, an attack can be accomplished from anywhere in the world through the Internet remotely and without great effort, the universe of those equipped for even the most esoteric attacks is several orders of magnitude larger. Ubiquitous networks not only expand the pool of possible attackers, they also dramatically expand the means of attack. The most nettlesome computer security issues are principally network attacks: Intrusions, malicious software, inappropriate access, loss of data, and denial of service attacks. Throughout the remainder of this chapter, nearly every technical security issue finds its most common expression in the network infrastructure.

National security experts have identified the following layers of security, all of which have some direct influence on information security, broadly understood:

- Physical security—protection of physical objects
- Personal security—protection of people
- Operations security—protection of operational or administrative activities
- Communications security—protection of primary means of communications (such as phones, radio)
- Network security—protection of network components and content
- Information security—protection of information and information assets[11]

As will be discussed in the section Security Controls—Major Concepts, HIPAA follows this model and addresses security controls through physical, administrative (Personal and Operations), and technical security (Communications, Network, and Information).

Characteristics of Information Security

Security under HIPAA generally means the technical and managerial practices, along with corresponding tools, that protect both a system and information from unauthorized access and misuse. More broadly, security often is defined as the state whereby systems are generally working for their intended purposes and that they are reliable and resistant to intentional attacks and unintentional misuse. Reliability is important for security as is becoming increasingly evident for operational effectiveness and patient safety. Many security professionals introduce security with a standard set of elements, with terminology arising from its initials, CIA:

Confidentiality—information can only be accessed by authorized individuals, and in turn it is not made available or disclosed to unauthorized individuals. This idea is closely related to privacy but is narrower in scope, because it only addresses user access; not the raft of legal and policy issues surrounding privacy. Confidentiality means that only those with a "need to know" can access certain information.

Integrity—information is complete and uncorrupted and has not been modified by unauthorized individuals. More broadly, integrity can refer to the quality of the information, its readability, and usefulness. For example, poor handwriting that results in an inaccurate transcription of a diagnosis or prescription constitutes an integrity problem that information systems are designed to address.

Availability—information can be accessed by users when needed and is correctly formatted for use. One of the main reasons for implementing IT in the first place is to expand availability of information to those who do not have physical access to paper records. The World Wide Web, EHR systems, and e-mail have all expanded availability of information. Security failures can result in interruptions of this service usually by disrupting machines or networks.

Improving security means enhancing one or more of these hallmarks of well-running systems. In some cases, tradeoffs are made between two or more elements. For example, limiting user access to certain files can improve confidentiality, but often at the cost of availability. Another important security property is not immediately apparent in the systems performance, but is equally important in terms of overall security:

Accountability—information access and usage can be attributed to unique individuals. When a clinician signs changes to a patient record, she is ensuring accountability. When a user accesses an application and leaves an auditable trail regarding his activities (e.g., records viewed, created, modified, or deleted), the system has tools to ensure accountability. These mechanisms are not only important in their own right, they are instrumental for improving the CIA and security of any application or system.

National Institute of Standards and Technology

The National Institute of Standards and Technology (NIST) has been designated as the principal information security and assurance agency for the civilian-sector federal government. NIST has published a series of guidance documents in its 800 series for planning, implementing, and evaluating information security technologies and practices. Recently, it has weighed in on HIPAA requirements in its *NIST Special Publication 800-66: An Introductory Resource Guide for Implementing the Health Insurance Portability and Accountability Act (HIPAA) Security Rule*. NIST suggests that effective information security (here called "computer security") has the following characteristics:

1. Computer security should support the mission of the organization.
2. Computer security is an integral element of sound management.
3. Computer security should be cost-effective.
4. Computer security responsibilities and accountability should be made explicit.
5. System owners have computer security responsibilities outside their own organizations.
6. Computer security requires a comprehensive and integrated approach.
7. Computer security should be periodically reassessed.
8. Computer security is constrained by societal factors.[12]

HIPAA Security Rule

Unlike the HIPAA Privacy Rule, which concerns all identifiable patient data whether in paper or electronic form, the Security Rule addresses only electronic patient data—Electronic Protected Health Information (E-PHI). Nonetheless, the Security Rule actually addresses a wider range of issues than the Privacy Rule, several of which have little direct relation to privacy (e.g., disaster recovery, integrity controls). The Security Rule provides for flexibility and diversity of approaches by allowing covered entities to plan and develop individual security programs within broad guidelines. Yet this needed flexibility comes at the cost of vague standards of care. The Security Rule tries to ameliorate this lack of clarity by distinguishing between "required" and "addressable" standards for specific controls. Yet this distinction amounts to less than what first meets the eye. Nearly every required control is oriented toward process and general objectives, and there is little guidance on the details or substance of these processes. Many addressable controls, however, are much more granular in their approach, but even there clear standards are hard to come by. The required provisions of the Security Rule could be summarized as follows: A covered entity must assess the value and feasibility of implementing a series of controls appropriate for its environment and document its strategic and tactical decision-making process. Although there is likely to be some emerging consensus regarding how certain required controls such as risk assessment and incident response procedures are implemented, whether a specific control actually meets HIPAA requirements is likely to remain unclear for several more years. We should anticipate that only a body of enforcement actions by CMS or through the courts will eventually establish guidance for compliance with HIPAA security standards.

Risk Assessment and Management

The Security Rule requires that each covered entity adopt security practices that it considers reasonable given the level of risk and institutional capabilities. By discussing information security in terms of risk assessment, HIPAA is well within the mainstream. An entire industry has grown up around ISO 17799, OCTAVE, NIST, and a surfeit of other risk assessment methodologies.[13] Table 13-1 lists NIST's approach. Risk management starts with a formal risk assessment in order to establish an effective security strategy and then incorporates controls and metrics throughout a security systems life cycle. CMS describes the relationships between the two concepts thus:

Risk analysis is the assessment of the risks and vulnerabilities that could negatively impact the confidentiality, integrity, and availability of the electronic PHI held by a covered entity, and the likelihood of occurrence. Risk management is the actual implementation of security measures to sufficiently reduce an organization's risk of losing or compromising its electronic PHI and to meet the general security standards.[14]

TABLE 13-1. NIST security risk assessment methodology

SDLC Phases	Phase Characteristics	Support from Risk Management Activities
Phase 1—Initiation	The need for an IT system is expressed and the purpose and scope of the IT system is documented	• Identified risks are used to support the development of the system requirements, including security requirements, and a security concept of operations (strategy)
Phase 2—Development or Acquisition	The IT system is designed, purchased, programmed, developed, or otherwise constructed	• The risks identified during this phase can be used to support the security analyses of the IT system that may lead to architecture and design trade-offs during system development
Phase 3—Implementation	The system security features should be configured, enabled, tested, and verified	• The risk management process supports the assessment of the system implementation against its requirements and within its modeled operational environment. Decisions regarding risks identified must be made prior to system operation
Phase 4—Operation or Maintenance	The system performs its functions. Typically the system is being modified on an ongoing basis through the addition of hardware and software and by changes to organizational processes, policies, and procedures	• Risk management activities are performed for periodic system reauthorization (or reaccreditation) or whenever major changes are made to an IT system in its operational production environment (e.g., new system interfaces)
Phase 5—Disposal	This phase may involve the disposition of information, hardware, and software. Activities may include moving, archiving, discarding, or destroying information and sanitizing the hardware and software	• Risk management activities are performed for system components that will be disposed of or replaced to ensure that the hardware and software are properly disposed of, that residual data is appropriately handled, and that system migration is conducted in a secure and systematic manner

Source: NIST. Risk Management Guide for Information Technology Systems. Special Publication 800-30, Table 2-1.
SDLC, system development life cycle.

HIPAA emphasizes both risk assessment and risk management as cornerstones of an effective security program. This section discusses several steps for developing a risk assessment and management process.

Organization and System Purpose

For information security in general and HIPAA in particular, it is best to think of systems broadly, as encompassing one or more IT applications, administrative processes, and underlying infrastructures. Articulating the purpose of these systems sets the stage for assessing risk. System purpose indicates which of the CIA security elements are most critical in a particular instance. It can also help determine the data collection needs of the organization or system. It is both good privacy practice under FIPP and general security practice to collect and maintain the least amount of data, the "minimum necessary," required to achieve the system's business purposes.

Threats

Threats are external dangers to an asset and exist whether an organization implements any security controls or not. The most common and well-known threats arise from malicious code, such as viruses and worms. The most extensive family of threats relate to intrusion—including those resulting from exploitation of system vulnerabilities by external hackers and using these to take control of software or hardware or to intercept network traffic. The two categories of malicious code and intrusion are the archetypes of computer insecurity. Other threats are just as serious, albeit less visible, such as those arising from equipment malfunction, physical theft, environmental hazard, and inappropriate use by system insiders.

Vulnerabilities

Unlike threats, defenders have some say in the type and scope of its vulnerabilities. Vulnerabilities are the holes in a system—administrative, technical, and otherwise—that subject an organization to threats. Security controls are directed toward addressing one or more of these vulnerabilities, and it is common for accounts of vulnerabilities to be mirror images of recommended controls. For instance, failure to lock server closets is a vulnerability, and the corresponding control would be to lock server closets as a matter of practice. It is not difficult to see that vulnerabilities are often simply the absence of certain controls.

Calculation of Risk—Likelihood, Damage

The standard approach to addressing risk is to multiply the likelihood of an incident by the amount of damage such an event would cause. Unfortunately, there is a dearth of data in nearly every organization; neither the likelihood nor damage of most information security events are settled quantities. At best, most risk-assessment methodologies can identify a few quantitative metrics and somewhat more qualitative accounts of risk factors. More effective incident reporting and widespread information sharing may begin to give security professionals a better sense of the likelihood of attacks. On the other side of the equation, damages for security/privacy incidents are likely to become increasingly apparent as HIPAA enforcement actions and related litigation establish a body of compliance and liability.

Risk Mitigation—Reducing Likelihood

Risk mitigation, the main part of risk management, includes controls of two primary types: Reducing likelihood of attacks and limiting damage from such attacks. In both cases, security controls are linked to identified threats and vulnerabilities and implemented according to the requirements of the system and an overall security strategy.

Reducing likelihood of attacks by preventing them is the first line of defense. One way to think of this is as prevention, and such prevention usually begins at the network perimeter through firewalls and intrusion detection (more on those below) and works its way inside to vulnerabilities on individual machines and applications.

Risk Mitigation—Limiting Damage

All systems break on occasion. A secure system is resilient—when it breaks, the damage is manageable, not catastrophic. This is especially important for HIPAA security. A broken system—an intrusion, theft, or virus—is not by itself a violation of HIPAA security. It becomes a problem when the incident results in a loss or disclosure of PHI. There is a well-traveled adage about most perimeter security: Such security is hard and crunchy on the outside, soft and chewy on the inside. Good information security requires that the inside be hardened by controlling the type and scope of damages that could result from a security incident.

Cost Effectiveness of Controls and Priorities

It is nearly as difficult to measure the cost effectiveness of controls as it is to quantify risk. Whereas it is sometimes clear what a control will cost—in money, personnel resources, attention of management—assessing the effectiveness of controls against that investment is difficult. One general rule for information security is that strong policies, incident response capabilities, and training of users and administrators are usually among the most cost-effective controls and best security investments.

On occasion one hears the following business "wisdom": That which cannot be measured will be ignored. Risk assessment and management struggle with a growing necessity to measure the value of security investments. In the absence of good data, most security professionals focus their concerns on the impact of known threats and vulnerabilities on the enterprise. The practice of risk assessment now relies on the experience and analogical reasoning of security professionals, and it is usually a combination of the knowledge of best practices and intuitive understandings of risk thresholds. The field moves so rapidly, security professionals are generally in a perpetual state of surprise regarding the next bundle of threats and the impacts on our respective organizations. We are always in danger of fighting the last war and are therefore wary of rigid methodologies and purely statistical reasoning. Although there is reason to believe that the quality of risk data will improve, it would be surprising if security decision making becomes noticeably more formal than it is today.

Security Controls—Major Concepts

Given these threats and risks, there are several actions that security officials can take.

Access Control

There is no more important concept in the HIPAA Security Rule than access control, which means ensuring that only authorized individuals are allowed to access (i.e., read, create, or modify) E-PHI. The emphasis on access control resonates for privacy practices, standards in FIPP, and even more directly approaches to security involving MLS. The treatment of PHI under HIPAA is in many ways analogous to the treatment of classified information at defense and intelligence organizations grounded in MLS. HIPAA seems to focus first on the protection of confidentiality and integrity, and secondarily addresses other security concerns. Similar to classified models, HIPAA emphasizes the role of human resource-related requirements of workforce clearance, separation of duties, need to know, and minimum necessary. Both privacy and security rules are in effect access control standards with a few additional items included as needed to preserve information and systems integrity.

In information security practice, access control consists of two processes: **Authorization**, the right of a user to access an electronic system, and **authentication**, the process by which an authorized user proves her identity. The former process is principally administrative in nature, and even in cases in which authorization is handled through automation it is almost always a human decision to grant access to a system. The latter is usually technical in nature, including things such as passwords and ID cards. HIPAA requires that access to E-PHI be granted only on a "need to know" basis and that this authorization be made by administrative management. Not every user needs to access every part of a system or record, and good security seeks to limit access by mapping job functions to access roles. This type of authorization process is known as role-based access, and it requires careful planning and granular controls. Most systems currently use a somewhat less rigorous approach, identity-based access, which generally gives full access to any user that meets a threshold test for need to know.

Authentication is the more technical side of the access process. It uses one or more factors to ensure the identity of users. The factors are often referred to as:

- Something you know [e.g., passwords, pass numbers, personal identification numbers (PINs), query and response mechanisms]
- Something you have (e.g., keys, tokens, credit cards)
- Something you are (e.g., fingerprints, facial or voice recognition)

Authentication is strongest when it utilizes more than one factor, resulting in "multi-factor" authentication. For example, a token combined with a PIN would be much stronger than one factor or the other by itself. It would be possible to guess a PIN or steal a token, but to accomplish both would be more difficult for any potential thief. Nonetheless, passwords remain not only the primary form but only form of authentication for most applications. Nearly everyone in the field agrees that this is unfortunate, but the specific inadequacies of passwords are subject to debate. Security professionals disagree on whether passwords should be assigned from a central source, required to follow difficult syntactic rules (e.g., interchanging alphanumeric characters) given minimum or maximum length, or changed regularly by users. About the only controls on which there is wide agreement are, first, that applications should lock users out after some small number of unsuccessful authentication attempts. This is an effective defense against attackers compromising a system by guessing passwords, using a dictionary, or what is called a brute-force attack in which every possible letter/numeral/character combination is shuffled through. Second, there is an increasing preference for "pass-phrases:" several words in a phrase used as the basis for a password. Recent empirical studies have demonstrated that pass-phrases are easier to remember and harder to guess or otherwise crack.[15]

Authentication is one of the few areas where the Security Rule requires a specific control—each user must have a unique ID for access to E-PHI. Implementing this standard is more difficult in practice than it might first seem. There are a myriad of applications capable of storing E-PHI including word processing documents and spreadsheets, many of which can be protected by requiring password access. These applications (such as Microsoft Access and Excel) can require that passwords be used to open documents, but there can only be one password per file. If more than one person is authorized to access the file, the only option is to share one identity and password, a seeming violation of HIPAA. Still, even a shared password provides some protection and seems preferable to leaving a file on a server or workstation open for any user to access. This example illustrates security limitations in many frequently used applications and that even the most innocuous security policy (such as unique user IDs) could have unintended consequences that diminish actual security.

Physical Controls

Under HIPAA, physical security is broadly understood to include safeguards against unauthorized access to physical locations, physical storage of data, and to the many threats posed to data from environmental hazards such as flood and electrical surges. Physical and environmental security refers to measures taken to protect systems, buildings, and related supporting infrastructure against threats associated with the environment.

As in most areas, physical security under HIPAA is principally an access control issue. The obligation is to control access first to high-risk areas—server rooms, networking closets, etc.—and then to consider lower-risk areas that might house workstations or other devices. There are a number of unremarkable controls that organizations can implement—key and automated locks, guards, video surveillance, and escorts of visitors are good examples. The second objective is to prepare for physical hazards, in order to prevent or mitigate damage and improve recovery efforts. Interestingly, the Security Rule considers in some detail disaster recovery and business continuity planning, a subject matter with little apparent relationship with the privacy concerns in HIPAA. This consideration indicates that the Security Rule was established to cover all major areas of security, and not simply those supporting privacy. Disaster response is a critical component of any security program because systems under stress are often the most vulnerable to attack. Moreover, several controls intended primarily to assist disaster recovery also serve other important security purposes. For example, the Security Rule emphasizes the need for data backup and recovery. In many organizations, backups are used first to help recover systems from a failure—sometimes caused by physical hazards but more often by hardware or software failures. Data backup procedures have other secondary, privacy-enhancing benefits, including the critical role of backup data in investigating security and privacy compromises. Thus, a good security control applies both to physical and electronic threats, serving multiple purposes of prevention, mitigation, and recovery.

Encryption

Encryption is the best-known and perhaps most important information security element. As was discussed in the introduction to Information Security, its use reaches back thousands of years and its sophistication and application have dramatically increased with each new communications technology. The art and science of encryption (known as cryptography) refers to the process of rendering communications unintelligible to all but intended recipients. In simple terms, a readable message (called plaintext or cleartext) is encrypted according to a certain algorithm. In its encrypted form (ciphertext), the message can be stored or transmitted without its being read and then decrypted back into plaintext by an authorized user or recipient. Cryptography uses all manner of techniques for rendering a message unreadable. There are substitution ciphers (encryption algorithms) whereby letters in the message are replaced by other letters—"a" becomes "q" or "2" for example—the Caesar cipher being an early example of this type of cipher. When multiple alphabets are used for one encrypted message—"a" becomes "q" and then "g" then "l"—it is called a polyalphabetic cipher, a technique first developed in Renaissance Italy. One can move characters around in a message—"cat" becomes "tca"—called a transposition cipher, or one can move whole blocks of characters, a block cipher. It has been common practice to use a combination of all of these in the most sophisticated algorithms and to express these through mechanical or electronic devices. Thomas Jefferson invented and patented one of the first cylindrical mechanical ciphers, and there is probably no more famous device in all of cryptography than Nazi Germany's electronic cipher, Enigma, which was ultimately broken by the Allies. Breaking codes, or cryptanalysis, goes as far back in time as making them and it uses sophisticated statistical models to indicate patterns in ciphertext. A skilled cryptologist can map patterns on the frequency of use of certain letters in a language. The mere fact that, in English, "e" is used more than "g" which is more common than "x" has enormous implications for cryptology, and it is surprising to many of us how effective frequency analysis is in breaking many codes.

Because cryptography is hard, devising a secure cipher is a substantial feat. Rather than require a unique algorithm for each instance of encryption, most encryption utilizes a limited number of tested and well-known algorithms with an unlimited number of possible keys. There is a direct analogy to lock and keys in the physical world. It would be impossible for locksmiths to reengineer locking mechanisms for every door, so instead they use a small number of designs, each of which will accommodate a large number of keys. Cryptography works much the same way, as nearly every crypto-system relies on one of a small number of ciphers spinning the same wool into a boundless variety of cloth. Thus, one of the fundamentals of cryptography is that messages must remain secure even if a potential code breaker understands the cipher intimately. Encryption standards (such as AES, DES, and others) are widely publicized and analyzed in the cryptographic community and do not rely on secrecy for security. This presumption against security through secrecy is increasingly a principle in information security.

Contemporary cryptographic algorithms fall into two major categories: Symmetric and asymmetric. In symmetric algorithms, encryption and decryption are mirror images of each other—the same key that is used to lock the door is also used to unlock it. This is often called private key cryptography, and as the name implies its security depends on the ability of the cryptographers to keep keys away from unauthorized individuals. Access to keys may be restricted through authorization and authentication of users, but private key cryptography has severe limitations when there are many intended recipients. How can a message be encrypted so that many users can read it without distributing the same private key to everyone, thus making it trivially easy for unintended recipients to procure the key? Or without having to encrypt the message over and over, and distributing different private keys to each intended recipient?

The answer is a minor miracle of cryptography and the discovery that has made information security across networks such as the Internet possible: Public key cryptography. In symmetric cryptography, the key used to encrypt a message is roughly identical to the key needed to decrypt the message's ciphertext. During the 1970s, several researchers working independently explored the possibilities of using a different key for each of these tasks. It is difficult to overstate how the resulting approach to what became known as asymmetric cryptography surprised and transformed the field. Why this is so may not be readily apparent to many readers without some explanation. Cryptography is essentially a product of mathematics, and most mathematical operations are symmetric in nature—addition is the reverse of subtraction, multiplication of division, etc.—and roughly as difficult to perform in one direction as the other. Yet there are certain operations that are more difficult to perform in one direction than in the reverse, specifically factoring large numbers into prime numbers. Multiplying a set of prime numbers is a trivially easy calculation, yet it has been known for centuries that factoring large numbers into constituent primes is exceptionally difficult. Asymmetry in math can be straightforwardly translated into asymmetry of cryptography and a pair of keys created—a public key and a private key. Whereas it may be easy to derive the public key with knowledge of the private key, the reverse is nearly impossible. In practice, public keys are made available to all users, and private keys are kept by each key holder only.

An example will demonstrate how asymmetric cryptography works and how it has dramatically expanded the scope of security. Before public key cryptography, Alice would send a message to Bob by using a key to encrypt the message and then ensure that Bob has the same key for decrypting it. The security of the message is a function of how well Alice distributes the key to Bob yet to no one else, or at least to no other unintended recipients. It is difficult enough to secure one key; imagine if Alice needs to send secret messages to many people and on a daily basis. Managing all of these keys can quickly become a near impossible task. Using asymmetric cryptography, Alice can now choose to encrypt the message using Bob's public key— available through, say, a directory of keys—but only Bob can decrypt the message, because he is the only person with the private key paired with his public key. If another person received the encrypted message, even with full knowledge of the public key, decrypting would be practically impossible without the corresponding private key. Consequently, Alice can send as many secure messages as she wants easily to anyone with a public key pair, and she need not distribute keys or send any additional information about herself or the nature of the message. She can also broadcast messages much easier by encrypting according to the public keys of each intended recipient without compromising security by overusing one key or needing to issue multiple keys.

Although public key cryptography has made security in complex environments such as the Internet possible, challenges remain. To maintain security, a public key system must assure the correspondence between public and private keys and between key pairs and key holders. There are myriad opportunities to impersonate key holders, alter information about keys, or otherwise disrupt the operation of the system using public keys. Security and assurance cannot be effectively maintained without an organization and processes trusted by users, an "infrastructure." The sophistication and complexity of assuring public key systems, a Public Key Infrastructure, has become one of the principal challenges for information security practitioners.

Network Security

Network security is one of the cornerstones of practical information security. In fact, many people erroneously consider information security and network security to be synonymous. Without local networks and the overarching network infrastructure, the Internet, threats to information confidentiality, integrity, and availability would be far less serious. By the same token, it is the centrality and ubiquity of the network that has made the most recent advances in IT possible.

There are manifold uses of networks—Web sites, local area networks, e-mail, distributed applications, etc.—and the range of security requirements is just as diverse. Networks that support Web pages may also support applications handling millions of electronic medical records. Designing a network architecture that provides maximum flexibility for the former while providing strong protections for the latter has become an increasingly challenging and complex task. The rise of the Internet has provided impetus for network security and improved tools to accomplish the task.

Network security begins (and, unfortunately for some organizations, ends) with perimeter defense. The most common source of viruses, worms, malicious software, and hacking intrusions is the vast expanse of the Internet. Like medieval cities, every secure organization first attempts to keep intruders out of its internal domain and the assets residing therein. The equivalent of a wall or mote is established on the perimeter, and it is the network firewall. There are all varieties of firewalls on the market and in use today, but most first filter incoming packets. A network firewall sits on the perimeter of the network and monitors packets [the constituent elements of communications across the Internet Protocol (IP) traffic—including source, destination, types of packets, attachments, ports, and conceivably any component of traffic]. The firewall is the point of egress for the network and it can accept, reject, or tag traffic based on a set of predefined policies. For example, the firewall may reject all traffic received from a certain source IP address, or it may only reject traffic from that IP address with certain types of attachments or directed toward certain ports on a destination machine inside the network. This example reveals the major problem with firewalls—the complexity of possible network issues (e.g., new viruses emerge daily) and how this can be expressed in policy. To address this, firewalls have become more sophisticated, checking certain types of transactions, say, to open sessions on certain ports or adjusting policies to levels and types of traffic. Still, the problem of fine tuning policy to the security needs of the organization, that is, writing policies that secure organizational assets without choking off network operations, has if anything grown worse. The recurring problem in all aspects of information security is establishing policy and procedures that are capable of capturing the complexity and unpredictability of most security threats and the need for flexibility and robustness of an organization's assets.

Perimeter defense is important, but most good security assumes that some threats and intruders will succeed in penetrating the network. Thus, most organizations use some type of intrusion detection system to indicate intrusions and to trace unauthorized access. Intrusion detection can take many forms. It can be driven principally by operational practice by periodically checking access logs or system files. For most organizations, these processes are augmented by technological tools that monitor network and in some cases application performance for indications of unauthorized access or activity. These tools can be quite effective in monitoring systems, yet they face a problem that corresponds to firewalls above. It is difficult to fine tune performance to capture the majority of intrusions without registering an overabundance of false positives. Again, there is no magic bullet technology here, and a great deal of attention must be paid by security professionals to adjusting security tools to the requirements of the organization.

The role of cryptography in network security continues to grow. One of the first widespread uses for public key encryption was the protection of the confidentiality of e-mail through an application called Pretty Good Privacy (PGP). Nearly everyone who uses the Internet for e-commerce uses one of the most successful encryption protocols, Secure Sockets Layer (SSL), from time to time. Web sites can establish encrypted sessions between Web servers and browsers without requiring users to install plug-ins or reconfigure their client machines. For network engineers, the challenge is creating secure network connectivity to those outside the protected bounds of the physical network, either because users are accessing the network from a remote site or using, say, a wireless technology. Many organizations have established encrypted channels known as Virtual Private Networks (VPNs) that can provide security to those outside the network space. The HIPAA Security Rule recommends encryption of E-PHI during transmission, and each of the above technologies can be used to achieve greater security.

Similar to nearly every security measure, encryption involves certain tradeoffs. Encrypted e-mail and VPNs protect confidentiality and message integrity but at the cost of ease of monitoring. If the outside world cannot read a message that has been encrypted, it is just as difficult for those monitoring the network. Encrypted traffic can inflict as much damage on a network through malicious code or intrusion, and it is substantially more difficult to detect such attacks if the communications are encrypted and unintelligible to sensors. VPNs, for example, solve one major problem (unauthorized interception of traffic) yet push the weakest security link back to the identity of the user. If the system does not use strong authentication of users, VPNs become the ideal means for intruders to cover their tracks. Security is a weakest link problem. If one problem is solved by, for example, locking doors, security vulnerabilities do not therefore evaporate. The principal vulnerability simply shifts to the next weakest link or links. If the doors are locked, that means it is probably time to check the security of the windows, and once having done that, the roof and air vents might need a once over.

Conclusion

As in nearly every area of IT, security tools are advancing rapidly. The sophistication of the threat environment demands the vigilance of information security professionals. However, the underlying structure of HIPAA privacy and security is unlikely to change a great deal. The practical requirements of risk management, access control, and security monitoring are the hallmarks of good security, and information security practice.

References

1. National Research Council. Networking Health: Prescriptions for the Internet. Washington, DC: National Academies Press; 2000.
2. Warren S, Brandeis LP. The Right to Privacy. Harvard Law Review; 1890.
3. Rosen J. The Unwanted Gaze: The Destruction of Privacy in America. New York: Random House; 2001.
4. Goffman E. The Presentation of Self in Everyday Life. New York: Anchor; 1959.
5. National Academy of Science. For the Record: Protecting Electronic Health Information. Washington, DC: National Academies Press; 1997. Available at: http://books.nap.edu/html/for/.

6. Goldman J, Hudson Z. Exposed: A Health Privacy Primer for Consumers. 1999. Available at: http://www.healthprivacy.org/usr_doc/33806.pdf.

7. Notice of Privacy Practices. Baltimore, MD: Johns Hopkins Medicine; April 14, 2004. Available at: http://www.hopkinsmedicine.org/patients/JHH/PROVIDER. pdf. Accessed Jan 25, 2006.

8. Kahn D. The Code Breakers: The Story of Secret Writing. New York: Macmillan; 1967.

9. Taylor T. Comparison paper between the Bell and LaPadula model and the SRI model. Proceedings of the 1984 Symposium on Security and Privacy. April 1984, pp 195–202.

10. Raymond E. The Cathedral and the Bazaar. Sebastopol: O'Reilly; 2001.

11. Whitman M, Mattord H. Management of Information Security. Boston: Thomson; 2004.

12. National Institute of Standards and Technology. An Introduction to Computer Security: The NIST Handbook. Special Publication 800-12; 1995.

13. National Institute of Standards and Technology. Risk Management Guide for Information Technology Systems. Special Publication 800-30; 2002.

14. Center for Medicare and Medicaid Services. (HIPAA Guidance.) Available at: http://questions.cms.hhs.gov.

15. Anderson R. Security in Clinical Information Systems. 1996. Available at: http://www.cl.cam.ac.uk/users/rja14/policy11/policy11.html.

14
Computer-based Documentation: Past, Present, and Future

KEVIN B. JOHNSON and S. TRENT ROSENBLOOM

Clinical structured entry and reporting, which involves the generation of the contents of medical documents through selection from a set of predefined and standardized categorical concepts, comprises an apotheosis among approaches to computer-assisted documentation. Structured entry and reporting systems are designed to enhance the process of clinical documentation by simultaneously presenting useful categorical concepts in a user interface and capturing input into the interface as machine-readable data.[1] Major goals of structured entry and reporting include producing raw data that enhance patient care by facilitating reminders and alerts while providing an infrastructure for clinical research. Documentation in a structured entry and reporting tool is achieved as a user navigates through lists of relevant concepts and gives them status (e.g., present/absent). A structured entry and reporting tool for documentation of medical encounters allows a healthcare provider efficiently to select concepts pertinent to the encounter type.[2] In parallel with the clinician generating a document, the structured entry and reporting tool can capture data suitable for research and for real-time clinical decision support and can generate a human-readable report. In the setting of a successful structured entry and reporting tool, post hoc manual abstraction of clinical information from the generated documents is generally unnecessary.

These tools have been called a variety of names. MEDLINE has no major heading for this tool, lumping papers into either the major heading "computerized medical record systems" or "documentation methods." Manuscripts use terms such as "structured reporting," "structured note capture," "computer-based documentation," and "structured data entry" to name a few. For the purposes of this chapter, we will use the term computer-based documentation (CBD) systems, defined as tools that capture data about a clinical encounter or event for the primary purpose of generating a summary of the encounter.

The authors believe that during clinical practice, healthcare providers will be best served by a spectrum rather than a monolithic type of CBD mechanisms. The mechanisms can be categorized according to the machine readability of their content, including handwritten notes scanned into computers and made available as images; free-text notes typed or transcribed into a computer-readable format; semistructured template-based notes of the type described in this report; and fully structured, more meticulously captured coded notes such as those already provided by many vendor systems (e.g., Logician by General Electric, EpicCare by Epic Systems, and elements of Practice Partner software from Physician Micro Systems). Relevant strengths and weaknesses of each note-capture mechanism vary. Fully structured coded notes, for example, facilitate data collection for research and real-time decision support but can be cumbersome to use during patient encounters and may lack the flexibility and expressivity required for general medical practices. Handwritten notes, by contrast, are extremely flexible and permit a high degree of expressivity but may be limited in their legibility and accessibility for data processing and analysis. Transcribed notes permit facile documentation into a format possibly useful for machine-based natural language processing for content extraction and summarization but are expensive to produce and require a time delay for the transcription process to occur. It is likely that each note-capture mechanism will find a clinical niche, with different clinicians and different sites each using the type that best fits the practice situation of the moment and that will vary during the course of a day.

This chapter provides an overview of the history of these tools, including many of the early successes and failures. We will then characterize current CBD tools, followed by a look into the future of these tools.

A History of CBD

Overview

Experiments with clinical structured entry and reporting began in the 1960s, when Warner Slack first reported the use of the Laboratory Instrument Computer (LINC) to document a physical examination.[3] Early computer-based history taking was conducted with the patient directly interacting with the system. Over the ensuing 20 years, work in the area has taken two forms: A group of researchers interested in improving the patients' ability to document their clinical findings and symptoms on a computer, and a group of researchers focusing on improving the provider's interaction with a computer to complete documentation while in the examination room. For the purposes of this review, we will focus only on the provider as the completer of documentation.

Capitalizing on early work done in the area of patient history taking, Greenes and colleagues[4] at the Laboratory of Computer Science at Massachusetts General Hospital and Harvard Medical School, developed a system designed for a physician to interact in real time with a computer to generate an encounter summary. The publication based on this project fully described many of the challenges that exist even in today's CBD environments. The system consisted of multiple components. The authors built a hierarchically organized structured vocabulary encompassing the concepts needed to manage adult outpatients in a hypertension clinic (see Figure 14-1). The authors constructed a template for an encounter summary, to which they mapped each concept. The authors displayed the hierarchical lists as a series of screens on a computer terminal. Each answer that was selected at each level generated corresponding text in a final encounter summary. The application supported typing narrative information at specific points in the interaction with the data structure.

Figure 14-2 shows a summary generated by this system. In addition to generating an encounter summary, the computer stored a coded version of the note. A separate application used an identical user interface to formulate a query of specific concepts. This application returned all notes satisfying that query, rather than generating an encounter summary. An evaluation of this application covered many key attributes that remain important to these tools today, including recording time as a function of experience, adequacy of the controlled vocabulary (by looking at the frequency and types of comments included), a usability survey, and the impact of having a prior note on needing the remainder of the medical record. These investigators noted the challenge of "subject matter development," noting that the process was arduous but speculating that it might become less so as domain areas overlap with one another.

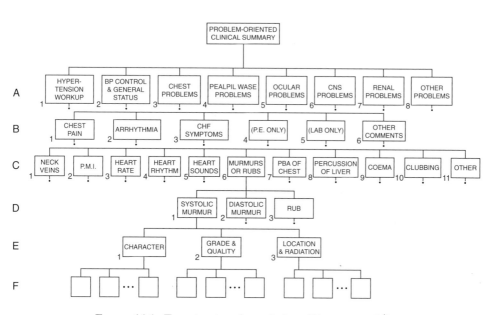

FIGURE 14-1. Tree-structured vocabulary (Greenes et al.[4]).

PATIENTS NAME: ▬▬▬▬▬▬▬
UNIT NO. ▬▬▬▬▬
SEX: M
AGE: 43
SINGLE MAILMAN

HYPERTENSION CLINIC – SUMMARY OF CURRENT STATUS
– 6-2-69

HYPERTENSION WORKUP
_____

(11-4-68):
    DATE FIRST NOTED: ABOUT 10 YEARS AGO (AT AGE 33).
(11-4-68):
    ETIOLOGIC IMPRESSION (CURRENT):
    IDIOPATHIC
        SUPPORTING FINDINGS: FAMILY HISTORY OF ESSEN-
        TIAL HYPERTENSION
        CREATININE CLEARANCE 139 L. IVP BILATERAL DOU-
        BLE COLLECTING SYSTEMS – OTHERWISE NORMAL.
        URINARY VMA 23. URINARY 17-OH CORTICOSTE-
        ROIDS 11.9. URINARY 17-KETO CORTICOSTEROIDS
        5.2.
(2-25-69):
    ETIOLOGIC AND FUNCTIONAL STUDIES: 3 HR PC BLOOD
    SUGAR 13.0. DATE: 2-24-69.

BP CONTROL & GENERAL STATUS
_____

(3-24-69):
    GENERAL:
    FEW MINOR COMPLAINTS. FEELS MODERATELY WELL.
(3-24-69):
    MEASUREMENTS:
    BP. RIGHT ARM. LYING: 200/122
    BP. RIGHT ARM. SITTING: 160/104
    WEIGHT (LB):193
    PULSE (BEATS/MIN): 68 REGULAR
(3-24-69):
    MEDICATIONS:
    CONTINUE ALL MEDS. AS BEFORE
(3-24-69):
    DIET:
    REDUCED CALORIE DIET
(3-3-69):
    HYPERTENSION STATUS:
        FAIRLY WELL CONTROLLED, OBESITY, WEIGHT SINCE
        LAST VISIT STABLE, ATE SALTY FOOD 3 DAYS AGO,
        HAS FELT VERY TIRED SINCE THEN

CHEST
_____

(3-3-69):
    NO CHEST PAIN
(12-16-68):
    NO CONGESTIVE HEART FAILURE SYMPTOMS
(3-24-69):
    PE: HEART SOUNDS NO CHANGE. PERCUSSION AND
    AUSCULTATION OF THE CHEST NORMAL. EDEMA:
    NONE
(2-24-69):
    LAB: ELECTROCARDIOGRAM: MODERATE LVH. NON.
    SPECIFIC ST & T WAVE CHANGES, DATE: 2-24-69.

FIGURE 14-2. Output generated by the system of Greenes et al.[4]

Radiology was one of the earliest specialties in which physicians directly interacted with a computer to generate a report. Brolin's MEDELA system[5] was one of the first such systems described in the literature. This radiology reporting system was one of the earliest systems actually used in practice by physicians. MEDELA was a terminal system that used a branching logic to project different frames on a terminal corresponding to numbers typed into a small numeric keypad. As the branching logic progressed, sentences were typed on an automatic typewriter. Systems such as this allowed providers to augment and improve the expressiveness of computer-based reporting by allowing typing on the same typewriter where automatic sentence typing has occurred. MEDELA was fairly advanced in its time both because of its use of three different technologies (a typewriter, a terminal, and a keypad) and because of its heavy reliance on graphical pictures to allow efficient traversing of a branching logic (see Figure 14-3).

Lessons learned by these systems continue to be relevant today. The main advantage of these systems was that the branching logic allowed some structure and more flexibility than predecessor systems or paper-based data forms. Similarly, the branching logic allowed for some level of decision support by selecting questions that were based on prior answers and excluding other questions that were no longer relevant. For example, these systems were able to prompt the user to select the reason for the study, which was used to tailor the CBD system's output and to ensure that questioning was appropriate for the study type. Early CBD systems were able to prompt the user to enter the gender of the patient, and use that information to avoid questions relating to anatomic or physiologic issues unique to the other gender.

These systems also included only the descriptive terms and diagnoses that were suitable for each examination, and utilized domain knowledge to arrange this information in ascending order of frequency. All of these efforts were designed to decrease the number of screens necessary to

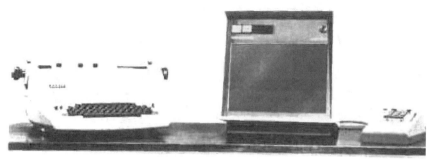

Figure 14-3. MEDELA terminal, consisting of an automatic typewriter, a display unit, and a small keyboard. (*Source*: Figure 1 from Brolin.[5])

navigate a structured vocabulary. For example, the neurologic examination included in MEDELA had 129 frames containing 4256 alternatives from which the radiologist needed to only give attention to 3 or 4 frames to complete a given report.

Other systems of the time included the systems MARS,[6] SIREP,[7] RADIATE,[8] and RAPORT.[9] Each of these systems used roughly similar approaches to generate a document.

After it was determined that many radiologists disliked using the typewriter,[10] a new interactive system was developed at the Johns Hopkins Hospital.[11] This system linked together a reporting terminal, a computer and a printer, a video screen, and a keyboard as shown in Figure 14-4. The physician touched a glass surface onto which a slide of radiological phrases was projected. In a manner similar to the MEDELA system, each phrase triggered both text generation and the display of a new slide onto the glass touchscreen. Once the report was completed, the radiologist pressed a key to generate the report. This system generated comprehensible, though "stilted" reports, used less secretarial (transcription) time, but did not result in high satisfaction among users.

Although these early systems in general had favorable reviews there were occasional concerns about their effect on medicine. For example, Irwin and Tillitt[12] were concerned that, in radiology, resident training might be stifled by tools that automatically generated concise studies thereby decreasing

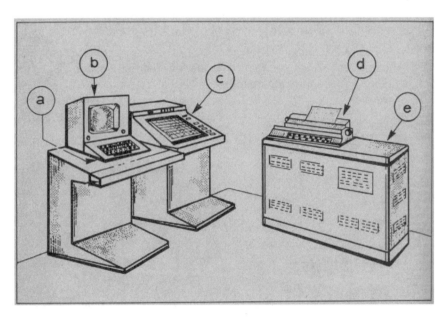

FIGURE 14-4. Structured radiology reporting system developed at Johns Hopkins Hospital (SIREP). (*Source*: Jeans et al.[7])

the need to understand how to create a well-packaged and succinct dictation. Another concern was that the technology forced a highly constrained vocabulary, thereby limiting the personalization and detail (and therefore the sophistication) of radiology reports.[4,5,7] In the area of radiology, there were concerns that these reports would detract from the reviewing of the film and potentially cause delays in the reporting process.[5] However, early data showed a decrease in the stenographic requirements in overtime spent using transcription without any decrease in note quality, suggesting a cost savings from these systems.[7]

From the first reports about the use of CBD in medicine, clinicians anticipated tradeoffs from its use in the examination room. There are numerous potential benefits to be achieved by using a computer to document a patient encounter. In addition to providing an easily searched medical record and ensuring more accurate online information, direct entry of encounter summaries allows them to be available immediately to other clinicians if the patient presents for health care at another site. For example, if a patient is seen in a primary care clinic and later sees a cardiologist or visits the emergency department, the data from the primary care visit will be available to healthcare providers at these other sites. Working with a computer during a patient visit also may provide a medium for interaction between physicians and patients, who can review their laboratory results and other medical information with their physician.[6] Computer systems also can provide feedback to ensure responsible care delivery through the use of reminders for screening studies and immunizations.[3,7] In pediatric practice, the types of anticipatory guidance, screening tests, and immunizations vary, depending on the age of the patient. Some pediatric clinicians use forms customized according to the patient's age to enter this information during health-maintenance visits. Newer computer systems often facilitate data entry by using similar online age-appropriate forms.[13] Systems also can provide online tutorials describing topics that should be discussed.[13] This is particularly important in a practice where residents in training may learn about primary care content from these prompts and may benefit from the reinforcement they provide during the encounter.

Although the potential benefits of encouraging clinicians to interact with a CBD system may seem compelling, the effects that a computer and direct data entry at the point of care have on patient–clinician interaction have been a concern. Early (primarily European) studies conducted in settings planning to adopt CBD tools noted concerns about the psychosocial aspects of the visit,[14–16] whereas many studies in actual settings did not substantiate this concern.[17–21] Studies also noted concerns about patient privacy being reduced by having sensitive information available in a computer.[15,16,18,20] Investigators such as Cruickshank predicted that patient acceptance would improve over time, and more recent studies in the United States support this prediction.[19,22] Since this time, studies objectively evaluating how computers impact the ambulatory encounter have noted that computers increase the duration of the encounter,[13,19] and change the patterns of communication as physicians focus on keying in information.[23,24] Studies also have suggested that patients have more confidence in physicians who use computers during the visit.[15,19] As a result of concerns about physicians having inadequate skills to use computers in the examination room, some groups have begun conducting workshops to teach skills and issues to enhance computer use during the ambulatory patient encounter.[25,26] Although this sort of workshop is used only in a limited number of sites, it is likely to find increased support as more technology is applied to the ambulatory setting.

Present-day Systems

Following the early leads in radiology, a number of structured entry and reporting systems have been developed and tested for use in specific clinical domains. Examples include the ARAMIS system that collects national data about patients with rheumatoid arthritis[27]; the endoscopy documentation tool, CORI[28,29]; Wirtschafter[30] and Shortliffe's[31] independent works developing chemotherapy documentation and decision support systems; an ophthalmology documentation system called NEON[32]; and Musen's T-HELPER[33] which advises community physicians if their patients meet criteria for enrollment in HIV-related clinical trials or modification of medical therapies. In addition, Weed's PROMIS system,[34] which was designed as a general use problem-oriented medical record, found its greatest use for documentation of obstetric and inpatient care.

Many of these clinical niche structured entry and reporting systems were developed to allow clinicians to document and store into research databases relevant patient information. The systems' user interfaces generally contained ad hoc mixtures of form fields that could be completed using mouse clicks, touchscreens, or keyboard entry, and spaces for text entry of unstructured information. Documentation of complex clinical cases has only rarely been demonstrated to be as efficient as more traditional documentation methods. The success or failure of these systems was likely tied to the benefit realized by the users. Systems that depended on more generalist practitioners to document so that researchers could access the data failed,[32] whereas systems that succeeded often served users who were both clinicians and researchers.[28-31,33]

To widen the appeal of CBD, developers have integrated new incentives and data entry methods. For example, Johnson's Clictate assists healthcare providers' documentation of pediatric care using guideline-based templates (see Figure 14-5).[13] Several commercial and institutional products, such as those by Logician,[35] Epic Systems,[36] Physician Micro Systems,[37] and the Department of Veteran's Affairs[38,39] have successfully been adopted as components of comprehensive electronic health record systems that, as a whole,

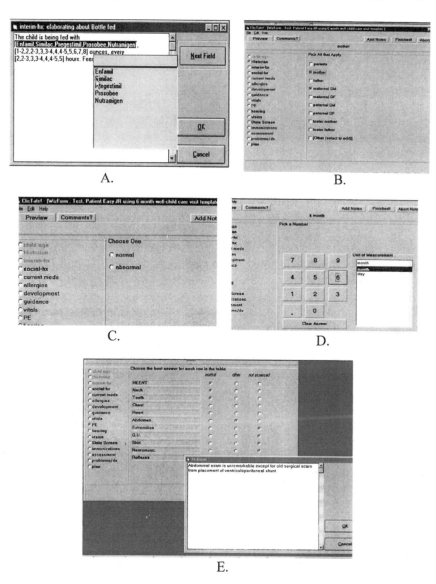

FIGURE 14-5. Clictate user interface components. These five examples illustrate the range of options used for data collection and include structured text (A), check boxes (B), radio buttons (C), a numeric keyboard (D), and a table (E). (*Source*: Johnson and Cowan.[13])

address workflow efficiency, automate coding, billing, and reimbursement, and provide patient-safety-related alerts. Many other commercial systems allow combined structured, semistructured, and unstructured entry of clinical documents from within the same tool. Examples include Dr. Notes,

SOAPware, and PracticeStudio. This hybrid approach enables users to balance documentation efficiency with the benefits that come from structured entry on a case-by-case basis. It is possible, however, that this approach may reduce the reliability and accuracy of the data captured by structured entry.

New technologies such as voice and handwriting recognition, tablet computers, and personal digital assistants have been advocated to users as alternate tools for entering data. Research on these new tools is still limited, and it is unclear if these data-input modalities will enable wider adoption.

Reasons for limited adoption remain largely speculative. Discussing the NEON tool for ophthalmology, Lum et al.[32] hinted that structured entry and reporting may be inefficient for ophthalmologists in general practice. McDonald suggests several additional factors that have attenuated clinician adoption of structured entry and reporting tools, including complexity and slow pace of navigating through user interfaces to find relevant content, inflexibility for documenting unforeseen findings, the lack of integration of clinical applications, and deficiencies in both coverage by and goals of the underlying data model.[40] Poon et al.,[2] in one of the few published outcomes studies specifically investigating the factors contributing to the local success of their structured entry and reporting tool, PEN-Ivory, identified optimal user interface characteristics that contributed to efficiency of input, integration, and navigation. Although PEN-Ivory operated with a vocabulary of 50,000 terms, Poon's study did not separately investigate the impact of the underlying terminology. Elkin et al.,[41,42] in their evaluations of structured problem list entry, have demonstrated that clinicians are willing to document using structured entry and reporting systems if the underlying terminology has terms that approximate frequently used phrases, suggesting that clinical terminologies may impact the usability of structured entry and reporting systems.

The Future of CBD

Since the early days of radiology and primitive CBD systems, there has been very little that has changed in the commercial products available for structured reporting. Why this is so is not clear. However, it is apparent that more recent technologic advances, such as the availability of personal digital assistants, tablet computers with built-in handwriting recognition technology, and low-cost speech recognition technology should result in improved tools for data capture at the point of care. Furthermore, other advances may well affect the architecture and functionality of these tools: Improving the terminology used by these tools; recent advances in natural language processing; and increased adoption of more primitive CBD tools.

Interface Terminology Support for Structured Entry

CBD systems, by definition, present users with terminologies of frequently documented or considered phrases that represent clinical entities of interest to health care and research. The terminologies that support structured entry and reporting systems are generally called "interface terminologies,"[43–45] but have elsewhere been called "colloquial terminologies,"[46] "application terminologies,"[47] and "entry terminologies."[48] Interface terminologies are specifically designed to support efficient structured entry and reporting interfaces by modeling the clinical concepts frequently used by healthcare providers as part of standard medical documentation tasks. Terms in clinical interface terminologies reflect common phrases and synonymy. Additionally, to optimize the efficiency of clinical documentation, concepts may contain what is called assertional medical knowledge, including relevant modifiers and corollary concepts. In Figure 14-6, an interface terminology modeling the concept chest pain would likely have a precomposed representation for chest pain that could be linked to modifiers for severity, pain character, and timing. Linking the modifiers to the concept in this way allows an associated structured entry and reporting system to display them together so that the user can easily select them if appropriate.

The classic example of a clinical interface terminology and the structured entry and reporting system it is designed to support are, respectively, MEDCIN and MediComp Systems. MEDCIN contains 215,000 concepts, has been in use since 1986, and was recently licensed by the Department of Defense for the Composite Health Care System II electronic health record system,[49] and underlies several commercial electronic health record structured entry and reporting modules. Initially developed in 1978 by Goltra as a clinical interface terminology overlying a database of clinical findings,

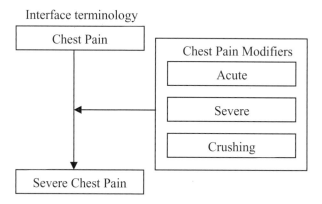

FIGURE 14-6. An interface terminology modifies the concept "chest pain" with linked modifier "severe" from a list of chest pain modifiers.

MEDCIN has since expanded to include concepts from clinical histories, physical examinations, tests, diagnoses, and therapies to enable coding of complete patient encounters.[50] MEDCIN concepts are precoordinated to allow "clinically precise phrasing"[50] while preventing nonsensical compositions and concept modification. Concepts are arranged consistently in multiple hierarchies, have associated normal and reference values, and are linked to more than 600,000 synonyms. MEDCIN also includes sanctioning logic, called "relationships," to enable the display of other concepts clinically relevant to the concept that the user is documenting. MEDCIN concepts also include logic to generate prose reports from categorically entered data. MEDCIN is currently linked to other terminologies, including CPT-4, ICD-9, ICD-10, and DSM-IV, but is not available in the UMLS. To date, scientific studies evaluating MEDCIN's terminological attributes such as domain coverage, concept clarity, and terminology usability are lacking.

Natural Language Processing

The basic tenet of structured data entry using an interface terminology is that data that are entered in a nonstructured tool cannot be easily converted into a computable form, as would be necessary to derive a level of service, generate orders, conduct clinical research, or monitor for specific conditions or circumstances. However, that tenet is challenged by recent advances in natural language processing.

One of the major barriers to the development and adoption of CBD, as described above, is the lack of an accepted standard nomenclature on which to build clinical phrases. This deficiency challenges our existing paradigm for CBD, in which some single set of phrases form the search space to generate a large number of documents. However, the inability to decide whether "heart" or "cardiac" should be the category in which one finds systolic murmur does not prevent us from understanding what systolic murmur means. Other contextual clues, such as whether it is found in the "family history" versus "physical exam" section of the note, or other words surrounding it, help to clarify its meaning. These heuristics are the basis of present-day medical language processing systems.

Although still early in their inception, these systems are becoming quite powerful. For example, the system developed by Friedman and colleagues,[51] called MedLEE, tries to analyze the structure of the entire sentence using patterns that are often found in medicine. For example, the pattern "finding in bodyloc cong bodyloc" is a well-formed pattern that will correspond to the phrase *pain in arms and legs*. This method, in addition to other error-recovery approaches and heuristics are combined within MedLEE.[52]

Medical language processing is by no means a trivial exercise. Text must first be processed using tools to separate words, phrases, and punctuation into individual units called tokens. Each token string must then be processed further, sometimes using stemming to generate canonical forms for

English variants (walked, walking, walk), using tagging to identify specific words (such as sections of the note) to help other processes or, in the case of patient names or identifiers, to hide that information. More complex systems parse complete sentences.

MedLEE has performed extremely well as a screening tool for chest radiographs, and more recently as a tool to identify cases related to medical errors. These results suggest that there is a role for medical language processing that may take pressure off other CBD systems to require controlled terminologies.

Extending the Reach of CBD Tools

Although CBD tools have evolved in many ways, systems implementers continue to be challenged by the potential complexity of encounter templates, defined as limited collections of clinical findings and impressions that guide the user through a given documentation task. Template developers may summarize the challenge in terms of developing a template that has acceptable performance (i.e., is tractable) across each section of the encounter summary.

Templates are generally designed to focus the user on those symptoms, signs, impressions, and plan elements that are most relevant to a particular problem. Template developers generally can constrain templates based on the presenting symptom(s) or based on the likely final diagnosis. Because a given symptom may have many causes, a comprehensive template based on a single symptom must include all pertinent symptoms and signs to support or exclude the possible diagnoses. For example, a sore throat can be caused by streptococcal pharyngitis (i.e., strep throat), a peritonsillar abscess, influenza, any one of a number of other viruses, allergic rhinitis, a myocardial infarction, or trauma. A template designed to encompass the workup for a sore throat must include the chief complaint—sore throat, and all symptoms and signs associated with these final diagnoses (e.g., fever, halitosis, rash, unilateral pain, rhinorrhea, sneezing, diaphoresis, chest pain). Although this approach permits great flexibility in documenting the presenting problem, it can increase the size and breadth of a template to the point where it becomes inefficient to use and complex to navigate.

Constraining a template based on a suspected diagnosis can lead to greater focus, but will also reduce its flexibility. For example, a developer could create a template for patients who likely have a final diagnosis of strep throat (see Figure 14-7). Such a template would contain all the common symptoms associated with strep throat, including sore throat, fever, hoarse voice, dysphagia, and perhaps skin rash. The template may also include specific questions about sick contacts, history of recurrent streptococcal infection, history of ear infections, and possibly history of rheumatic disease, and would continue with lists of frquently seen signs, including exudative tonsillitis, cervical lymphadenopathy, nasal turbinate congestion, and a scarlatiniform skin rash. The template may contain an assessment that

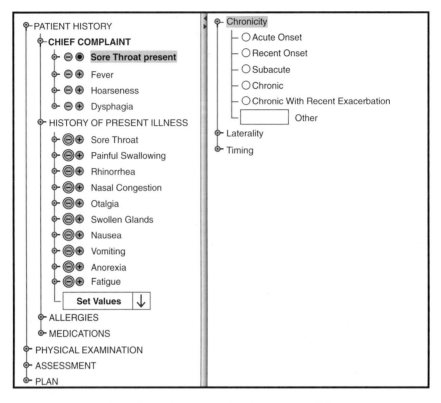

FIGURE 14-7. Strep throat template for structured data entry.

will almost always be either classic streptococcal pharyngitis; pharyngitis that is less likely to be streptococcal in origin, or no pharyngitis. The plan may include performing a rapid strep or streptococcal culture, administering antibiotics (penicillin or an equally efficacious one) and a statement about when to return to work or school.

For clinical encounters that precisely follow the sequence and content of the template, documentation using the CBD system may be relatively efficient. In such cases, the clinician can, in essence, just fill in the blanks. However, for cases in which the patient has symptoms that were not predicted by the template developers, or in which the healthcare provider suspects a diagnosis other than the one encompassed by the template, the CBD system can make it challenging to document the full nuance of the patient's case. For example, after having committed to using the template for strep throat, a healthcare provider using a traditional CBD system could choose from three methods to handle a new patient complaint of pleuritic chest pain and cough. First, the provider could document the additional symptoms outside the template structure, thus eliminating any benefits gained from the template. Second, the provider could select a new template with greater relevance to the current problem, but requiring redundant documentation. Third, the provider could choose not to document the new information. None of these approaches encourages efficient and complete documentation.

To address the challenge of balancing documentation flexibility with a constrained focus, a radically different model for template construction must be considered. One such model is found in the work of Shultz and colleagues.[53] In this model, users may dynamically merge multiple constrained templates and notes (i.e., templates containing patient-specific clinical information) as needed, to create new templates meeting broad documentation needs.

In Shultz's CBD system, Quill, users create individualized templates and can access other users' or generic domain-specific templates. In Quill, templates consist of collections of clinical findings and associated modifiers (e.g., the finding "Sore Throat" and its modifier "Chronicity") arranged in a customized sequence, often with common default values. Users generate notes by setting status to a template's findings and modifiers and by adding, removing, or rearranging findings as necessary. Additional information may be incorporated into the note at any point during its creation by locating and inserting the relevant finding. For example, if a patient complains of incidental ear pain during a strep throat workup, the healthcare provider can search for "Otalgia" and add it to the note's History of Present Illness section. Any time a user makes any of these changes, they have the option of storing it as a new template; by this means, template generation and note completion use the same processes. In the current example, the provider could store for future use the modified strep throat template that includes the finding otalgia.

In Quill, merging templates is identical to adding a new finding. Users merge templates by selecting and adding a new template to an existing one. The user may do this in preparation for future patient encounters while creating new templates, or dynamically while documenting a specific patient encounter. Merging templates creates a union of the two, in which the individual findings from each appear, but are not duplicated. The template superstructure (i.e., chief complaint, history of present illness, physical examination, vital signs) is maintained, and is used to ensure that the findings from each of the source templates are correctly placed in the final merged template.

In addition, notes may be merged. Similar to templates, notes are collections of findings, relevant modifiers, and customized sequence. Notes also include patient-specific clinical information (e.g., sore throat "is present," temperature is "102.4, Fahrenheit"). Merging notes allows healthcare providers to reuse previously gathered clinical information for a subsequent patient encounter, and may enhance the efficiency of clinical documentation. Quill allows notes to be merged to notes or to blank templates, creates a union in which the findings from each appear once, and the most recently added clinical data prevail, in case of a conflict. As with templates, merging notes may create new templates that the user may choose to store for future documentation needs.

Templates and notes may need to be merged under the following circumstances:

1. One provider wants to incorporate information from a prior encounter.
2. One provider wants to incorporate information from a collaborating provider.
3. One provider wants to incorporate elements from multiple templates.

In a model that permits merging templates and notes, a healthcare provider may maintain multiple focused templates designed around probable diagnoses. As clinical information suggesting additional problems becomes available, the provider can merge a different template without giving up previously documented findings. For example, after having already noted in a strep throat template the presence of a sore throat, fever, and nausea, the provider could merge a pneumonia template after the patient adds that he has a cough, sputum, and pleuritic chest pain. Merging also permits the provider to reuse a prior note containing the patient's physical examination and a note documenting the nurse's intake evaluation which includes the vital signs.

Quill represents a state-of-the-art, though as yet unevaluated approach to CBD that demonstrates a technical solution to many of the problems identified in earlier CBD systems.

Additional Features

As CBD tools become better integrated within electronic medical records systems, there has been wider consideration of how they fit into the workflow of clinical practice. Early radiology systems were designed with the assumption that these tools generated documents that served two purposes: The creation of an appropriately expressive summary of the findings, and the construction of documentation in support of billing. These systems communicated primarily with patient identification and radiology scheduling systems (or, in fact, took over the process of radiology scheduling) but rarely needed or could benefit from other interfaces for data input.

Today's generally available tools operate in concert with many other demands on clinician time, and could potentially receive data from or provide documentation to other computer tools. A recent survey of the American Medical Informatics Association's Clinical Working Group[54] asked early adopters of these systems to suggest additional features that could be provided by these systems. A summary of those recommendations is shown in Figure 14-8.

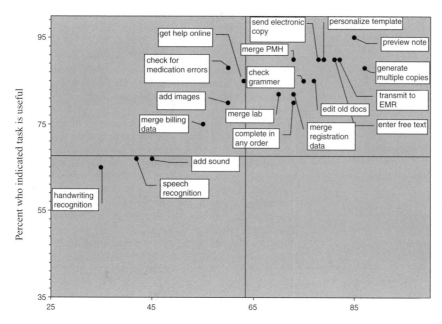

FIGURE 14-8. Summary of desired features in a CBD system.

Of interest in this figure are the features in the upper left quadrant. Survey respondents thought that CBD tools would be made more useful by allowing images and billing data to be added to the documentation environment and by providing system and content help such as recognizing potential medication errors. Of note, there were additional features listed in the upper right quadrant that are not uniformly present in these tools.

Essaihi and colleagues[55] recently published a "palette" of actionable items that are found in clinical guidelines (see Table 14-1). This palette seems particularly well suited to thinking through potentially new ways to integrate action with documentation. For example, more advanced CBD tools should link with electronic prescription writers, and should document not only that a medication has been started or stopped, but also any changes (increased dose, increased frequency) and the reason for the change, as a byproduct of generating the prescription. Procedures, such as administering immunizations, should result in a "procedure note" with the appropriate details (lot number, site administered, side effects, etc.) as well as a note stating that immunizations were given in the main note.

Undoubtedly, as clinical terminologies mature, the uses for data from CBD tools will help drive adoption. As adoption of these tools increases and spreads out of larger practice settings, market forces will steer the feature set of this technology and likely make it more usable in ways that have not been articulated thus far.

TABLE 14-1. Actionable items in clinical guidelines

Action Palette Item, as Noted by Essaihi et al.[55]	CBD Equivalent
Prescribe	Generate prescriptions, automatically document additions, deletions, and changes to medications list in the note.
Test	Order diagnostic tests, automatically document any ordered and resulted tests in the note.
Perform procedure	Create a new note using a procedure summary format, and document that the procedure was performed in the first note.
Refer/consult	Schedule patient to see another clinician for evaluation and treatment. Document the date and other details in the note.
Educate/counsel	Document any counseling done or handouts given to the patient during the visit. This may be done by linking Web download actions to the note, for example.
Dispose	As a byproduct of documentation, begin the discharge or admission process.
Monitor	Automatically summarize or link to disease-specific follow-up data, such as blood pressures, follow-up visits, laboratory tests.

References

1. Kahn CE Jr. Self-documenting structured reports using open information standards. Medinfo 1998;9(pt 1):403–407.
2. Poon AD, Fagan LM, Shortliffe EH. The PEN-Ivory project: exploring user-interface design for the selection of items from large controlled vocabularies of medicine. J Am Med Inform Assoc 1996;3(2):168–183.
3. Slack WV, Peckham BM, Van Cura LJ, Carr WF. A computer-based physical examination system. JAMA 1967;200(3):224–228.
4. Greenes RA, Barnett GO, Klein SW, Robbins A, Prior RE. Recording, retrieval and review of medical data by physician-computer interaction. N Engl J Med 1970;282(6):307–315.
5. Brolin I. MEDELA: an electronic data-processing system for radiological reporting. Radiology 1972;103(2):249–255.
6. Lehr JL, Lodwick GS, Nicholson BF, Birznieks FB. Experience with MARS (Missouri Automated Radiology System). Radiology 1973;106(2):289–294.
7. Jeans WD, Danton RM, Kilburn AR. An assessment of a computerized reporting system (SIREP). Br J Radiol 1980;53(629):421–427.
8. Templeton AW, Lodwick GS, Turner AH Jr. RADIATE: a new concept for computer coding, transmitting, storing, and retrieving radiological data. Radiology 1965;85(5):811–817.
9. Mani RL. RAPORT radiology system: results of clinical trials. AJR Am J Roentgenol 1976;127(5):811–816.
10. Fairman WL, Dickhaus EA. Technology evaluation: a case study of MARS (Missouri Automated Radiology System). Med Care 1977;15(1):79–82.
11. Wheeler TK, Rubery ED, Haybittle JL. A computer-based radiotherapy clinical record system using mark-sense forms. Br J Radiol 1976;49(586):863–867.
12. Irwin GA, Tillitt R Jr. A computer assisted radiological reporting system. Radiology 1976;118(2):329–331.
13. Johnson KB, Cowan J. Clictate: a computer-based documentation tool for guideline-based care. J Med Syst 2002;26(1):47–60.

14. Potter AR. Computers in general practice: the patient's voice. J R Coll Gen Pract 1981;31(232):683–685.

15. Cruickshank PJ. Computers in medicine: patients' attitudes. J R Coll Gen Pract 1984;34(259):77–80.

16. Cruickshank PJ. Patient stress and the computer in the consulting room. Soc Sci Med 1982;16(14):1371–1376.

17. Solomon GL, Dechter M. Are patients pleased with computer use in the examination room? J Fam Pract 1995;41(3):241–244.

18. Rethans JJ, Hoppener P, Wolfs G, Diederiks J. Do personal computers make doctors less personal? Br Med J (Clin Res Ed) 1988;296(6634):1446–1448.

19. Ornstein S, Bearden A. Patient perspectives on computer-based medical records. J Fam Pract 1994;38(6):606–610.

20. Ridsdale L, Hudd S. Computers in the consultation: the patient's view. Br J Gen Pract 1994;44(385):367–369.

21. Legler JD, Oates R. Patients' reactions to physician use of a computerized medical record system during clinical encounters. J Fam Pract 1993;37(3): 241–244.

22. Makoul G, Curry RH, Tang PC. The use of electronic medical records: communication patterns in outpatient encounters. J Am Med Inform Assoc 2001;8(6):610–615.

23. Greatbatch D, Heath C, Campion P, Luff P. How do desk-top computers affect the doctor-patient interaction? Fam Pract 1995;12(1):32–36.

24. Warshawsky SS, Pliskin JS, Urkin J, et al. Physician use of a computerized medical record system during the patient encounter: a descriptive study. Comput Methods Programs Biomed 1994;43(3–4):269–273.

25. Liaw ST, Marty JJ. Learning to consult with computers. Med Educ 2001;35(7): 645–651.

26. Paperny DM. Computers and information technology: implications for the 21st century. Adolesc Med 2000;11(1):183–202.

27. Bruce B, Fries JF. The Stanford Health Assessment Questionnaire: a review of its history, issues, progress, and documentation. J Rheumatol 2003;30(1): 167–178.

28. CORI: Clinical Outcomes Research Initiative Publications List. http://cori.ohsu. edu. Last Access Date 1/1/2004.

29. CORI: Clinical Outcomes Research Initiative. http://cori.ohsu.edu. Last Access Date 1/1/2004.

30. Wirtschafter DD, Scalise M, Henke C, Gams RA. Do information systems improve the quality of clinical research? Results of a randomized trial in a cooperative multi-institutional cancer group. Comput Biomed Res 1981;14(1):78–90.

31. Shortliffe EH. Update on ONCOCIN: a chemotherapy advisor for clinical oncology. Med Inform (Lond) 1986;11(1):19–21.

32. Lum F, Schein O, Schachat AP, Abbott RL, Hoskins HD Jr, Steinberg EP. Initial two years of experience with the AAO National Eyecare Outcomes Network (NEON) cataract surgery database. Ophthalmology 2000;107(4):691–697.

33. Musen MA, Carlson RW, Fagan LM, Deresinski SC, Shortliffe EH. T-HELPER: automated support for community-based clinical research. Proc Annu Symp Comput Appl Med Care 1992:719–723.

34. Stratmann WC, Goldberg AS, Haugh LD. The utility for audit of manual and computerized problem-oriented medical record systems. Health Serv Res 1982;17(1):5–26.

35. Logician Ambulatory. http://www.medicalogic.com/products/logician. Last Access Date 12/15/2005.
36. Epic Systems Corporation. Available at: http://www.epicsys.com/.
37. Physician Micro Systems, Inc. Practice Partner Patient Records. http://www.pmsi.com. Last Access Date 12/15/2005.
38. Brown SH, Hardenbrook S, Herrick L, St. Onge J, Bailey K, Elkin PL. Usability evaluation of the progress note construction set. Proc AMIA Symp 2001:76–80.
39. Brown SH, Lincoln MJ, Groen PJ, Kolodner RM. VistA: U.S. Department of Veterans Affairs national-scale HIS. Int J Med Inf 2003;69(2–3):135–156.
40. McDonald CJ. The barriers to electronic medical record systems and how to overcome them. J Am Med Inform Assoc 1997;4(3):213–221.
41. Elkin PL, Mohr DN, Tuttle MS, et al. Standardized problem list generation, utilizing the Mayo canonical vocabulary embedded within the Unified Medical Language System. Proc AMIA Annu Fall Symp 1997:500–504.
42. McKnight LK, Elkin PL, Ogren PV, Chute CG. Barriers to the clinical implementation of compositionality. Proc AMIA Symp 1999:320–324.
43. Spackman KA, Campbell KE, Cote RA. SNOMED RT: a reference terminology for health care. Proc AMIA Annu Fall Symp 1997:640–644.
44. Rogers J. Interface Terminologies. Personal Communication. 2003.
45. Huff SM, Lau LM, Masarie FE, Morris J, Russler D. Panel Discussion: The impact of business issues on terminology adoption: clinical software developers' perspective. AMIA Fall Symposium, Washington, DC., 1999.
46. McDonald FS, Chute CG, Ogren PV, Wahner-Roedler D, Elkin PL. A large-scale evaluation of terminology integration characteristics. Proc AMIA Symp 1999: 864–867.
47. Rose JS, Fisch BJ, Hogan WR, et al. Common medical terminology comes of age. Part 1. Standard language improves healthcare quality. J Healthc Inf Manag 2001;15(3):307–318.
48. Chute CG, Elkin PL, Sherertz DD, Tuttle MS. Desiderata for a clinical terminology server. Proc AMIA Symp 1999:42–46.
49. Military Health System Information Management Program Review Board. 2000. Available at: http://www.tricare.osd.mil/charters/minutes/impr020900.htm.
50. Medicomp Systems. Available at: http://www.medicomp.com/.
51. Friedman C, Alderson PO, Austin JH, Cimino JJ, Johnson SB. A general natural-language text processor for clinical radiology. J Am Med Inform Assoc 1994; 1(2):161–174.
52. Friedman C, Hripcsak G, Shablinsky I. An evaluation of natural language processing methodologies. Proc AMIA Symp 1998:855–859.
53. Shultz E, Rosenbloom T, Kiepek W, et al. Quill: a novel approach to structured reporting. AMIA Annu Symp Proc 2003:1074.
54. Johnson KB, Ravich WJ, Cowan JA Jr. Brainstorming about next-generation computer-based documentation: an AMIA clinical working group survey. Int J Med Inform 2004;73(9–10):665–674.
55. Essaihi A, Michel G, Shiffman RN. Comprehensive categorization of guideline recommendations: creating an action palette for implementers. AMIA Annu Symp Proc 2003:220–224.

15
Health Text Analysis*

PETER L. ELKIN

Knowledge representation in health care has taken a diverse and varied approach to its evolution and view of the ultimate solution. An understanding of the content of the health record is essential to our development of an intelligent electronic health record (iEHR). Information retrieval of detailed health information requires a formal understanding of the content of the record. This understanding, in turn, will fuel the decision support systems (e.g., Guideline Management and Alert software) which will enhance patient safety and improve the efficiency of the practice of medicine and its associated disciplines to be delivered through the EHR system (EHR-S).

The earliest efforts were database driven where records were entered using structured data entry with small controlled lists of concepts. The next step in the evolution of these systems was the development of free text entry of data elements which were matched and reviewed by clinicians and a final "coded" entry was entered into the clinical record. These two approaches were combined to allow both preselected and novel entry of clinical statements. As the field progressed, several knowledge bases of controlled health terminologies were developed. These were later combined into the Unified Medical Language System (UMLS).[1] In the late 1990s, the focus shifted to the development of description logic-based reference terminologies. These two approaches were combined to allow both preselected and novel entry of clinical statements. Since that time, this theme has been heard resounding from an increasingly large group of scientists. These terminologies continue to evolve today.

Classification has long been an important feature of information retrieval through the coding of health text. In 1839, William Farr stated in his First Annual Report of the Registrar-General of Births, Deaths, and Marriages in England, "The nomenclature is of as much importance in this depart-

---

* This work was supported in part by a grant from the National Library of Medicine LM6918-A104.

ment of inquiry, as weights and measures in the physical sciences, and should be settled without delay."[2]

Today, the need for controlled vocabularies to support health record systems has been widely recognized (see Chapter 12). Classifications provide systems with the means to aggregate data. This aggregation of data can be done at multiple levels of granularity and therefore can enhance the clinical retrieval of a problem-oriented record, data pertaining to a classification for billing purposes, or outcomes data for a given population. However, maintenance of large-scale classifications has become a burdensome problem as the size of term sets has escalated (ISO 15188). These corpora of structured knowledge have become larger and larger [Systematized Nomenclature of Medicine Clinical Terms (SNOMED-CT) v1.0 has approximately 340,000 concepts and 800,000 terms], and it has become difficult to fit the terms from a domain into a pick list, or even a searchable list, for direct data entry. This has given greater relevance to the use of health text processing technologies. Also, direct data entry of health data is time consuming and many clinicians already dictate their records which are later transcribed. Without a well-structured backbone, classifications cannot scale to provide the level of accuracy required by today's EHR and epidemiologic applications, as evidenced by the importance of vocabularies in the many standards discussed in Chapter 12.

The solution rests with standards.[3] Over the past ten or more years, Medical Informatics researchers have examined the structure and content of existing classifications to determine why they seem unsuitable for particular needs, and they have proposed solutions. In some cases, proposed solutions have been carried forward into practice and new experience has been gained.[4] As we enter the twenty-first century, it seems appropriate to pause to reflect on this experience, and publish a standard set of goals for the development of comparable, reusable, multipurpose, and maintainable controlled health vocabularies (ISO 12200, ISO 12620).

History of Classification

The present coding practices rely on data methods and principles for terminology maintenance that have changed little since the adoption of the statistical bills of mortality in the mid-seventeenth century.[5] The most widely accepted standard for representing patient conditions, International Classification of Diseases–Clinical Modification (ICD-9-CM),[6] is a direct intellectual descendent of this tradition. ICD-9-CM relies overwhelmingly on a tabular data structure with limited concept hierarchies and no explicit mechanism for synonymy, value restrictions, inheritance, or semantic and nonsemantic linkages. The maintenance environment for this healthcare classification is a word processor and its distribution is nearly exclusively paper-based.

The first edition of the Physicians' Current Procedural Terminology (CPT) appeared in 1966. In the United States (US), CPT, although copyrighted by the American Medical Association, is the coding system used by Medicare and virtually all third-party payers, including workers compensation and Medicaid. As part of the Medicare Part B physician payment schedule, CPT codes are associated with the Resource-Based Relative Value Scale and used to determine payment for services. The CPT code set is Level I of the Centers for Medicare and Medicaid Services Common Procedure Coding System. The CPT code set, currently in its fourth edition, contains numeric modifiers, notes, guidelines, and an index designed to provide explanatory information and facilitate the correct usage of the coding system. The American Medical Association is currently working to develop the next generation of CPT (i.e., CPT-5).

Significant cognitive advances in disease and procedure representation took place in 1928 at the New York Academy of Medicine, resulting in industry-wide support for what became the Standard Nomenclature of Diseases and Operations. The profound technical innovation was the adoption of a multiaxial classification scheme.[7,8] Now a pathologic process (e.g., Inflammation) could be combined with an anatomic site (e.g., Oropharynx Component: Tonsil) to form a diagnosis (e.g., Tonsillitis). The expressive power afforded by the compositional nature of a multiaxial terminological coding system tremendously increased the scope of tractable terminology and additionally the level of granularity that diagnosis could be encoded about our patients.[7]

The College of American Pathology (CAP) carried the torch further by creating the Systematized Nomenclature of Pathology, and subsequently SNOMED. In these systems, the number, scope, and size of the compositional structures has increased to the point where an astronomical number of terms can be synthesized from SNOMED atoms. One well-recognized limitation of this expressive power is the lack of syntactic grammar, compositional rules, and normalization of both the concepts and the semantics. Normalization is the process by which the system knows that two compositional constructs with the same meaning are indeed the same (e.g., that the term "Colon Cancer" is equivalent to the composition of "Malignant Neoplasm" and the site "Large Bowel"). These are issues addressed by CAP in their efforts to make SNOMED a robust reference terminology for health care.[9]

Other initiatives of importance are the Clinical Terms v3 (Read Codes), which are maintained and disseminated by the National Health Service in the United Kingdom, and the Galen effort, which expresses a very detailed formalism for term description. The Read Codes are a large corpus of terms, which is now in its third revision that is hierarchically designed and is slated for use throughout Great Britain. CAP and the National Health Service have merged the content of SNOMED-Reference Terminology (RT) and Clinical Terms version 3 into a derivative work (announced April 1999), which is named SNOMED Clinical Terms.

In 2003, Tommy G. Thompson, then US Secretary of Health and Human Services, expressed his support for the use of information systems to improve the quality of health care. He said that his first priority was to develop incentives to use SNOMED-CT and electronic medical records to fully integrate health information among medical institutions and various computer systems. To bring this vision to fruition, the terminologies used must provide adequate coverage of today's most common clinical problems. Health and Human Services and other federal agencies have contracted with the College of American Pathologists, which publishes SNOMED-CT, so that until at least July 2008 healthcare organizations that have reporting responsibility to the US government may use the terminology at no cost.

Classifications as opposed to nomenclatures need to exist where the patterns of aggregation needed for a purpose are not adequately supported by the hierarchies of a reference terminology (the operative reference terminology). Classifications must be exclusively derived as a set of precoordinations from the postcoordinations of a reference terminology.

Unified Medical Language System

Over the past decade, the National Library of Medicine (NLM) has sponsored an effort to compile approximately 43 vocabularies into a metathesaurus. This metathesaurus serves as a compilation of these individual terminologies and also supports translation between them.[10–12] This is done by using concept-level identifiers, which denote synonymy at the concept level. The structure is tabular, but supports the hierarchies, which already exist within the source vocabularies. Dozens of laboratories under contract to the NLM have participated in the development and content enhancement over the years.[13] At present, the metathesaurus holds approximately 1,000,000 concepts and approximately 2,800,000 unique strings. Because the UMLS contains sources, which were optimized for nonclinical purposes, such as the MeSH terminology—the controlled vocabulary powering PubMed—the UMLS has been criticized for not being more clinically relevant. For example, the MeSH terminology was derived to support query into the MEDLINE database, which holds the Medical Literature, which is quite a different purpose than entry of controlled terms into a patient's problem list. Nevertheless, the volume of content and the access to this rich source of synonymy provides a powerful resource for providing a comprehensive problem list entry tool.[14]

The Large Scale Vocabulary Test Trial

This large national trial was designed to determine the extent to which a combination of existing machine-readable health terminologies covered the concepts and terms submitted from a diverse set of national collaborators using the Internet and the UMLS knowledge sources, lexical programs, and a lexical server.[15] In this trial, a Web-based interface to the UMLS knowledge sources server served participants who searched more than 30 vocabularies in the 1996 UMLS metathesaurus combined with three planned additions to the metathesaurus. They were to determine whether the concepts, for which they desired controlled representation, were present in the above sources. For each item submitted to the Web interface, the user was asked to select the closest match from a candidate exact match or a list of potential partial matches. The interface recorded a profile of the sessions with the interface, including the terms searched for, the concept selected, and whether it was judged to be an exact match, a broader than, narrower than, associated with, or unrelated term. The terms submitted were made available to the NLM and to each of the participants. A team of subject experts reviewed records to identify matches missed by the participants and to correct obvious errors in relationships designated above.

The results showed that the UMLS matched exactly 58% of the concepts submitted, 41% were partial or related concepts, and 1% were unable to be matched. Sixty-three participants submitted 41,127 terms, which represented 32,677 normalized strings. More than 80% of the terms submitted came from a patient's medical record and were related to patient conditions. A broad spectrum of medical specialties were represented in the dataset. The review increased the exact matches from 55% to 58%. The percentage of exact matches varied from 45% to 71% by medical specialty. Individual vocabularies from within the UMLS metathesaurus contains between less than 1% to 63% of the terms and less than 1% to 54% of the concepts. Only SNOMED International and the Read Codes contained more than 60% of the terms and more than 50% of the concepts. The authors concluded that the majority of terminology needed to record patient conditions already exists. They further state that the metathesaurus, which is a compilation of multiple vocabularies, matched significantly more concepts exactly, than any individual contributing vocabulary.

National Drug File–Reference Terminology

In fiscal year 2001, the Department of Veterans Affairs (VA) Veterans Health Administration (VHA) provided health care to 4.1 million veterans and dependents in the form of 43 million outpatient visits, 573,000 inpatient admissions, and 167 million prescriptions (as 30-day equivalents). VHA has developed and deployed a variety of electronic tools to assist clinicians, including VISTA (Veterans Integrated Service and Technology Architecture), CPRS (Computerized Patient Record System), BCMA (Bar Code Medication Administration), and others.

VHA is continually looking for ways to use information technology (and other tools) to improve care quality, promote patient safety, and reduce costs. Reference terminologies and terminology services that permit retrospective and real-time aggregation, and sophisticated decision support are important areas under investigation. Formal terminologies are also being evaluated as a way to reduce maintenance and mapping effort. VHA's initial reference terminology project is National Drug File–Reference Terminology (NDF-RT), a formalization of the NDF. Other reference terminologies will be deployed under the VHA Enterprise Reference Terminology project.

NDF-RT uses a Description Logic[16]-based reference model that includes a defined set of abstractions denoting levels of description for drug products (based on work performed within the HL7 Vocabulary Technical Committee); a set of hierarchical and definitional relationships; and sets of nondefinitional properties used at each hierarchical level to capture associated details. The model includes hierarchies for chemical structure, mechanism of action, physiologic effect, and therapeutic intent. As of October 2003, NDF-RT has completed its final phases of expert review by doctors of clinical pharmacology and has been made available to interested parties (Mayo has access to the most recent version of the NDF-RT). The most recent version of NDF-RT includes 4202 active ingredients (including salt forms) and 108,112 National Drug Codes level products. Role definition counts (including inferred roles) are 118,504 mechanism of action roles; 119,095 physiologic effect roles; 123,379 may treat roles; 52,827 may prevent roles; and 5522 may diagnose roles.

Research Efforts

Until the 1920s, logic and mathematics was considered spiritual not scientific. Since the time of Pythagoras, mathematics was considered a revelation of the divine order. In *Principia Mathematica*, Russell and Whitehead demonstrated that mathematics was logical. Logical positivism was then applied to science and psychology.

Chomsky published, in 1955 in mimeograph form and in press in 1975, his seminal work, *The Logical Structure of Linguistic Theory*.[17] This work expressed the view that language was a predictable, systematic, and logical cognitive activity that required a meta-model of language to effectively communicate. He demonstrated that the behaviorists' stimulus-response model could not account for human language. This idea, that language is processed, led to the application of computer science to free text (natural language) processing. Computational linguistics (CL) is the field of computer science that seeks to understand and to represent language in an interoperable set of semantics. CL overlaps with the field of Artificial Intelligence and has often been applied to machine translation from one human language to another.

Researchers have succeeded, to varying degrees, to create CL algorithms for retrieving clinical texts. In 1994 Sager published a paper entitled, "Natural Language Processing and the Representation of Clinical Data."[18] Here, Dr. Sager showed that for a set of discharge letters, a recall** of 92.5% and a precision*** of 98.6% could be achieved for a limited set of preselected data using the parser produced by the Linguistic String Project at New York University.[19-21]

Researchers have also succeeded, to varying degrees, at representing the concepts underlying clinical texts. In 1999, Wagner, Rogers, Baud, and Scherrer reported on the Natural Language generation of urologic procedures.[22,23] Here they used a conceptual graph technique to apply translations for 172 rubrics from a common conceptual base among French, German, and English. They demonstrated that the GALEN model was capable of technically representing the concepts well; however, the language generation was often not presented in a form that native speakers of the target language would find natural. Trombert-Paviot et al.[24] reported the results of the use of GALEN in mapping French procedures to an underlying concept representation. Wroe et al.[25] in 2001 reported the ability to integrate a separate ontology for drugs into the GALEN model. Rector, in his exposé "Clinical Terminology: Why Is It So Hard?" discusses the importance of and ten most challenging impediments to the development of compositional systems capable of representing the vast majority of clinical information in a comparable manner.[26] In 2001, Professor Rector published one workable method for integrating information models and terminology models.[27]

In 2004, Friedman et al.[28] reported a method for encoding concepts from health records using the UMLS. In this study, the investigators used their system, MedLEE, to abstract concepts from the record and reported a recall of 77% and a precision of 89%. In 2001, Nadkarni[29] provided a description of the fundamental building blocks needed for Natural Language Processing (NLP). He discussed their method for lexical matching and part of speech tagging in discharge summaries and surgical notes. Lowe developed MicroMeSH, an early MUMPS-based terminology browser which incorporated robust lexical matching routines. Lowe, working with Hersh, reported

---

** Recall = proportion of relevant texts retrieved by the algorithm. Also called "sensitivity."
*** Precision = proportion of texts retrieved by the algorithm that are relevant. Also called "positive predictive value."

the accuracy of parsing radiology reports using the Sapphire indexing system.[30] They reported good sensitivity and were able to improve performance by limiting the UMLS source vocabularies by section of the report.

Beyond representing clinical concepts, tools are needed to link text provided by clinicians to the concepts in the knowledge representation. Cooper and Miller[31] created a set of NLP tools aimed at linking clinical text to the medical literature using the MeSH vocabulary. Overall, the composite method yielded a recall of 66% and a precision of 20%. Berrios[32] reported a vector space model and a statistical method for mapping free text to a controlled health terminology. Zou et al.[33] reported a system, IndexFinder, which was principally a phrase representation system. Srinivasan et al.[34] indexed MEDLINE citations (titles and abstracts) using the UMLS. Their method took the output of a part-of-speech tagger and fed the SPECIALIST minimal commitment parser, the lexicon used by the UMLS system. The output of this stage was matched to a set of grammars that yielded a final match.

NLM recently developed MetaMap.[35] It has the capacity to be used to code free text (natural language) to a controlled representation which can be any subset of the UMLS knowledge sources. MetaMap uses a five-step process that begins by using the SPECIALIST minimal commitment parser which identifies noun phrases without modifiers. The next step involves the identification of phrase variants. These variants are then used to suggest candidate phrases from within the source material.[36] Linguistic principals are used to calculate a score for each potential match. Brennan and Aronson[37] used MetaMap to improve consumer health information retrieval for patients.

The Mayo Experience

The clinical problem list is an important source of information about a patient. It is a regulatory requirement,[38] as well as a recommended method of communicating the state of a patient's health.[39] Given physicians' dislike for structured data entry (see Chapter 12), an attractive feature of an EHR-S is the ability to link the physician's free-text-entered problem with an underlying structured vocabulary.[40] The author of the current chapter and colleagues at the Mayo Clinic have worked for the past several years in providing that feature, resulting in the Mayo Vocabulary Server. Figures 15-1, 15-2, and 15-3 show the flow of data through the system that addresses not only the problem list, but the entire clinical record.

The Mayo problem list vocabulary was a clinically derived lexicon created from the entries made to Mayo Clinic's Master Sheet Index and the problem list entries made to the Impression/Report/Plan section of the Clinical Notes System.[41] We reduced needless repetition—lexical variants, spelling errors, and qualifiers (administrative or operational terms). Qualifiers

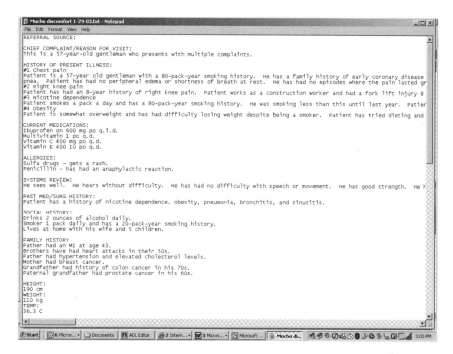

FIGURE 15-1. Free text health record. There is an implied structure but no readily computable structure to the information.

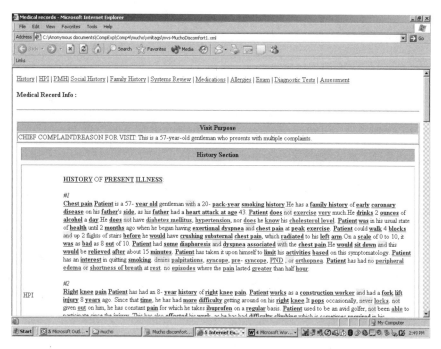

FIGURE 15-2. A fully encoded health record. In color, concepts representing positive assertions are colored blue (the majority), whereas concepts representing negative assertions are colored red, and uncertain assertions are colored green.

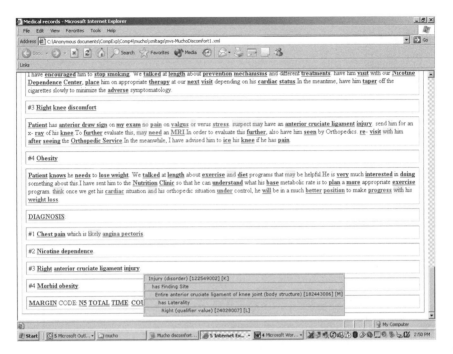

FIGURE 15-3. Phrases are built into compositional expressions consisting of a dyadic parse tree. Each concept is linked to other concepts in the tree by relationships (verbs) or Boolean operators. The standard logical Boolean set of And, Or, Not is expanded to include Maybe, to represent uncertainty.

were recoordinated with other terms, at run-time, which greatly increased the number of input strings, which the system is capable of recognizing (i.e., more than 1.4 million strings are now recognized, whereas the original lexicon could only recognize approximately 8000 strings).

In this work, the authors demonstrated a high degree of redundancy from within this clinically derived lexicon. By breaking out qualifiers from modifiers and then by removing the qualifiers from the terms within the lexicon, the authors have been successful in eliminating significant redundancy (41.6%). Relatively few problems with recoordination of the original, now composite terms (e.g., "*Family History of* Adenocarcinoma of the Prostate") were encountered. This is facilitated by the relatively simple rules for reconstruction of qualifier-term compositions, which change the administrative or temporal meaning of a canonical term. This is as opposed to modifiers, which change the meaning of a term in a clinical sense and have complex rules of interaction. For example, one could not have a patient with Stage I, Metastatic Breast Cancer.

As a result of using qualifiers as separate terms, the software can recognize approximately 1.4 million different input strings (composite terms).

This is a significant increase from the 7953 terms researchers had the ability to recognize initially. This represents an approximately 200-fold increase in the number of terms that would be able to be recognized as input strings to the problem manager system. The power of this conceptual modality is exemplified but not limited to this increase in the conceptual power of the system. There also exists considerable benefit in having a smaller database of terms to maintain and a greater assurance that duplication does not by design exist within the terminology. In a usability trial at the Mayo Clinic's Usability Laboratory, seven clinicians were introduced to 11 different scenarios, and all reported that they found the compositional expressions generated by the system to be clinically useful.

The authors have begun to examine the basis for compositionality by working toward a set of definitions that serve to organize workers' thoughts regarding composition. In this preliminary work, the authors defined the different types of composition.[41] Using these definitions, the authors presented methods of both server-based and client-based composition. Many of the obstacles involved in the creation of composition were presented. The authors also suggested mechanisms for minimizing these obstacles. The authors have presented a simple representational schema for compound concepts involving qualifiers (concepts that change the meaning of another concept in a temporal or administrative sense) and other terms. The authors submit that the interaction between modifiers (concepts that change the meaning of another concept in a clinical sense) are much more complicated.[42] One mechanism for addressing this complication is to involve the user in the decision-making process (User-Directed Compositionality).

Compositionality[42] in a Mayo Usability Study was found to be an essential part of the problem manager's functionality.[43] The greatest utility stemmed from the addition of modifiers and qualifiers (e.g., Acute, Left, Severe) to primary terms. It was also clear that users expressed no trepidation when selecting compound terms. Users found the rapid access to common qualifiers and modifiers very helpful and, as developers, the authors appreciated the concomitant decrease in the number of user-directed subsearches.

By forging a better understanding of the way that modifiers interact with other terms, the authors can improve the accuracy and usability of our postcoordinated terms. The better a system can become at anticipating which postcoordinated terms the users will find most acceptable, the greater will be the overall level of acceptance.

In the 1998 article "A Randomized Controlled Trial of Automated Term Composition," we reported the results of a trial using an early compositional technique to match a set of randomly selected clinical problem statements.[44] From a corpus of approximately 1,000,000 unique terms entered into the Impression/Report/Plan section of the clinical notes system in the calendar year 1997, the authors randomly selected 1000 terms. The authors then further randomized these 1000 terms into two groups of 500 (Sets A and B). The authors constructed two copies of the same term-matching interface, one without ATC (alpha) and one with ATC (beta). The authors took four expert indexers and assigned them to one of the following tasks. The first reviewer (R_1) compared set A using the alpha program and then set B using the beta program [$R_1(A_{alpha} + B_{beta})$]. The second compared set A using the alpha program and then set B using the alpha program [$R_2(A + B)_{alpha}$]. The third compared set B using the beta program and then set A using the beta program [$R_3(B + A)_{beta}$]. The fourth compared set A using the beta program and then set B using the alpha program [$R_4(A_{beta} + B_{alpha})$].

The program with ATC (beta) mapped 540 of the 1000 concepts correctly (54.0%). The same program without ATC mapped only 276 of the 1000 concepts correctly (27.6%). Therefore, the program with ATC was significantly (numerically and statistically) more effective at matching concepts in our problem lists than the same search engine without ATC ($P < .0001$; McNemar method). Reviewers numbered one and four achieved these results from the comparison of the alpha program with the beta program.

Automated term composition ATC provided significantly better coverage of a randomly chosen set of patient problems diagnosed at the Mayo Clinic during the 1997 calendar year, compared with the same information retrieval system without ATC. The use of SNOMED-RT yielded considerably better results than the UMLS with coverage rates of 80% of unique concepts and 95.12% of concepts as they are found in medical problem lists generated by clinicians. The accuracy of the mappings has been found to be 98.2% to 98.4% and the accuracy of retrieval is 99.8%.

To test the system further, we took a random sample of 100 Web pages from the 6000 Web pages on the Mayo Clinic's Health Oasis Web site.[45] The Web pages were divided into four datasets, each containing 25 pages. These were humanly reviewed by four clinicians to identify all of the health concepts present (R_1D_A, R_2D_B, R_3D_C, R_4D_D). The Web pages were simultaneously indexed using the SNOMED-CT beta release. The indexing engine had been previously described and validated. A different clinician reviewed the indexed Web pages to determine the accuracy of the automated mappings compared with the human identified concepts (R_4D_A, R_3D_B, R_2D_C, R_1D_D). This review recognized 13,220 health concepts. Of these, 10,383 concepts were identified in the initial human review (78.5% ± 3.6%). The automated process identified 10,083 concepts correctly (76.3% ± 4.0%) from within this corpus. The computer identified 2420 concepts that were not identified by the clinician's review but were, upon further consideration, important to include as medical concepts. There was on average a 17.1% ± 3.5% variability in the human reviewers' ability to identify the important medical concepts within Web page content. Concept-based indexing provided a positive predictive value of finding a medical concept of 79.3% compared with keyword indexing, which only has a positive predictive value of 33.7% ($P < .001$). The authors found that SNOMED-RT is a reasonable ontology for Web-page indexing. Concept-based indexing provides a significantly greater accuracy in identifying medical concepts compared with keyword indexing.

Whereas problem lists are important for patient care, it is important to retrieve sets of patients for many purposes: Finding patients for whom new guidelines dictate a recall of patients; better financial management; data mining for discovering relationships in data; finding patients to recruit into studies; and many others. Today, ICD-9-CM is the most frequently used method of retrieving clinical records. However, this method provides a coarse net. *Concept-based Indexing* may provide more granular data representation for—and therefore retrieval of—clinical records.[46] To date, there are no data to show that a clinical reference terminology is superior to a precoordinated terminology—one that allows no composition—in its ability to provide access to the clinical record.

In this study, we compared the sensitivity, specificity, positive likelihood ratio, positive predictive value, and accuracy of SNOMED-RT versus ICD-9-CM in retrieving 10 diagnoses from a random sample of 2022 episodes of care.

We randomly selected 1014 episodes of care from the inpatient setting and 1008 episodes of care from the outpatient setting. Each record had associated with it, the free text final diagnoses from the Master Sheet Index at the Mayo Clinic and the ICD-9-CM codes used to bill for the encounters within the episode of care. The free text diagnoses were coded by two expert indexers (disagreements were addressed by a staff clinician) as to whether queries regarding one of five common or five uncommon diagnoses should return this encounter. The free text entries were automatically coded using the Mayo Vocabulary Processor. Each of the 10 diagnoses was exploded in both SNOMED-RT and ICD-9-CM and, using these entry points, a retrieval set was generated from the underlying corpus of records. Each retrieval set was compared with the gold standard created by the expert indexers.

SNOMED-RT produced significantly greater specificity in its retrieval sets (99.8% versus 98.3%, $P < .001$ McNemar test). The positive likelihood ratios were significantly better for SNOMED-RT retrieval sets (264.9 versus 33.8, $P < .001$ McNemar test). The positive predictive value of a SNOMED-RT retrieval was also significantly better than ICD-9-CM (92.9% versus 62.4%, $P < .001$ McNemar test). The accuracy defined as 1 − [the total error rate (FP + FN)/total # episodes queried (20,220)], with total error rate = false positive + false negative, was significantly greater for SNOMED-RT (98.2% versus 96.8%, $P = .002$ McNemar test). Interestingly, the sensitivity of the SNOMED-RT-generated retrieval set was not significantly different from ICD-9-CM, but there was a trend toward significance (60.4% versus 57.6%, $P = .067$ McNemar test). However, if we examine only the outpatient practice, SNOMED-RT produced a more sensitive retrieval set than ICD-9-CM (54.8% versus 46.4%, $P = .002$ McNemar test).

Our data clearly show that information regarding both common and rare disorders is more accurately identified with automated SNOMED-RT indexing using the Mayo Vocabulary Processor than it is with traditional handpicked constellations of codes using ICD-9-CM. SNOMED-RT provided more sensitive retrievals of outpatient episodes of care than ICD-9-CM.

The methods discussed so far have addressed the direction of text to controlled vocabulary. The mirror question concerns *coverage*: To what extent does the chosen controlled vocabulary cover the given clinical domain? We performed an evaluation of the content coverage of SNOMED-CT for clinical problem lists.[46] Concept-based indexing is purported to provide more granular data representation for clinical records.[47] One area of the health record that is important for codification is the patient's problem list. In this study, we evaluated the content coverage of SNOMED-CT for the most common problems seen at the Mayo Clinic.

In this study, we compared the sensitivity, specificity, positive likelihood ratio, positive predictive value of SNOMED-CT in providing content coverage for the information stored in patient problem lists.

We selected the 5000 most common nonduplicated (unique text strings) from the Mayo Mastersheet Index associated with episodes of care from both the inpatient and the outpatient setting. Each record had associated with it, the free text final diagnoses from the Master Sheet Index at the Mayo Clinic. The free text diagnoses were coded by two physicians (disagreements were addressed by an expert clinician/terminologist) as to whether the terminology (SNOMED-CT) was able to represent the problem. The free text entries were also automatically coded using the Mayo Vocabulary Server. Reviewers also had available to them a SNOMED-CT browser to allow them to look up any nonexact matches. Each problem was compared with the gold standard created by the expert indexers.

SNOMED-CT had a coverage of 92.3% for 4996 common problem statements which served as the test set for this study. SNOMED-CT correctly identified 4568 terms (48.9% required a compositional expression to exactly represent the concept), 36 terms were not believed to be sensible expressions or were misspelled and were not matched by SNOMED-CT, nine were believed to not be sensible but were matched by SNOMED-CT and 383 terms were believed to be sensible but did not match exactly to SNOMED-CT. In this study, SNOMED-CT had a sensitivity (recall) of 92.3%, a specificity of 80.0%, and a positive predictive value (precision) of 99.8%. After correction for missing or erroneous synonymy in SNOMED-CT, the Mayo Vocabulary Server (MVS) engine had a sensitivity (recall) of 99.7%, a specificity of 97.9%, and a positive predictive value (precision) of 99.8%. The positive likelihood ratio**** increased to 47.5 and the negative predictive value was 97.0%. The inter-rater reliability for their judg-

---

**** Positive likelihood ratio = sensitivity/(1–specificity). A value of 1 means no discrimination (ability to cover a free text term); values more than 20 are excellent.

ment regarding SNOMED-CT was 91.8% with a kappa of 0.49, and for the engine was 94.3% with a kappa score of 0.79.

We concluded that SNOMED-CT has good coverage of the terms used frequently in medical problem lists. Improvements to synonymy and the addition of missing modifiers would lead to the greatest return on investment toward improved coverage of common problem statements. Compositional expressions are required to exactly represent a significant portion of common problem statements.

Content coverage studies provide valuable information to potential users of terminologies. We have detailed the VA NDF-RT ability to represent dictated medication list phrases from the Mayo Clinic. NDF-RT is a description logic-based resource created to support clinical operations at one of the largest healthcare providers in the US.

Medication list phrases were extracted from dictated patient notes from the Mayo Clinic. Algorithmic mappings to NDF-RT using MVS were presented to two non-VA physicians. The physicians used a terminology browser to determine the accuracy of the algorithmic mapping and the content coverage of clinical drug names. We performed a similar study to evaluate coverage of NDF-RT. The 509 extracted documents on 300 patients contained 847 medication concepts in medication lists. NDF-RT covered 97.8% of the concepts. Of the 18 phrases that NDF-RT did not represent, 10 were for OTCs and food supplements, 5 were for prescription medications, and 3 were missing synonyms. The MVS engine properly mapped 809 of 847 phrases with an overall sensitivity (precision) of 95.4% and positive likelihood ratio (recall) of 35.3. This study demonstrates that NDF-RT has more general utility than its initial design parameters dictated.[48]

Discussion

As we move into the genomic age, it becomes even more imperative that we provide tools and resources needed for a computable understanding of phenomic information. Personalized medicine will require a more granular understanding of the specific details regarding our patient's problems. It will no longer be enough to know that our patient has hypertension or even hypertension and diabetes mellitus, but we will need to know that our patient has type II diabetes mellitus with the metabolic syndrome and that they are markedly obese and have specific dietary and exercise habits that are limited by osteoarthritis of the right knee joint. This level of detail when coupled with treatment history and a comprehensive medication history including what has worked (and to what degree) in the past and a detailed adverse reaction history will pave the way for a safer practice of medicine. Indeed, more information will lead to best practice which will no longer mean meeting a minimal standard of care, but instead asymptotically approaching an ideal standard of health practice signaling a climate in which patients can expect a more comprehensive and safer healthcare environment.

The next steps include widespread implementation of current NLP systems which will need built-in mechanisms for feedback to improve our algorithms as well as our ontologies in support of accurate and complete representation of health data. Through a collaborative, iterative approach, we can reach our goal of a scientific computable understanding of health phenomics.

References

1. http://www.nlm.nih.gov/umls. Accessed June 16, 2005.
2. Great Britain. General Register Office. Annual Report of the Registrar General for England and Wales. London: H.M. Stationary Office; 1839. Reprinted in Irish University Press Series of British Parliamentary Papers. Health: General. Shannon: Irish University Press; 1968.
3. Masys DR. Of codes and keywords: standards for biomedical nomenclature. Acad Med 1990;65:627–629.
4. Solbrig HR. Final Submission to the CorbaMED Request for Proposals on Lexical Query Services (CorbaLex), OMG. 1998. Available at: http://www.omg.org/cgi-bin/doc?formal/99-3-6.pdf or http://www.omg.org/cgi-bin/doc?formal/99-3-1.pdf. Accessed June 16, 2005.
5. Great Britain. General Register Office. Annual Report of the Registrar General for England and Wales. London: H.M. Stationary Office; 1839. Reprinted in Irish University Press Series of British Parliamentary Papers. Health: General. Shannon: Irish University Press; 1968–.
6. Evans DA, Cimino JJ, Hersh WR, Huff SM, Bell DS, for the Canon Group. Toward a medical-concept representation language. J Am Med Inform Assoc 1994;1:207–217.
7. Cote RA, Rothwell DJ. The CLASSIFICATION-nomenclature Issues in medicine: a return to natural language. Med Inform 1989;14(1):25–41.
8. Bernauer J, Franz M, Schoop D, Schoop M, Pretschner DP. The compositional approach for representing medical concept systems. Medinfo 95;8:70–74.
9. Musen MA, Wieckert KE, Miller ET, Campbell KE, Fagan LM. Development of a controlled medical terminology: knowledge acquisition and knowledge representation. Methods Inf Med 1995;34(1–2):85–95.
10. Tuttle MS, Olson NE, Keck KD, et al. Metaphrase: an aid to the clinical conceptualization and formalization of patient problems in healthcare enterprises. IMethods Inf Med 1998;37(4–5):373–383.
11. Tuttle MS, Chute CG. Adding your terms and relationships to the UMLS Metathesaurus. In: Clayton PD, ed. Proceedings of the 15th Annual Symposium on Computer Applications in Medical Care. New York: McGraw Hill; 1991: 219–223.
12. McCray AT, Sponsler JL, Brylawski B, Browne AC. The role of lexical knowledge in biomedical text understanding. In: Stead WW, ed. Proceedings of the 11th Annual Symposium of Computer Applications in Medical Care. Washington, DC: IEEE Publications; 1987:103–107.

13. Lindberg DAB, Humphreys BL, McCray AT. The Unified Medical Language System. Methods Inf Med 1993;32:281–291.

14. Elkin PL, Cimino JJ, Lowe HJ, et al. Mapping to MeSH: the art of trapping MeSH equivalents from within narrative text. In: Greenes RA, ed. Proceedings of the 12th Annual Symposium on Computers in Medical Care. Washington, DC: IEEE Publications; 1988:185–190.

15. Humphreys BL, McCray AT, Cheh ML. Evaluating the coverage of controlled health data terminologies: report on the results of the NLM/AHCPR large scale vocabulary test. J Am Med Inform Assoc 1997;4(6):484–500.

16. Baader F, Calvanese D, McGuinness D, Nardi D, Patel-Schneider P, eds. The Description Logic Handbook: Theory, Implementation and Applications. Cambridge, UK: Cambridge; 2003.

17. Chomsky N. The Logical Structure of Linguistic Theory. New York: Plenum; 1975.

18. Sager N, Lyman M, Bucknall C, et al. Natural language processing and the representation of clinical data. J Am Med Inform Assoc 1994;1(2):142–160.

19. Sager N. Syntactic analysis of natural language. In: Advances in Computers. Vol 8. New York: Academic Press; 1967:153–188.

20. Grishman R, Sager N, Raze C, Bookchin B. The linguistic string parser. In: AFIPS Conference Proceedings. Vol 41. Montvale NJ: AFIPS Press; 1973: 427–434.

21. Sager N, Gishman R. The restriction language for computer grammars of natural language. Commun ACM 1975;18:390–400.

22. Wagner JC, Rogers JE, Baud RH, Scherrer JR. Natural language generation of surgical procedures. Int J Med Inform 1999;53(2–3):175–192.

23. Wagner JC, Rogers JE, Baud RH, Scherrer JR. Natural language generation of surgical procedures. Medinfo 1998;9(pt 1):591–595.

24. Trombert-Paviot B, Rodrigues JM, Rogers JE, et al. Galen: a third generation terminology tool to support a multipurpose national coding system for surgical procedures. Stud Health Technol Inform 1999;68:901–905.

25. Wroe CJ, Cimino JJ, Rector AL. Integrating existing drug formulation terminologies into an HL7 standard classification using OpenGALEN. Proceedings/ AMIA Annual Symposium. 2001:766–770.

26. Rector AL. Clinical terminology: why is it so hard? Methods Inform Med 1999; 38(4–5):239–252.

27. Rector AL. The interface between information, terminology, and inference models. Medinfo 2001;10(pt 1):246–250.

28. Friedman C, Shagina L, Lussier Y, Hripcsak G. Automated encoding of clinical documents based on natural language processing. J Am Med Inform Assoc 2004; 11(5):392–402.

29. Nadkarni P, Chen R, Brandt C. UMLS concept indexing for production databases: a feasibility study. J Am Med Inform Assoc 2001;8:80–91.

30. Huang Y, Lowe H, Hersh W. A pilot study of contextual UMLS indexing to improve the precision of concept based representation in XML-structured clinical radiology reports. J Am Med Inform Assoc 2003;10:580–587.

31. Cooper GF, Miller RA. An experiment comparing lexical and a statistical method for extracting MeSH terms from clinical free text. J Am Med Inform Assoc 1998;5:62–75.

32. Berrios DC. Automated indexing for full text information retrieval. Proc AMIA Symp 2000:71–75.

33. Zou Q, Chu WW, Morioka C, Leazer GH, Kangarloo H. IndexFinder: a method of extracting key concepts from clinical texts for indexing. Proc AMIA Symp 2003:763–767.

34. Srinivasan S, Rindflesch TC, Hole WT, Aronson AR, Mork JG. Finding UMLS metathesaurus concepts in MEDLINE. Proc AMIA Symp 2002:727–731.

35. Aronson AR, Bodenreider O, Chang HF, et al. The NLM indexing initiative. Proc AMIA Symp 2000:17–21.

36. Aronson AR. Effective mapping of biomedical text to the UMLS metathesaurus: the MetaMap program. Proc AMIA Symp 2001:17–21.

37. Brennan PF, Aronson AR. Towards linking patients and clinical information: detecting UMLS concepts in e-mail. J Biomed Inform 2003;36(4–5):334–341.

38. Joint Commission on Accreditation of Healthcare Organizations. 2005–2006 Standards for Ambulatory Care. Oakbrook Terrace, IL: JCAHO; 2005.

39. Weed L. The problem-oriented record: its organizing principles and its structure. League Exch 1975;(103):3–6.

40. Chute CG, Elkin PL. A clinically derived terminology: qualification to reduction. J Am Med Inform Assoc 1997;(suppl):570–574.

41. Elkin PL, Tuttle M, Keck K, Campbell K, Atkin G, Chute CG. The role of compositionality in standardized problem list generation. Medinfo 1998;9(pt 1): 660–664.

42. Elkin PL, Brown SH, Lincoln MJ, Hogarth M, Rector A. A formal representation for messages containing compositional expressions. Int J Med Inform 2003;71(2–3):89–102.

43. Elkin PL, Mohr DN, Tuttle MS, et al. Standardized problem list generation, utilizing the Mayo canonical vocabulary embedded within the Unified Medical Language System. Proc AMIA Annu Fall Symp 1997:500–504.

44. Elkin PL, Bailey K, Chute CG. A randomized controlled trial of automated term composition. Proc AMIA Symp 1998:765–769.

45. Elkin PL, Ruggieri A, Bergstrom L, et al. A randomized controlled trial of concept-based indexing of web page content. Proc AMIA Symp 2000:220–224.

46. Elkin PL, Ruggieri AP, Brown SH, et al. A randomized controlled trial of the accuracy of clinical record retrieval using SNOMED-RT as compared with ICD9-CM. Proc AMIA Symp 2001:159–163.

47. Elkin PL, Brown SH, Husser C, et al. An evaluation of the content coverage of SNOMED-CT for clinical problem lists. In review at BMJ, at this time.

48. Brown SH, Elkin PL, Rosenbloom ST, et al. VA national drug file reference terminology: a cross-institutional content coverage study. Medinfo 2004;11(pt 1): 477–481.

16
Digital Imaging

Khan M. Siddiqui and Eliot L. Siegel

Picture archiving and communication systems (PACS) have revolutionized the practice of radiology and medical imaging during the past 10–15 years. Digital imaging, communication, and information technologies offer many advantages over conventional paper- and film-based operation. With the advent of digital imaging, plate and detector technology, and various other imaging modalities, it is possible to enhance diagnostic value. Through computer and display capabilities, it is also possible to manipulate and enhance digital images for value-added diagnosis. On a broader scale, digital imaging, communication, and information technologies can be used to understand healthcare delivery workflow, a process that can result in more timely and accurate service delivery and reductions in operating costs.[1]

With all these benefits, digital imaging, communication, and information technologies are gradually changing the method of acquiring, storing, viewing, and communicating medical images and related information. One natural development along this line is the emergence of digital radiology departments and a digital healthcare delivery environment. A digital radiology department has two components: A radiology information system (RIS) and a digital imaging system (PACS). The RIS is a subset of the hospital information system (HIS) or computer-based patient record (CPR) and encompasses many text-based computing functions, including transcription, reporting, ordering, scheduling, tracking, and billing. A PACS deals with image-based computing functions, such as acquisition, archiving, communication, retrieval, interpretation, processing, distribution, and display. When an RIS and PACS are combined with the CPR, a totally filmless and paperless healthcare delivery system becomes a possibility. However, removing film and paper takes away the conventional method for distributing radiology information throughout the hospital or healthcare enterprise. Because the goal of any radiology department is to deliver timely and accurate interpretations to requesting clinicians, the digital department needs an integrated digital method through which results can be delivered.[2]

Digital Image Availability in Clinical Practice

Before digital imaging, healthcare providers used film-based medical image review. Film-based image review was plagued by limited availability of past studies, lost images, lost time, decreased productivity, and resulting delays and potential deleterious effects in patient care. Digital imaging has addressed these hindrances to image access and allows images to be transmitted, managed, and used electronically via computers and the Internet. The result is new efficiencies and productivity for providers and health systems—and a major step forward in reducing medical errors.[3]

Digital medical images can be conveyed instantaneously throughout the hospital or the healthcare system. Images can be accessed via personal computer, laptop, or personal data assistant from virtually anywhere—the physician's office, emergency room, operating room, or even the physician's home. This reduces delays by cutting time spent searching for files, film, or patient information among various departments. Physicians can view images when they want and where they want, providing greater flexibility.

This flexibility and easy access produces savings in both time and money. Researchers from the University of Montreal Hospital found that a digital imaging archive and RIS cut the median time between image acquisition and interpretation by as much as 40%.[4] A digital clinic and patient information system shared by several Boston-area hospitals was reported to save an estimated $1 million annually, in part, by reducing time spent searching for files and in the process of admitting patients. Projected income revenues from better patient retention as a result were between $3 and $4 million annually.[5]

The clinical information system in use at the MedStar Health hospital system in the Washington, DC/Baltimore, MD area provides immediate access to imaging files dating from 1997 to the present. The system also allows staff to retrieve—in less than 5 seconds—video of previously recorded procedures, cardiac catheterizations, or full-motion echocardiography.[6]

Another advantage of digital imaging is that once a new scan is completed, it can be viewed immediately by all physicians involved with the patient's care. In addition, images can be integrated with other electronic information—such as patient histories, physician notations, and laboratory data. Physicians can order imaging tests electronically, rather than by submitting requests on paper or over the phone. This reduces time and costs for transcription, delivery, and order clarification. At Brigham and Women's Hospital in Boston, physicians can order imaging tests via a secure Internet site. In so doing, the time required to order such tests is reduced by 85%.[7]

One study at a major university hospital found that the transition to digital imaging reduced report turnaround times for radiology orders from 7 hours 37 minutes to 4 hours 21 minutes (43%). In turn, reduced turnaround time helped reduce the average lengths of patients' stays as well as overall costs.[8] One hospital system found that the seamless integration of medical images with complete treatment information improved clinical workflow and helped stretch resources to meet staff shortages.[9]

Technologies

Digital Imaging and Communications in Medicine

Digital Imaging and Communications in Medicine (DICOM) has been a major motivator in the success story of PACS and radiologic information technology (IT).

A Brief Background on the DICOM Standard

The introduction of digital medical image sources in the 1970s and the use of computers in processing these images after their acquisition led the American College of Radiology (ACR) and the National Electrical Manufacturers Association (NEMA) to form a joint committee to create a standard method for the transmission of medical images and associated information. This committee was formed in 1983, and 2 years later produced ACR–NEMA Standards Publication No. 300-1985. Before this standard was issued, most devices stored images in a proprietary format and transferred files of these proprietary formats often over a proprietary network or on removable media. Although initial versions of the ACR–NEMA effort (version 2.0 was published in 1988) created standardized terminology, an information structure, and a file encoding method, most of the promise of a standard method of communicating digital image information was not realized until the release of version 3.0 in 1993. Version 3.0 was accompanied by a name change, Digital Imaging and Communications in Medicine (DICOM), and numerous DICOM enhancements have followed to deliver on the promise of standardized communications.[10]

The earliest DICOM standard specified a network protocol utilizing Transmission Control Protocol (TCP)/Internet Protocol (IP), defined the operation of service classes beyond the simple transfer of data, and created a mechanism for uniquely identifying information objects as they are acted upon across the network. DICOM was also structured as a multipart document to facilitate extension of the standard. In addition, DICOM defined information objects not only for images but also for patients, studies, reports, and other data groupings. With version 3.0, the standard was ready to deliver on its promise of not only permitting the transfer of medical images in a multivendor environment, but also facilitating the development and expansion of PACS and interfacing with medical information systems.

Scope of DICOM

The DICOM Standards Committee creates and maintains international standards for communication of biomedical diagnostic and therapeutic information in disciplines that use digital images and associated data. The goals of DICOM are to achieve compatibility and improve workflow efficiency between imaging systems and other information systems in healthcare environments worldwide. DICOM is a cooperative standard. Therefore, connectivity works because vendors cooperate in testing through scheduled public demonstrations, over the Internet, and during private test sessions. Every major diagnostic medical imaging vendor in the world has incorporated the standard into product designs, and most are actively participating in the enhancement of the standard. Most of the related imaging and imaging-related IT professional societies throughout the world have supported and are participating in the enhancement of the standard as well.

DICOM is used or will soon be used by virtually every medical profession that uses images within the healthcare industry. These include, but are not limited to, cardiology, dentistry, endoscopy, mammography, nuclear medicine, ophthalmology, orthopedics, pathology, pediatrics, radiation therapy, radiology, and others. DICOM is even used in veterinary medical imaging applications. DICOM also addresses the integration of information produced by these various specialty applications in the CPR. It defines the network and media interchange services allowing storage and access to these DICOM objects for CPR systems.

Technology Overview

The DICOM standard addresses multiple levels of the International Organization for Standardization (ISO) Open System Interconnection network model and provides support for the exchange of information on interchange media. DICOM currently defines an Upper Layer Protocol that is used over TCP/IP (independent of the physical network), messages, services, information objects, and an association negotiation mechanism. These definitions ensure that any two implementations of a compatible set of services and information objects can communicate effectively.

Independence from the underlying network technology allows DICOM to be deployed in many functional areas of application, including but not limited to communication within a single site (often using various forms of Ethernet), between sites over leased lines or virtual private networks, within a metropolitan area (often using Asynchronous Transfer Mode), across dial-up or other remote access connections (such as by modem, an integrated services digital network, or digital subscriber lines), and via satellite (with optimized protocol stacks to account for increased latency).

At the application layer, the services and information objects address five primary areas of functionality:

- Transmission and persistence of complete objects (such as images, waveforms, and documents)
- Query and retrieval of such objects
- Performance of specific actions (such as printing images on film)
- Workflow management (support of worklists and status information)
- Quality and consistency of image appearance (both for display and print)

DICOM does not define architecture for an entire system; nor does it specify functional requirements beyond the behavior defined for specific services. For example, storage of image objects is defined in terms of what information must be transmitted and retained, not how images are displayed or annotated. An additional DICOM service is available to specify how images should be presented with annotations to the user. DICOM can be considered as a standard for communication across the "boundaries" between heterogeneous or disparate applications, devices, and systems.

The services and objects that are defined in DICOM are designed to address specific, real-world applications, such as the performance of an imaging study on an acquisition device. DICOM is therefore not a general-purpose tool for distributed object management. In general, information is transferred "in bulk" according to a "document" paradigm. By contrast, general-purpose standards for distributed object or database management generally provide lower level, more specific access to individual attributes. Although the DICOM standard does provide so-called "normalized" services for patient and study management, these have not proven popular, and the "composite," document-oriented services have prevailed. This is likely a consequence of the natural division of functionality between different vendors, devices, and applications. For example, the ability to "set" or "change" a patient's name is generally implemented in a proprietary and centralized manner. To safely distribute responsibility for such a change across boundaries between different applications requires more underlying support than DICOM currently possesses (such as support for transactions and two-phase commitment).

Current pressing needs in DICOM development (as indicated by the priorities set by its various working groups) are to address issues relating to new modality technology, structured and coded documents for specific clinical domains, workflow management, security, and performance. These issues are being successfully addressed using the conventional "underlying" DICOM technology. Where there are interfaces with standards based on other technologies (such as Health Level-7 [HL7] version 2.x and 3), the focus for harmonization is on a shared "information model." It may be that in the future the nature of the underlying technology will be revisited, whether to make use of more sophisticated off-the-shelf distributed object management tools, such as Common Object Request Broker Architecture, or less sophisticated but widely used encoding tools, such as Extensible Markup Language (XML). However, the current priority is to address improvements in functionality to better meet the needs of the end user rather than to adopt an alternative encoding and distribution technology. This priority is continually reinforced by the need to remain compatible with the installed base of equipment.

When specific new technology is required, as in support of new features such as security and compression, the strategy is to adopt proven international, industry, or de facto standards. Network confidentiality and peer authentication in DICOM thus are provided by the use of either Transport Layer Security (an Internet standard) or Integrated Secure Communication Layer (an ISO-based standard). Rather then develop medical image-specific compression schemes, DICOM adopts standards developed by the ISO/International Electrotechnical Commission Joint Technical Committee 1/SC 29/WG 1, such as the Joint Photographic Experts Group (JPEG) and JPEG 2000 standards. For interchange media, standard file systems compatible with conventional software (such as ISO 9660 and Universal Disk Format) are used.

DICOM's Relationship to Other Standards

Throughout the development of DICOM, much attention was devoted to establishing working relationships with other standard initiatives throughout the world. The initial version of the standard leveraged prior work by the American Society for Testing and Materials. The TCP/IP standard was adopted in 1993. In the 1990s, cooperation with the European Committee for Standardization (CEN) resulted in a number of jointly developed supplements. CEN has created and approved a normative reference to the DICOM standard in EN 12052, an official European Norm. In parallel, the convergence of a Japanese interchange media format with DICOM required much joint work, in which the Japan Industries Association of Radiological Systems had a major role. In the United States, DICOM participated in the early coordination efforts for healthcare standards with the American National Standards Institute–Health Information and Surveillance Systems Board, from which DICOM adopted a harmonized patient name structure, and started progressively to define links with HL7. This cooperation entered into a very active phase with the creation in 1999 of a joint DICOM–HL7 working group. DICOM established a Type A liaison with the ISO Technical Committee (TC) 215 at its creation in 1999. ISO TC215 has decided not to create an imaging working group but, instead, to rely on DICOM for biomedical imaging standards. It is anticipated that ISO will create and approve a standard that will reference the DICOM standard, as CEN has done. In 2003, the DICOM Standards Committee became a member of the E-Health Standardization Coordination Group, a group endorsed by the International Telecommunication Union with the objective of promoting a stronger coordination among the key players in the e-health standardization area.

The DICOM committees are also focusing their attention on the evolution of standards linked to the Internet. Their strategy is to integrate Internet recommendations as soon as they are stable and largely disseminated in consumer commercial products. In this evolution, much care is taken to ensure that the consistency of the DICOM standard is maintained with its large installed base. DICOM already uses standard healthcare enterprise intranets. The e-mail exchange of DICOM objects (using a standard Multipurpose Internet Mail Extensions type) is also possible, and Web access to DICOM-persistent Objects (WADO) service has been defined in a joint effort with ISO TC215. It is clear that the use of DICOM objects and services in frequently used IT applications will grow in the future, given the widely agreed upon need to create electronic health records.

Finally, DICOM has a strong relationship with the Integrating the Healthcare Enterprise (IHE) initiative, in which profiles of standards are defined to address a number of healthcare workflow and enterprise integration challenges.

DICOM's Organizational Structure

DICOM is a standards organization administered by the NEMA Diagnostic Imaging and Therapy Systems Division. The complete bylaws of the DICOM Standards Committee are available on the NEMA Web site (www.nema.org). Working groups of the DICOM Committee perform the majority of work on the extension of and corrections to the standard. Working groups are formed by the DICOM Committee to work on a specific classification of tasks. Once formed, they petition the DICOM Committee to approve work items for which the working group will execute the plan delineated in the work item. Once the output of a work item (generally a supplement or correction proposal) has been completed, it is submitted to the Base Standards Working Group for their review. Supplements to the standard then go through a public comment period, after which the DICOM Committee authorizes the supplement for letter ballot by DICOM members. Letter ballots require approval by two-thirds of those voting and return of more than half of the ballots sent out. Because the working groups perform the majority of work on the extension of and corrections to the standard, the current status and future directions of the DICOM standard are best represented by review of each working group.

The DICOM 3.0 Standard

The current DICOM standard (2004) includes 18 parts following the ISO directives (Table 16-1). Two fundamental components of DICOM are the information object class and the service class. Information objects define the contents of a set of images and their relationship, and the service classes describe what to do with these objects. The service classes and information

TABLE 16-1. Parts of the current DICOM standard (2004)

Part 1	Introduction and Overview
Part 2	Conformance
Part 3	Information Object Definitions
Part 4	Service Class Specifications
Part 5	Data Structures and Encoding
Part 6	Data Dictionary
Part 7	Message Exchange
Part 8	Network Communication Support for Message Exchange
Part 9	Point-to-point Communication Support for Message Exchange (Retired)
Part 10	Media Storage and File Format for Data Interchange
Part 11	Media Storage Application Profiles
Part 12	Media Formats and Physical Media for Data Interchange
Part 13	Print Management Point-to-point Communication Support (Retired)
Part 14	Grayscale Standard Display Function
Part 15	Security Profiles
Part 16	Content Mapping Resource
Part 17	Explanatory Information
Part 18	Web Access to DICOM Persistent Objects

object classes are combined to form the fundamental units of DICOM: Service-object pairs (SOPs).

DICOM does not define or depend on any particular PACS architecture. Instead, the standard specifies services that apply at the boundaries between PACS and imaging components. In some PACS, the use of DICOM may be confined to the periphery of the systems and used solely for acquisition of images from modalities. In others, DICOM services may be used internally within the PACS between PACS subsystems. In addition, the DICOM file format may be used internally on short-term storage or long-term archive media, or images may be stored internally in a proprietary form and transformed to and from DICOM datasets as required.

The key to the successful use of DICOM services in a multivendor environment is the correct matching of DICOM services and roles (Table 16-2). "Role" in this case means that a device is either a "user" of a particular service (Service Class User [SCU]) or a "provider" of a service (Service Class Provider [SCP]).

Specifying generic image storage services is not sufficient to achieve interoperability between applications. It is necessary to define in detail the contents of images for each modality. The DICOM standard thus specifies Information Object Definitions (IODs), which describe the data structures that contain image data and associated information. In DICOM, the combination of Service Class and an IOD is referred to as an SOP class. A device may support the user (SCU) or provider (SCP) role for one or more SOP classes.

TABLE 16-2. DICOM services

DICOM	Typical PACS Uses
Service	
Image Storage	Transfer images from modality to PACS archive
	Transfer images from PACS archive to workstation
Query/retrieve	Query archive from workstation
	Retrieve images from archive to workstation
Modality worklist	Supply scheduling information to modalities
	Provide modalities with demographics for image header
	Facilitate matching received images with requests and old studies
Modality performed procedure step	Update schedule when procedure step has commenced
	Notify PACS when procedure step is complete
	Advise PACS of list of images comprising procedure step
Storage commitment	Allow modality to delete local images when PACS has confirmed they are stored
Interchange media storage	Record images on media for transfer to another institution, physician, or PACS
	Receive images from outside sources (modalities or PACS)
	Internal long-term archive format to reduce risk of obsolescence of storage media

Source: Adapted from DICOM 2004, available at http://medical.nema.org.[11]

DICOM Conformance Statements

Specifying and implementing a PACS using DICOM components requires an understanding of the DICOM conformance statement. The standard specifies that the manufacturer of any device claiming conformance shall provide a conformance statement that describes the capabilities of the device. To facilitate comparison, each conformance statement has a standard structure. Conformance statements can be directly obtained from the vendor and are usually made available on vendors' Web sites.

DICOM conformance is voluntary. No official body has authority to enforce conformance with the standard. No certification or testing authority verifies claims of conformance. Conformance to the standard does not guarantee interoperability between devices but does allow assessment of the feasibility of interoperability between devices. The purpose of the conformance statement is to allow the user to determine which features of the standard are supported by a particular implementation and what extensions and/or specialization are added by that implementation. By comparing the conformance statements of two implementations, a knowledgeable reader should be able to determine whether interoperability is possible.

The conformance statement specifies which SOP classes the device supports and in which roles. One can determine from the conformance state-

TABLE 16-3. General contents of DICOM conformance statement

1. The implementation model of the application entities (AEs) and how these relate to both local and remote real-world activities
2. The proposed (for association initiation) and acceptable (for association acceptance) presentation context used by each AE
3. The SOP classes and their options supported by each AE and the policies with which an AE initiates or accepts associations
4. The communication protocols to be used in the implementation
5. A description of any extensions, specializations, and publicly disclosed privatizations to be used in the implementation
6. A description of any implementation details that may be related to DICOM conformance or interoperability

Source: Adapted from DICOM 2004, available at http://medical.nema.org.[11]

ment whether a device supports the service necessary to meet the user's requirements and whether two devices are compatible, in that they support the necessary SOP classes in complementary roles.[1,11] The general contents of a conformance statement are listed in Table 16-3.

Integrating the Healthcare Enterprise

Even with the DICOM and HL7 standards available, there is still a need for consensus on how to use these standards for smoothly integrating heterogeneous healthcare information systems. IHE is neither a standard nor a certifying authority. Instead, it is a high-level information model for driving adoption of HL7 and DICOM standards. IHE is a joint initiative started in 1997 by the Radiological Society of North America (RSNA) and the Healthcare Information and Management Systems Society (HIMSS). The mission was to define and stimulate manufacturers to use DICOM- and HL7-compliant equipment and information systems to facilitate daily clinical operation. The IHE technical framework defines information models and vocabulary for using DICOM and HL7 to complete a set of well-defined radiologic and clinical transactions for specific tasks. These common vocabulary and models would then help healthcare providers and technical personnel to understand one another better and thereby achieve smoother system integration.[12–17]

IHE Technical Framework and Integration Profiles

The IHE Technical Framework is a detailed, rigorously organized document that provides a comprehensive guide to implementing the defined integration capabilities. The Technical Framework delineates standards-based transactions among systems (generically defined as IHE actors) required to support specific workflow and integration capabilities. There are four key concepts in the IHE technical framework: Data model, IHE actors, transactions, and Integration Profiles.

Data model. The data model is adapted from HL7 and DICOM and shows the relationship between the key frames of reference (for example, Patient, Visit, Order, and Study) defined in the framework.

IHE actors. Information systems or applications that produce, manage, or act on information are represented as functional units called IHE actors. Each actor supports a specific set of IHE transactions. A given information system may support one or more IHE actors.

Transactions. Transactions are exchanges of information between actors using messages based on established standards (such as HL7, DICOM, and W3C). Each transaction is defined with reference to specific standards and additional detailed information, including use cases. This is done to add greater specificity and ensure a higher level of interoperability between systems.

Integration Profile. An Integration Profile is the organization of functions segmented into discrete units. It includes actors and transactions required to address a specific clinical task or need. IHE Integration Profiles provide a common language, vocabulary, and platform for healthcare providers and manufacturers to discuss integration needs and the integration capabilities of products. IHE Integration Profiles organize sets of IHE actors and transactions to address specific patient care needs. Integration Profiles offer a convenient way for vendors and users to reference the functionality defined in the IHE Technical Framework without having to restate all of the detail regarding IHE actors and transactions. They describe clinical information and workflow needs and specify the actors and transactions required to address them. Additional information can be obtained from the IHE, RSNA, and HIMSS Web sites (www.ihe.net, www.rsna.org/IHE, and www.himss.org, respectively). As of early 2005, IHE has defined Integration Profiles for a set of 12 clinical needs in radiology (Table 16-4) and a set of four needs in the IT infrastructure domain (Table 16-5).

IHE Integration Statements

IHE Integration Statements are documents prepared and published by vendors to describe the intended conformance of their products with the IHE Technical Framework. They identify the specific integration capabilities a product is designed to support in terms of the key concepts of IHE: Actors and Integration Profiles. Links to the Web sites of companies that publish IHE Integration Statements for their products are provided at www.ihe.net/resources/ihe_integration_statements.html.

TABLE 16-4. IHE-defined integration profiles for clinical needs in radiology (2005)

Scheduled Workflow	Defines the flow of information for the key steps in a typical patient imaging encounter (registration, ordering, scheduling, acquisition, distribution, and storage)
Patient Information Reconciliation	Defines an efficient method to handle the reconciliation of information for cases in which procedures are performed on unidentified or mistakenly identified patients
Consistent Presentation of Images	Makes it possible to ensure a consistent view of images and annotations across different displays and media
Presentation of Grouped Procedures	Enables management of cases in which images for multiple procedures are acquired in a single acquisition step (for example, spiral CT of the chest and abdomen)
Postprocessing Workflow	Extends the scheduled workflow profile to support workflow steps such as computer-aided detection (CAD), image processing, and image reconstruction
Reporting Workflow	Addresses the need to schedule, distribute, and track the status of key reporting tasks such as interpretation, transcription, and verification
Evidence Documents	Allows nonimage information such as observations, measurements, CAD results, and other procedure details to be stored, managed, and made available as input to the reporting process
Key Image Note	Allows the addition of textual notes and pointers to key images in a series
Simple Image and Numeric Reports	Implement a standard way of creating, managing, storing, and viewing reports that include images, text, and numerical values
Charge Posting	Makes detailed information about procedures performed available to billing systems to allow consistent and timely billing of technical and professional charges
Basic Security	Establishes the first level of enterprise-wide security infrastructure for meeting privacy requirements (such as those of the Health Insurance Portability and Accountability Act) by managing cross-node security and consolidation of audit trails
Access to Radiology Information	Establishes a mechanism for sharing radiologic images and information across department boundaries

Source: Adapted from Integration Profiles: The Key to Integrated Systems. http://www.ihe.net/resources/ihe_integration_profiles.cfm.

TABLE 16-5. IHE-defined integration profiles for the IT infrastructure domain (2005)

Patient Identifier Cross-referencing	Allows an institution to maintain in a single location all the identifiers used by its various information systems for each patient
Retrieve Information for Display	Provides a simple mechanism for obtaining and displaying documents and key patient-centric information
Enterprise User Authentication	Allows for a single user sign-on across multiple systems
Patient Synchronized Applications	Allow for maintaining patient context across multiple applications

Source: Adapted from IHE Frequently Asked Questions, http://www.ihe.net/About/ihe_faq.cfm.

Picture Archiving and Communication Systems

A PACS consists of image and data acquisition, storage, and display systems integrated by digital networks and application software. Such a system can be as simple as a film digitizer connected to a display workstation with a small image database or as complex as an enterprise image management system. PACS design should emphasize system connectivity. A general multimedia data management system that is easily expandable, flexible, and versatile in its operation calls for both integrating various HISs and building a sound PACS infrastructure. From a management point of view, a hospital- or enterprise-wide PACS is an attractive option, because it provides economic justification for implementation of the system. Proponents of PACS are convinced that the ultimately favorable cost/benefit ratio should not be evaluated as a balance of the resources of the radiology department alone but should extend to the entire hospital or enterprise operation. From an engineering point of view, the PACS infrastructure is the sum of the basic design concepts needed to ensure that the system includes features such as standardization, open architecture, expandability, connectivity, reliability, fault tolerance, and cost effectiveness.[1,2]

PACS Infrastructure

The PACS infrastructure design provides the necessary framework for the integration of distributed and heterogeneous imaging devices and makes intelligent database management possible. It offers an efficient means of viewing, analyzing, and documenting study results and furnishes a method for effectively communicating study results to referring healthcare providers. The PACS infrastructure consists of a basic framework of hardware components integrated by a standardized, flexible software system for communication, database management, storage management, job scheduling, interprocessor communication, error handling, and network monitoring. The infrastructure as a whole is versatile and can incorporate rules to reliably perform not only basic PACS management operation but also more complex research, clinical service, and education requests. The software modules of the infrastructure embody sufficient understanding and cooperation at a system level to permit the components to work together as a system rather than as individual networked computers.

Hardware components include patient data servers, imaging modalities, and PACS controllers with database, archive, and display workstations connected by communication networks for handling efficient data and image flow in the PACS. Image and data stored in PACS can be extracted from the archive and transmitted to application servers for various uses. Figure 16-1 shows basic components and data flow for a generic PACS.

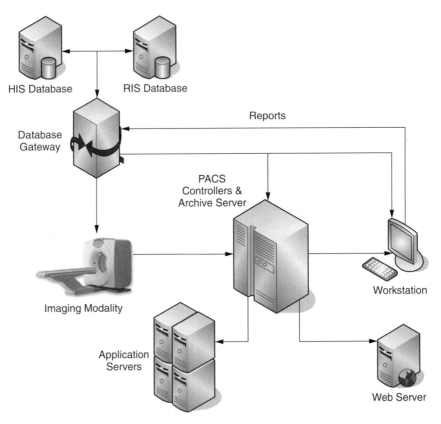

FIGURE 16-1. Basic components and data flow for a generic PACS. HIS, hospital information system; RIS, radiology information system; PACS, picture archiving and communication system.

PACS Implementation Solutions

Self-initiated Solution

Most early PACS implementations were initiated by university hospitals and academic departments and by research laboratories for major imaging equipment manufacturers. In this model, a multidisciplinary team is assembled by the radiology department or hospital. This team becomes a system integrator, selecting PACS components from various vendors. The team develops system interfaces and writes the PACS software according to the clinical requirements of the hospital.

This allows the team to continuously upgrade the system with state-of-the-art components. The system can be upgraded without a dependence on the schedule of the vendor. However, substantial commitment is required on the part of the hospital to assemble and support the work of a multidisciplinary team. In addition, because the system developed by the team will be one of a kind and made from components from different vendors, service and maintenance will be quite difficult. As PACS technology has matured, fewer institutions select this model for implementation.

Two-team Effort Solution

A team of experts drawn from outside and inside the hospital is assembled to write detailed specifications for the PACS for a defined clinical environment. A vendor is contracted to implement the system. This model is a team effort between the hospital and vendors.

The primary advantage of the two-team model is that although the PACS specifications are tailored to a specific clinical environment, the responsibility for implementation is delegated to the vendor. The hospital acts as a purchase agent and does not have to develop the details of or oversee the installation. A hospital team tends to be overambitious and underestimates the technical and operational difficulties in implementing certain clinical functions. However, the vendor may lack necessary elements of clinical expertise and thereby overestimate the performance of each component. As a result, the completed PACS may not meet overall specifications. The cost of contracting with a vendor to develop a specified PACS is also high, because only one such system is built. This model has been gradually replaced by the partnership model.

Turnkey Solution

In this model, the vendor develops a generic, one-for-all PACS and installs it in a department for clinical use. This model is market driven. Some vendors see potential profit in developing a specialized turnkey PACS to promote the sale of other imaging equipment.

The advantage of this model is that the cost of delivering a generic system tends to be lower. One disadvantage is that if the vendor needs a couple of years to complete the production cycle, fast-moving computer and communication technologies may render the system obsolete. It is doubtful that a generalized PACS will fulfill requirements for every specialty in a department or every radiology department.

Partnership Solution

In this solution, the hospital and a vendor form a partnership to share the responsibility. It is most suitable for a large-scale implementation. With the recent availability of PACS implementation data from initial installations, health centers are learning to take advantage of the desirable and discard the undesirable features of PACS for their own daily operational environments. As a result, the boundaries between implementation solutions have gradually merged into the partnership solution. The health center forms a partnership with a selected manufacturer or a system integrator, which is then responsible for PACS implementation, maintenance, service, training, and upgrade. The arrangement can be through a long-term purchase agreement with a maintenance contract or by leasing the system.

Application Service Provider Solution

A system integrator provides all PACS-related services to the client, which can be an entire hospital or a single practice group. No IT requirements are imposed on the client. The Application Service Provider solution is attractive for smaller practices trying to move toward filmless imaging or a smaller subset of PACS implementations (for example, off-site archiving, disaster recovery, DICOM Web server development, or Web-based image databases).[1,2]

Current PACS Architectures

There are three basic PACS architectures: Stand-alone, client-server, and Web-based. From these three basic architectures, variations and hybrid design types have evolved.

Stand-alone PACS Model

The three major features of the stand-alone model are:

1. Images are automatically sent to designated reading and review workstations from the archive server.
2. Workstations can also query and retrieve images from the archive server.
3. Workstations have short-term cache storage.

Advantages:

1. If the PACS server goes down, imaging modalities or acquisition gateways have the flexibility to send directly to the end-user workstation so that the radiologist can continue reading new cases.
2. Because multiple copies of an imaging study are distributed throughout the system, there is less risk of losing data.
3. Some historical PACS examinations will be available in workstations, because they have a local storage cache.
4. The system is less susceptible to daily changes in network performance because PACS examinations are preloaded onto the local storage cache of end-user workstations and available for viewing immediately.
5. Examination modification to the DICOM header for quality control can be made before archiving.

Disadvantages:

1. End-users must rely on correct distribution and prefetching of PACS examinations, which is not possible all the time.
2. Because images are sent to designated workstations, each workstation may have a different worklist, which makes it inconvenient to read and review all examinations at any workstation in one setting.
3. End-users depend on the query/retrieve function to retrieve ad hoc PACS examinations from the archive, which can be a complex function compared with the client-server model.
4. More than one radiologist may attempt to interpret and report a single examination simultaneously at different workstations.

Client-server Model

The three main features of the client-server model are:

1. Images are centrally archived at the PACS server.
2. End-users select images via the archive server from a single worklist at the client workstation.
3. Because workstations have no cache storage, images are deleted locally after they have been interpreted.

Advantages:

1. Any PACS examination is available on any end-user workstation at any time, making it convenient to read or review.
2. No prefetching or study distribution is needed.
3. No query/retrieve function is needed. The end-user simply selects the examination from the worklist on the client workstation, and images are loaded automatically.
4. Because the main copy of a PACS examination is loaded on the PACS server and is shared by the client workstations, radiologists will be made

aware when they are reading the same examination at the same time and thus can avoid duplicate readings.

Disadvantages:

1. The PACS server can be a single point of failure if adequate disaster recovery and redundancy are not built in. If it goes down, the entire PACS is down. In this case, end-users will not be able to view any examinations on the client workstations. Newly acquired examinations must be held back from archiving at the modalities until the server is back up.
2. Because there are more database transactions in the client-server architecture, the system is exposed to the potential for more transaction errors.
3. The architecture is very dependent on network performance.

Web-based Model

The Web-based PACS model is similar to the client-server architecture with regard to data flow. However, the main difference is that the client software is a Web-based application.

Advantages:

1. The client workstation hardware can be platform independent as long as the Web browser is supported.
2. The system is a completely portable application that can be used both onsite and at home with an Internet connection.

Disadvantages:

1. The system may be limited in the amount of functionality and performance by the Web browser.

Enterprise PACS and CPR with Images

An enterprise PACS is for very large-scale implementation. It is becoming more and more popular in today's enterprise healthcare delivery system. Figure 16-2 shows the generic architecture. In the generic architecture, the three main components are PACS at each hospital in the enterprise, the enterprise data center, and the enterprise CPR.

Enterprise-level healthcare delivery emphasizes sharing of enterprise integrated resources and streamlining operation. In this respect, if an enterprise consists of several hospitals and clinics, it is not necessary for every hospital and clinic to have similar specialist services. A specific service, such as radiology, can be shared among all entities in the enterprise, resulting in the concept of a radiology expert center relying on the operation of teleradiology. Under this setup, all patients registered in the same enterprise can be referred to the radiology service center for examinations. The patient being cared for then becomes the focus of the operation. A single unique

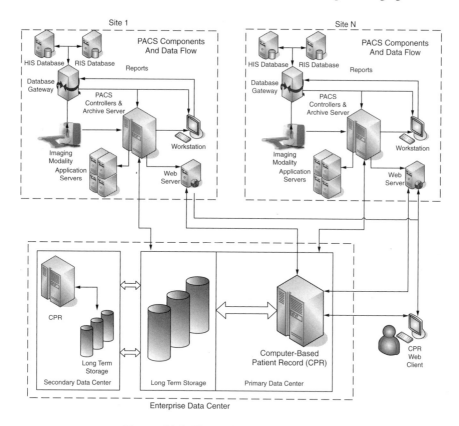

FIGURE 16-2. Enterprise PACS and CPR.

patient index would be sufficient for any healthcare provider to retrieve the patient's comprehensive record. For this reason, the data management system would not be the conventional HIS, RIS, or other organizational information system. Instead, the CPR concept would prevail.

The traditional HIS is hospital operation oriented. Sometimes several separate data information systems must be invoked simultaneously, using various log-ons, before complete patient information can be retrieved during a visit. CPR enables the concept of single sign-on. In this operation, the CPR server would have necessary linkages connected to all information systems involved. Using the patient's name or unique identifier, the healthcare providers at the CPR client can seamlessly retrieve all relevant information on the patient across different systems in the enterprise. The majority of current CPR systems are still limited to textual information. To be optimally effective for healthcare delivery, images must be incorporated into the CPR server.

Enterprise PACS, therefore, should have a means of transmitting relevant patient images and related data to the CPR server, and the CPR server should have the infrastructure design to distribute images and related data in a timely manner to the healthcare providers at the point of care.[1,2]

PACS: Hidden Costs

One of the major allures of "going PACS" is the cost savings widely said to be generated after implementation. However, early adopters were dismayed when hidden costs and unanticipated expenses bit large chunks out of those projected savings. The actual hardware and software turned out to be the least expensive parts of PACS.[18]

Additional expenses that affect savings include film services, information systems, and storage costs. The combination of these factors makes the savings much less than originally projected. However, better awareness of those costs, careful preplanning by customers, and vendor service innovations in second- and even third-generation PACS have made buyers more experienced and savvy about the potential financial pitfalls.

Some cost-associated problems still exist, especially as the market expands to smaller facilities. Customers at midsized community hospitals still may not be completely aware of all the elements involved, including important factors such as infrastructure upgrades. Conscientious vendors should tell such institutions exactly what is needed, whether this involves a network upgrade to their local area network or custom integration work with their existing RIS.

Vendors should also provide readiness assessments. These involve, among other elements, a modality review to determine what additional costs might be incurred in upgrading modalities to DICOM standards and an assessment to estimate the complexity and cost of making the network meet PACS requirements. Assessments should also involve determining a site's readiness at a cultural level. The creation of a project team to implement PACS is crucial. If the institution is not prepared on the project side, then achieving an adequate return on investment can be difficult.

Unrealized returns on investment, particularly compared with rosy projections of immediate cost savings, have generated much of the reported customer dissatisfaction with PACS. With good management and a vendor who steps up to help the customer be adequately prepared, however, more and more successful installations are being implemented.

Beyond the Department

Sometimes customers enter the process with a focus that is far too narrow, producing a distorted image of costs and savings. PACS adoption was originally viewed as a departmental project—specifically, the radiology department, where the greatest percentage of savings could be expected in the elimination of film-associated costs. But those kinds of savings alone could never justify the cost of purchasing and implementing a PACS. A broader outlook was necessary to see PACS as an enterprise-wide operation.

Initially, most people underestimated the potential impact of PACS in areas outside of radiology, and the burden of unanticipated costs lies in precisely those areas. PACS purchasers focused only on radiology were quite surprised to find themselves with enterprise-wide problems. Many "filmless" radiology departments, for example, found that they still had to print film copies and get these copies physically to other departments—effectively negating the benefits of the digital transition. It soon became clear that the question was not what is needed to integrate PACS into the radiology department but how to introduce PACS to the rest of the hospital.

Today PACS is recognized as an enterprise-wide proposition. Both vendors and customers now take a broader view of implementation. Many vendors once advocated a "one size fits all" approach, in which all facilities could be fitted with the same solution. Different facilities clearly have diverse styles, budgets, structures, and cultures and, therefore, have different needs. As PACS technology becomes more mainstream—spreading out to midsized institutions and radiology centers—a more individualized approach is taking hold. This change tends to reduce inaccurate cost estimates and insufficient budgets. Many of the problems encountered can be avoided with careful preplanning.

Planning Ahead

General recommendations that have been made about planning for PACS include:

- *Research*—Know what you want from PACS and a prospective vendor. Gain a complete understanding of your operations—both departmental and enterprise—from a preimplementation and postimplementation perspective.
- *Budge*—Budgets should be kept reasonably flexible. Budgets carved in stone tend to be simplistic and restrictive.
- *Modality assessment*—Determine the age and DICOM conformance of your modalities.
- *Network infrastructure*—Determine your current network's capabilities and future requirements. Network distribution must include all elements as far along the chain of participants as the referring physicians' offices and homes. Plan for secure connectivity from the hospital or imaging facility down to the referring physicians. Poor planning in this important area will incur additional costs and require additional networking and security capabilities.
- *Install a PACS team*—This team should anticipate any ancillary costs, which can become quite large and wreak havoc on budgets and estimates.

Part of the team's job is to plan carefully for the future in regard to integration of infrastructure components, modalities, and clinical databases.

- *Return on investment factoring*—Determine your projected return on investment by factoring in cost reductions and productivity gains. PACS is not just about how much money you can save on specific items such as film.
- *Service agreement*—Determine what kind of service contract you want. You may hear pros and cons about such contracts. Some have complained that it adds unnecessary cost to the PACS package. A hardware service contract may not be essential, but a software service contract is seen as almost a requirement, because most software service agreements include software obsolescence. Down the road, the costs of software upgrades can far exceed the cost of the agreement.

Problems

Without proper planning, specific problem areas and associated costs could include:

- *Film*—Additional costs could involve maintaining film backup or continuing usage of film storage costs.
- *Storage*—As your facilities perform more examinations and modalities evolve, more data are created. Customers need to budget for and install more storage capacity to handle data. For example, if a customer buys additional imaging equipment that creates more data, that same data requirement would have to be balanced on the storage side of PACS. Without such planning, bottlenecks can occur. Another strategy could be to purchase only limited storage and buy more when needed, because the cost of storage has a rapid downward trajectory.
- *Off-site viewing*—Infrastructure upgrade costs must be taken into account, especially for image-enabling outside of the facility. Overlooking this element invites substantial trouble. When customers intend to enable images outside of the facility setting, they soon realize they need better monitors and workstations—necessitating an unplanned upgrade for a costly major network infrastructure.

Customers are sometimes faced with the unexpected prospect of rebuilding an entire infrastructure to support an enterprise-wide system. The common response is to sacrifice or diminish expectations. Instead of 20 workstations, they try to get away with 10—essentially taking necessary equipment out of the equation. The hospital ends up buying a bare-bones system, which tops out after 6 months, leaving the hospital stuck with the need to upgrade this already large capital investment. The result is most often that the vendor and customer are mutually dissatisfied and in adversarial positions. Everyone must sacrifice, and no one is happy.

As a solution to this all-too-common situation, some vendors place diagnostic quality image capability on every personal computer without forcing an institution to revamp its infrastructure. This solution is one example of ways in which vendors are developing new strategies to accommodate customers and reduce ongoing PACS costs.

Another way is through the development of new service delivery models, such as the fee-for-service model, which is helping to bring PACS into smaller settings, such as community hospitals and imaging centers. Without such measures, many of these facilities would not be able to afford PACS.

Purchase Options

In the past, vendors typically provided a complete PACS package that included hardware, software, and an upgrade servicing agreement. Today, most facilities buy the hardware on their own, because the technology has come down in price. PACS vendors provide software licenses, installation services, and service agreements—typically as 5-year contracts—with payment made in "real time" or "fee for service" as opposed to upfront with the purchase.

The fee-for-service model adds a great deal of variability to the equation and also makes it difficult to forecast ultimate costs. In some cost-per-study models, a fixed portion is agreed upon, usually 70%–80% of the anticipated costs of the products and services. A variable portion agreement allows the institution to pay on a modified on-demand model, so that payment increases or decreases according to an agreed-upon metric based on hospital business, usage, or profits.

More and more customers are leaning toward a leasing arrangement. Some customers are becoming more comfortable with the idea of not owning equipment, now viewed not as a permanent acquisition but as a technologic asset that needs routine replacement. They may want the flexibility of being able to swap out certain elements of the PACS solution during the typical 5-year lifecycle. In addition, they find lease rates more attractive than tax-exempt financing or outright purchase options.

Eliminating Surprises

As the mainstreaming of PACS continues, vendors and customers improve their ability to forecast costs and savings and reduce those unhappy surprises that bedeviled early PACS adopters. More effective planning at the outset by customers—supported by vendors' implementation experiences—is the key to not busting the budget.

Institutional Impact: Productivity at the Baltimore Veterans Affairs Medical Center

Institutions worldwide have reported on the effects of the film-to-filmless transition on time, cost, and quality of product.[19-29] This section of the chapter describes the benefits, costs, savings, and cost-benefit analysis of filmless transition at the Baltimore Veterans Affairs Medical Center (BVAMC).[30,31]

BVAMC started its PACS implementation in the late 1980s and early 1990s. The goals of the project were to integrate with the VA's home-grown Clinical Patient Record System (CPRS) and then to-be-developed VistA imaging system. The system was in operation in the middle of 1993 in the new BVAMC and has since evolved and integrated with other VA hospitals in Maryland into a single imaging network—the VA Maryland Health Care System.

Benefits

Four significant benefits seen at the BVAMC are:

1. Reduction in routine workflow steps
2. Reduction in unread cases
3. Reduction in retake rates
4. Improvement in clinician workflow

One of the major benefits has been the virtual elimination of "unread" imaging studies. The unread imaging study rate decreased from 8% before PACS to approximately 0.3% in 1996. Remaining unread studies are now identified in a weekly audit with the HIS/RIS system and are subsequently interpreted or reinterpreted on PACS (see Figure 16-3).

Computed radiography has also contributed to reduction in retake rates resulting from unsatisfactory examinations. This reduction has been by 84%, from 5% in the film-based environment to 0.8% after transition to computed radiography and filmless operation (Figure 16-4).[32]

The transition to filmless operation has resulted in the elimination of a number of steps in the process in which imaging studies are made available for interpretation by the radiologists. This has reduced the interval from when a study is obtained until it is reported from several hours (and sometimes the following day) to less than 30 minutes (during the normal workday). This "real-time" reporting has had a positive impact on the quality of patient care and perception of radiology services by referring clinicians. This rapid reporting in conjunction with the purchase of an enterprise-wide digital dictation system has reduced the interval from when a study is performed until it is dictated from approximately 24 hours to 2

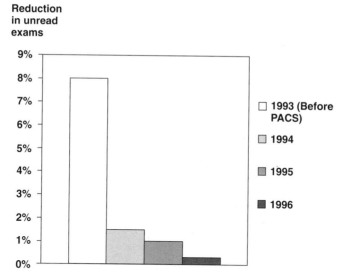

FIGURE 16-3. Reduction in lost or unread examinations at BVAMC. There was a 96% reduction in lost or unread examinations, but not a complete elimination of these within 3 years of the transition to filmless operation.

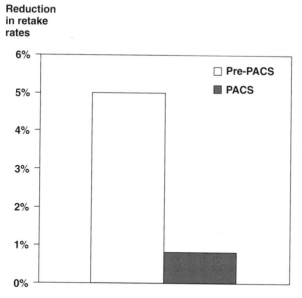

FIGURE 16-4. Image retake rates at BVAMC. The wide dynamic range of computed radiography and the ability to manipulate images at the workstation resulted in a reduction of 84% in image retake rates for the general radiography technologists. There was also a shift in the most common reason for retakes from "error in technique" (images too light or too dark) to problems with patient positioning.

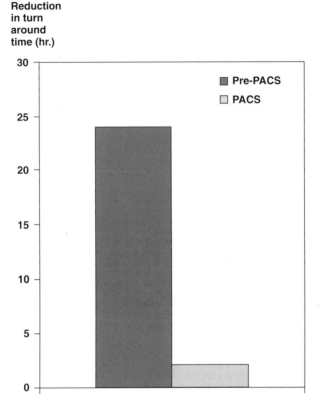

Reduction
in turn
around
time (hr.)

FIGURE 16-5. Workflow improvement at BVAMC. The combination of a reduction in workflow steps and rapid availability of images after they are obtained has reduced the time from image acquisition to transcription from approximately 24 hours to 2 hours.

hours (see Figure 16-5). Another result has been the positive effect on the quality of patient care and the perception of radiology services by referring clinicians. These benefits were associated with a strong (92%) preference for PACS versus film among the clinicians at the BVAMC when an initial survey was conducted within 2 years of the implementation of the PACS. Clinicians' perception of the biggest benefit of PACS on their practice was the fact that it saves them time and makes them more productive. In response to a formal survey in the mid-1990s, 98% of the respondents indicated that the PACS resulted in more effective utilization of their time.

Costs

The two major contributors to the cost of the system are the depreciation and the service contract. With regard to the best figure for capital depreciation, the Department of Veterans Affairs uses 8.8-year depreciation on medical equipment, whereas computer equipment is often depreciated using a 5-year time period. The other significant contributor to the cost of the PACS is the service contract, which includes all of the personnel required to operate and maintain the system. It also includes software upgrades and replacement of all hardware components that fail or demonstrate suboptimal performance. This includes replacement of any monitors that do not pass quality-control tests. No additional personnel are required other than those provided by the vendor through the service contract.

Savings

Savings in the radiology department were achieved in a number of different ways. Films are still used in two circumstances. Mammography examinations are still processed on film but are digitized and integrated into PACS after primary interpretation. Despite these uses, there has been a reduction of 95% of film-related costs based on the projected value in a conventional film-based department. Additional savings have also been realized and include reduction in film-related supplies, such as film folders, film chemistry, and processors.

One of the largest—and to some extent unexpected—savings associated with PACS has been the ability to recover space in the radiology department. The old film file room occupied approximately 2500 square feet, and this space has been used now for the PACS data center and as space for an additional magnetic resonance scanner.

The largest savings associated with PACS at the BVAMC have been in personnel costs. The personnel cost savings include radiologists, technologists, and clerical staff. An estimate was made that at least two more radiologists would have been needed to handle the 76% expected increase in workload at the BVAMC had the PACS not been installed. The efficiency of technologists has also improved by about 60% for cross-sectional imaging examinations, which translates to three to four additional technologists had the PACS not been implemented (see Figure 16-6).[33] Only one clerk is required to handle the limited amount of mammography studies and films and CDs created for outside facilities.

Economics for PACS for Entire Hospital

The hospital-wide savings associated with filmless operation are more difficult to quantify. The average clinician estimates that he or she saves approximately 50–70 minutes per day because of the improved image accessibility associated with the PACS, based on a survey conducted at BVAMC. Even with a reduction in the estimate of clinicians' time savings to a more conservative 10–12 minutes per day and applying this across the entire institution result in savings of approximately two to four clinician full-time

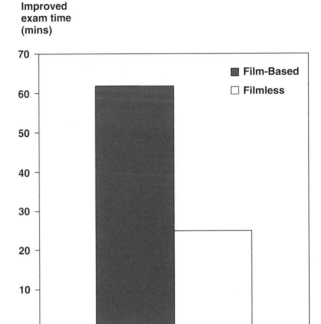

FIGURE 16-6. CT techs at BVAMC. Computed tomography technologists required 60% less time when studies were acquired and sent to PACS in comparison with the traditional film-based environment.

equivalent positions per year. This represents significant monetary savings in clinician time alone. A number of other even more difficult to quantify cost benefits are associated with the PACS. These include decreased waiting times for radiology reports as report turnaround has decreased from 24 hours to 2 hours as a result of implementation of a digital dictation system integrated with PACS. This carries with it the potential for positive effects on length of stay, clinician efficiency, accuracy in patient care, medicolegal risks, and savings associated with a decreased rate of lost studies.

Cost/Benefit Analysis

The BVAMC underwent a study by a group of investigators from Johns Hopkins University to identify a crossover point at which filmless operation becomes more cost beneficial than conventional film-based operation. The study found that in a conventional film-based environment the cost per unit examination was relatively flat as the volume of studies performed in the radiology department increased from 20,000 to 100,000 examinations per year (Fig. 16-7). As the number of studies increases, additional space,

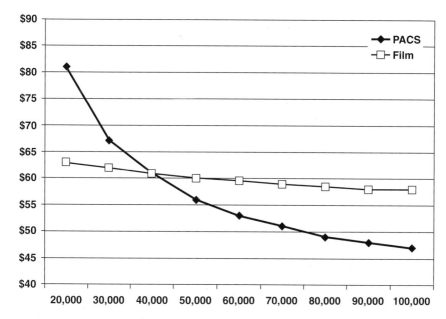

FIGURE 16-7. Cost per unit examination at BVAMC. The cost per unit examination is relatively flat as volume of studies performed in the radiology department increases from 20,000 to 100,000 studies per year; however, there is a rapid decrease in unit cost per study with a PACS. At 90,000 studies per year, there is an approximately 25% decrease in cost per unit study with a PACS in comparison with film. The "break even" point occurs at approximately 39,000 studies per year.

personnel, and supplies are needed. With filmless operation, there was a rapid decrease in unit cost per study because equipment costs for the system are fixed and do not increase substantially with added volume. At a volume of 90,000 studies per year, there was an approximately 25% savings in cost per unit study with filmless operation compared with film. The "break even" point between film-based and filmless operation occurs at approximately 39,000 studies per year. At volumes greater than that, the study found the filmless environment to be more cost effective than the film-based environment.[30,34]

References

1. Huang HK. PACS and Imaging Informatics: Basic Principles and Applications. Hoboken, NJ: John Wiley & Sons; 2004.
2. Dreyer KJ, Mehta A, Thrall JH. PACS: A Guide to the Digital Revolution. New York: Springer-Verlag; 2002.
3. Reiner BI, Siegel EL, Siddiqui K. Evolution of the digital revolution: a radiologist perspective. J Digit Imaging 2003;16:324–330.

4. Ridley EL. RIS-PACS integration delivers improved interpretation, reporting times. December 1, 2003. Available at: www.auntminnie.com/index.asp?Sec=sup&Sub=pac&Pag=dis&ItemId=60249. Accessed December 11, 2005.

5. Institute of Medicine. Networking Health: Prescriptions for the Internet, Institute of Medicine. Washington, DC: National Academy of Sciences; 2000:81.

6. Drazin E, Fortin J. Digital Hospitals Move Off the Drawing Board. iHealth Report. Oakland, CA: California HealthCare Foundation; 2003:9. Available at: www.chcf.org/documents/ihealth/DigitalHospitalsOffDrawingBoard.pdf. Accessed December 11, 2005.

7. Symonds W. How e-hospitals can save your life: when hospitals computerize patient care, they drastically reduce errors and costs. Business Week Online. December 11, 2000. Available at: www.businessweek.com/archives/2000/b3711079.arc.htm. Accessed December 11, 2005.

8. Hearings before the Subcommittee on Health of the House Committee on Ways and Means. March 6, 2002. Testimony by Donald Rucker, MD, Vice President and Chief Medical Officer, Siemens Medical Solutions Health Services Corporation. Available at: http://waysandmeans.house.gov//legacy/health/107cong/3-7-02/records/simens.htm. Accessed on December 11, 2005.

9. Medical Imaging Web site. Digital Imaging and Information Technology. Available at: www.medicalimaging.org/efficiencies/digital.cfm. Accessed December 11, 2005.

10. Digital Imaging and Communications in Medicine Web site. Available at: medical.nema.org. Accessed December 11, 2005.

11. DICOM Strategic Document version 4.0. 2004. Available at: medical.nema.org/dicom/geninfo/Strategy.htm. Accessed December 11, 2005.

12. Siegel EL, Channin DS. Integrating the healthcare enterprise: a primer. Part 1. Introduction. Radiographics 2001;21:1339–1341.

13. Channin DS. Integrating the healthcare enterprise: a primer. Part 2. Seven brides for seven brothers: the IHE integration profiles. Radiographics 2001;21:1343–1350.

14. Channin DS, Parisot C, Wanchoo V, et al. Integrating the healthcare enterprise: a primer. Part 3. What does IHE do for ME? Radiographics 2001;21:1351–1358.

15. Henderson M, Behlen FM, Parisot C, et al. Integrating the healthcare enterprise: a primer. Part 4. The role of existing standards in IHE. Radiographics 2001;21:1597–1603.

16. Channin DS, Siegel EL, Carr C, Sensmeier J. Integrating the healthcare enterprise: a primer. Part 5. The future of IHE. Radiographics 2001;21:1605–1608.

17. Channin DS. Integrating the healthcare enterprise: a primer. Part 6. The fellowship of IHE: year 4 additions and extensions. Radiographics 2002;22:1555–1560.

18. Harvey D. Diagnosing "hidden" PACS costs. Radiol Today 2004;5:8.

19. Langen HL, Bielmeier J, Wittenberg G, Selbach R, Feustel H. Workflow improvement and efficiency gain with near total digitalization of a radiology department [in German]. Rofo 2003;175:1309–1316.

20. Redfern RO, Langlotz CP, Abbuhl SB, Polansky M, Horii SC, Kundel HL. The effect of PACS on the time required for technologists to produce radiographic images in the emergency department radiology suite. J Digit Imaging 2002;15:153–160.

21. Nissen-Meyer S, Holzknecht N, Wieser B, et al. Improving productivity by implementing RIS and PACS throughout the clinic: a case study [in German]. Radiologe 2002;42:351–360.
22. Sacco P, Mazzei M, Pozzebon E, Stefani P. PACS implementation in a university hospital in Tuscany. J Digit Imaging 2002;15(suppl 1):250–251.
23. Gross-Fengels W, Miedeck C, Siemens P, et al. PACS: from project to reality. Report of experiences on full digitalisation of the radiology department of a major hospital [in German]. Radiologe 2002;42:119–124.
24. Hayt DB, Alexander S, Drakakis J, Berdebes N. Filmless in 60 days: the impact of picture archiving and communications systems within a large urban hospital. J Digit Imaging 2001;14:62–71.
25. Redfern RO, Horii SC, Feingold E, Kundel HL. Radiology workflow and patient volume: effect of picture archiving and communication systems on technologists and radiologists. J Digit Imaging 2000;13(2 suppl 1):97–100.
26. May GA, Deer DD, Dackiewicz D. Impact of digital radiography on clinical workflow. J Digit Imaging 2000;13(2 suppl 1):76–78.
27. Ouvry A. PACS implementation dramatically impacts people and radiology work processes. Proc SPIE Med Imaging 1997;3035:602–603.
28. Siegel EL, Reiner BI. Challenges associated with the incorporation of digital radiography into a picture archival and communication system. J Digit Imaging 1999;12(2 suppl 1):6–8.
29. Reiner B, Siegel E, Carrino JA. Workflow optimization: current trends and future directions. J Digit Imaging 2002;15:141–152.
30. Siegel EL, Reiner BI. Filmless radiology at the Baltimore VA Medical Center: a 9 year retrospective. Comput Med Imaging Graph 2003;27(2–3):101–109.
31. Siegel EL, Diaconis JN, Pomerantz S, et al. Making filmless radiology work. J Digit Imaging 1995;8:151–155.
32. Reiner B, Siegel E, Scanlon M. Changes in technologist productivity with implementation of an enterprisewide PACS. J Digit Imaging 2002;15:22–26.
33. Reiner BI, Siegel EL, Hooper FJ, Glasser D. Effect of film-based versus filmless operation on the productivity of CT technologists. Radiology 1998;207:481–485.
34. Saarinen AO, Wilson MC, Iverson SC, et al. Potential time savings to radiology department personnel in a PACS-based environment. Proc SPIE 1990;1234:261–269.

17
Clinical Adoption

NANCY M. LORENZI

Riley Jones stood by the coffee machine early one Monday, drinking in a mega dose of caffeine—the traditional drug of choice for computer types. As the project leader for the implementation of the new information system for the clinicians in the Medical Center, he was contemplating the anticipated hectic week ahead. His thoughts were interrupted by the loud and rather excited voice of John Molder, a physician, talking to someone outside his door.

"Did you see yesterday's *Times*? Look at this—three articles in just one issue! 'High School Students Change Grades in Local School Computer.' And, 'Security Flaw Found in Popular Internet Program.' And this one, too, 'Chain Stores Tracking and Selling Your Buying Profiles.' Now you want us to put all our patient information into this new computer system. Why don't we just take out ads in the *Times* and publish them!"

"Now come on, John, I'm sure it's not going to be all that bad." Riley recognized the voice of Bob Hobbs, one of the clinicians. Then he heard Bob say that he was going to call for a meeting of the administrative committee "to really look into security issues for our systems?"

Riley thought, "Wonderful! That's all I need right now—another meeting to prepare a presentation for, about another reason why 'they' will not use our systems. I should have gone into something quiet and peaceful." After pouring another cup of coffee, he went back to his office to begin his week with a lot less enthusiasm.

From Resistance to Adoption

The scenario above was constructed from numerous interactions with people in all areas of health care. These people are seeing the healthcare arena that they have known, loved, and mastered changing rapidly and dramatically before their eyes. Whereas a new information system may be fairly straightforward in a technical sense, we have to implement these new systems within complex organizations composed of equally complex individuals. It is often said that the only person that welcomes change is a wet baby. While this is probably an overstatement, it is a valid point that changes within organizations very often engender significant resistance.[1]

The levels of resistance to a new informatics system can vary widely both between and among specific groups. The term *resistance* can mean virtually anything: A less-than-enthusiastic response, a refusal to participate in training, actively organizing protests among colleagues, or actually sabotaging the system through either acts of omission or commission.

Resistance to change in healthcare organizations is certainly not limited to physicians; however, their dominant role makes their resistance especially telling. Physicians have readily accepted many changes in the practice of medicine over the past 50 years such as the use of new medical devices, new drugs, and new surgical procedures. Why then is informatics so often resisted? Any major new system is going to generate reasonable amounts of the FUD factor—fear, uncertainty, and doubt. However, here are some specific reasons that are quite relevant to physician resistance to informatics.[1]

- *Perceived **low personal benefits:*** Physicians often perceive, whether rightly or wrongly, that the informatics system will have little positive impact on making their job easier or improving patient care—two of their major concerns.
- *Fear of **loss of status:*** If the proposed system involves activities such as direct physician order entry, the physicians may perceive a loss of status in doing data entry as opposed to "barking out" orders for others to implement. In addition, tersely worded system-generated "alerts" can be an assault on the professionals' egos.
- *Fear of **revealing ignorance:*** The computer represents a whole new area of knowledge to many physicians and an area in which they may not be confident of their learning skills. To these physicians, accustomed to being viewed as assertive sources of knowledge, the informatics area can be perceived as a potential source of embarrassment, especially if "lesser" mortals appear more proficient.
- *Fear of an **imposed discipline:*** Many clinical systems impose a lack of flexibility that makes physicians feel that their needs, desires, and historic procedures are being made secondary to the "needs" of the new system. Through the intentional limitation of choices, physicians may be forced into the use of only "approved" protocols.
- *Fear of **wasted time:*** Physicians are notoriously time conscious and tend to resist the training or learning time necessary to become comfortable with informatics systems. In addition, they are highly sensitive to time required to use the system and are not necessarily charitable in judging whether the new system takes more or less time than previous methods.

The prospect of long-run benefits may well not outweigh the perception of reduced short-run efficiencies.

- *Fear of **unwanted accountability:*** Even those with a limited understanding of informatics realize that modern systems can be capable of accumulating significant databases that can be used to analyze the activities of individual system users. Those accustomed to being held accountable on only a few broad measures often fear the creation of an environment in which their performance can be quickly and easily monitored on a wide range of variables. At a more dramatic level, increased measurement and data raise the specter of potential increases in legal liability.
- *Fear of **new demands:*** A subtle—and often unrecognized—fear is a concern about what new informatics systems will do to the accustomed and comfortable ways in which physicians fill their time. One of the impacts of informatics upon other professions has been that computerized systems have increasingly assumed the burden of the routine, freeing the professional for the more complex and creative aspects of the professional role.

The breadth of the above concerns shows how difficult the problem of overcoming physician resistance can be. When dealing with a group of physicians, all of the above concerns can appear in varying combinations among individuals within the group.

One of the problems that a change agent faces is that it is easy to listen to resisters, but that sometimes taking their statements literally can be misleading. Whenever there is "talk" about resistance to *any* change, we must ensure that we have correctly identified the change(s) being resisted. The following four categories of resistance are often useful in analyzing specific situations:

- ***Resistance to environmental changes***—these are changes in the organization's general environment that will have impact on the way that the organization functions and possibly on its very survival.
- ***Resistance to general organizational or systems changes***—these are changes in the way the organization is structured or the broad systems that it uses to pursue its mission. These changes might result from either external or internal forces.
- ***Resistance to the changers***—in this case, it matters little what the change is. If "they" are for it, I am against it!
- ***Resistance to a specific change***—this is the type of resistance that a new or updated computer system might engender, based on its own merit or the process by which it is implemented.

Why is it so important to accurately identify the real source of the resistance? If we do not, we can waste time, money, and staff goodwill by using inappropriate solutions to the real problem. For example, high-quality training on how to use a new system can be a tool to combat the latter type of resistance, but it will do little good against the first three. The management lesson is to identify and fight the real problem first. If the real problem is resistance to what is happening in health care, deal with the problem at that level first.

Toward Adoption

Physician resistance to technology has been discussed in the literature for years.[2,3] Recently, during personal implementation experience, it is becoming more apparent that physicians are more than willing to adopt technology if it is both user friendly and if it fits within their work flow. If clinicians will use technology that meets their needs, then the process of buying/designing systems and introducing them must be carefully considered.

The aim of effective change management techniques is not to eliminate all resistance. This is typically impossible when a group of any size is involved. The aims are (1) to keep initial general resistance at reasonable levels, (2) to prevent that initial resistance from growing to serious levels, and (3) to identify and deal with any pockets of serious resistance that do occur despite the previous efforts. Unfortunately for the healthcare industry, many consultants are making a good living from being brought in to solve implementation crises that could have been reasonably prevented at the early stages. The following strategies have proven effective for us in many situations.[1]

Collecting Benchmark Data

One of the first steps in preparing to implement a new system is to gather accurate performance data for the existing system(s). A common form of resistance to a new system is the making of constant unfavorable comparisons to the old system. Although presenting factual data will not overcome emotional reactions, it is important that unfounded allegations about the new system not go unanswered.

Analyzing the Benefits

Early in the overall process, an accurate cost benefit analysis must be performed from the viewpoint of the physician users—and other major user groups as well. A very valid question for any user is "What's in it for me?" If the answer is, "Nothing," then why should the user embrace the system? This situation typically calls for a rethinking of the overall system design to ensure that there are some benefits for all the affected groups.

General Organizational Climate

If the general organizational climate is relatively negative, attack that problem directly through the use of sound organizational development techniques. Installing an informatics system—no matter how good it may be—will not solve this problem. In fact, the system may be doomed by the negative general climate.

Assess the Workflow

The current workflow will need to be assessed and, if needed, a redesign team can be established. This team could be an internal multidisciplinary team with people from the various parts of the organization, for example, clinic operations, the quality office, and the informatics department. This team could analyze the operations and recommended process improvements. This assessment must be completed before a new system is introduced so that the new information system is not "blamed" by the nonparticipants in the process.

Champions

An informatics system needs champions. The optimal approach is to identify several *medically respected* physicians to fulfill this champion role. These people should be integrated into the planning process from the beginning with their advice sought on virtually all aspects of the development and implementation process. A potentially useful—but also potentially dangerous—group is the subset of physicians that we call the *techie-docs*. These are the computer enthusiasts who often consider themselves to be experts in medical informatics, despite having relatively spotty knowledge in the area. This group can easily cause two types of problems: (1) they may advocate inappropriate—or even unfeasible—proposals that sound good to other physicians that know even less about informatics, and (2) they may not be that respected in an overall sense but keep getting appointed as the physician representatives to informatics committees. This is why we stress that informatics systems must have some *champions that are respected medically*.

General Ownership

Developing respected champions is only the first step in building general ownership in the system. The primary twin tools for general ownership are involvement and communication. The single best tool in building ownership is participation in the overall process—planning, design, selection, implementation, etc.—by those that the new system will affect. However, there is an important issue that arises in medical areas. In systems of any size, the participation often has to be representative rather than total.

Modern rapid-prototyping software development tools are an excellent means of developing ownership. Various groups can be shown rough system prototypes, and their inputs can be rapidly incorporated in successive stages of the prototype. Some minor changes can often be made "before their very eyes!" A common problem is that once the prototyping is done, a black hole develops in an information sense. The users became relatively excited about the project and then—nothing. It is important that they be kept aware that work is rapidly progressing on the system. It may be useful to even stage some brief presentations by the developers to highlight their progress.

Building Ownership

The danger is that the participation process often attracts the "amateur techies" in the organization, either by self-selection or by appointment. However, these people may not be high-clout people in the organization. It is critical to have some participation from key power people. In health-care organizations, this often translates as people who are highly respected *clinically*.

Rapid Implementation

As indicated above, a potential downside of involving people early to build ownership is the waiting period between the early involvement and the actual implementation. Within reason, it is a good strategy to concentrate resources on a limited number of projects to minimize the waiting period for system implementation. This will lessen the efforts needed to rebuild the ownership developed in earlier stages.

Realistic Expectations

No matter how good the new informatics system is, it will not improve the quality of the coffee. If the physicians are oversold on what the new system will do, the system is doomed to be regarded as at least a partial failure. This includes setting realistic expectations for the impacts on *initial productivity* during the early implementation stages. It is almost inevitable that productivity will initially decline, no matter how good the system and the preparations for its implementation.

Timely Training

Getting physicians to participate in informatics training in a traditional classroom sense is notoriously difficult. Any training must be brief, high-quality, closely timed to the point of need, and specifically directed to the physicians' needs. Reconcile yourself that there will have to be special sessions to pick up stragglers and that part of the training will have to be accomplished hands-on through the support process. Ego issues can also be important, especially for "senior" people who may be anxious about their lack of computer abilities. Private or small-group sessions often help considerably in these cases. Similarly, the style, pace, and depth of training may need to be adjusted for all the various user subgroups. Those doing the training should have outgoing, positive personalities. Good training does more than merely build skills. Ideally, education starts the selling process, participation adds enthusiasm, and training is the final opportunity to "close the sale."

Timely, Appropriate Training

Quality training can help significantly in reducing anxieties about using a new system. However, the timing is critical. Training that is either too early or too late will waste resources and raise frustrations, not alleviate them.

Extensive Support

With modern software tools, there is no excuse for developing systems without extensive contextual online user support written in language that the users can understand. Supplementary written support should also be provided in a format most comfortable for the users. For example, physicians might prefer a "cheat sheet" in the 3×5 card format that many use for various purposes.

When the system is first installed, ample on-site help should be available, to be subsequently replaced with good phone support as the initial demands dwindle. Time-conscious physicians demand prompt, high-quality support or they rapidly become discontented with the system.

System Stability

Physicians are busy people. Even if they are willing to invest the time to learn the system, they almost certainly will not be willing to spend the time to relearn the release of the month. Well-crafted software is relatively stable, at least in its user interface, and effective prototyping should sharply limit the number of changes necessary in the interface. There will be bugs but correcting them should not require constantly modifying the user interface.

Protecting Professional Egos

Although it is costly, skilled one-on-one or very small-group training may be an effective strategy for those physicians and other professionals most likely to be affected by computer phobia. This is especially important if these particular professionals are also highly respected medically by their peers within the organization.

Professionals have an understandable need for respect. Therefore, the dialogues present in informatics systems should be carefully reviewed for usefulness, clarity, and *respectful tone*. For example, alerts should be programmed as respectful questions rather than as terse declarative statements. Error messages must give useful instructions for correcting the situation. Although these suggestions may sound simple, they are often violated by informatics personnel who are used to functioning under another paradigm of human-computer interface.

Feedback Processes

Any aggressive change management strategy should contain multiple mechanisms for actively soliciting feedback at all stages of the change process. The alternative is to have rumors, half-truths, and even untruths flooding the grapevine. When feedback is solicited and obtained, it must be processed promptly and return feedback must be provided. Every issue cannot be resolved to everyone's satisfaction. This is life in the real world. Still, people must feel that both they and their concerns are regarded as important.

Having Fun

Smart change managers try to introduce an element of fun into the change management process whenever possible. Two techniques that we have seen used numerous times to stimulate the introduction of new clinical systems are lunch-time or end-of-day sessions with free pizza and soft drinks and sessions that feature some nonthreatening competition between the physicians and the system or between physicians using the system and physicians not using the system. The message is that facing the future doesn't have to be grim!

Table 17-1 is a checklist of the organizational strategies listed. This checklist is an opportunity to realistically assess your plans in accord with the known best organizational strategies. Once the assessment occurs, the next step is to clearly indicate what needs to change in your current process to better ensure success.

TABLE 17-1. Checklist of organizational strategies

| | How Does Your Organization Rate? | | | | |
| | On Target | | Needs Improvement | | Does Not Have |
Category	1	2	3	4	5
Have you collected benchmark data?					
Do you know the benefits of the new system?					
What is the general organizational climate?					
Are there realistic expectations?					
Do you have a process to assess the workflow?					
Do you have champions?					
Is there general ownership of the new system?					
Do you have plans to build ownership?					
Do you have a plan for rapid implementation?					
Will your training be timely and appropriate?					
Will you provide extensive support?					
Do your plans include protecting professional egos?					
What are your plans to ensure system stability?					
Do you have feedback processes planned?					
Do you have plans for having fun during or after implementation?					

System Diffusion

Information technology change strategy must focus on the specific desired outcomes for the total organization and every effort must be made to ensure that the changes and the organization's plans are the same, and to educate the organizational leaders on both the potential opportunities and threats that stem from the information technology efforts under consideration. The complexity of healthcare organizations often makes it impossible to implement new information systems simultaneously throughout the organization. Therefore, informatics systems must be implemented according to a specific strategy. E.M. Rogers developed a diffusion of innovation theory.[4] Rogers defined diffusion "as the process by which (1) an innovation; (2) is communicated through certain channels; (3) over time; (4) among the members of a social system." Although the diffusion of innovations seems very simple, the process is quite complicated. Rogers says that potential adopters of an innovation have to learn about an innovation and be persuaded to try it out before making a decision to adopt or reject the innovation. After adoption and implementation, the adopters decide to either continue using the innovation or stop using it. This theory is very important because it shows that adoption is not a momentary, irrational act, but an ongoing process that can be studied, facilitated, and supported.

Diffusion of innovations can seem very simple. A number of studies have focused on diffusion strategies.[5-8] Understanding the diffusion of innovative ideas is one of the key areas to successfully transforming health care. This is an overview of an applied diffusion process from the challenge through the process and from the embryonic product to the product becoming a transformation product in both its intended arena and beyond. Rogers also classified adopters on the basis of innovativeness. According to this theory, members of a population vary greatly in their willingness to adopt a particular innovation. People adopt in a time sequence, and they may be classified into adopter categories on the basis of when they first begin using a new idea.

The distribution of innovativeness within a population (see Table 17-2) will resemble a normal curve beginning with "Innovators" who lead in adopting an innovation, and make up about 2.5% of a population. Innovators are very venturesome. They are eager to try new ideas. Innovators are mobile and communicate outside of local peer networks. Communication networks among innovators are common. Innovators are able to cope with the high degree of uncertainty associated with an innovation early in the adoption process.

"Early Adopters" make up approximately 13.5% of a population and have the most opinion leaders. Potential adopters look to early adopters for advice and information about the innovation. The early adopter is considered by many as "the individual to check with" before using a new idea. Because early adopters are not too far ahead of the average individual in innovativeness, they serve as a role model. The early adopter is respected by his or her peers, and is the embodiment of successful and discrete use of new ideas.

TABLE 17-2. Innovativeness in a population

Innovativeness	Approximate Proportion of Population (%)
Innovators	2.5
Early adopters	13.5
Early majority	34
Late majority	34
Laggards	16

Most people will fall into either the <u>Early Majority</u> (34%) or the <u>Late Majority</u> (34%) categories. The early majority adopt new ideas just before the average member of a social system. This category gets its information largely from the early adopters. This further emphasizes the importance of the early adopter in the overall adoption process. The "early majority" interacts frequently with their peers, but seldom holds leadership positions. The early majority's unique position between the very early and the relatively late to adopt makes them an important link in the adoption process. They provide "interconnectedness" in the system's networks. The late majority adopt new ideas just after the average member of a social system. Adoption may be both an economic necessity and the answer to increasing network pressures. Innovations are approached with a skeptical and cautious air, and the late majority do not adopt until most others in their social system have done so. They can be persuaded of the utility of new ideas, but the pressure of peers is necessary to motivate adoption. Almost all of the uncertainty about a new idea must be removed before the late majority feel that it is safe to adopt.

"<u>Laggards</u>," who will resist adopting an innovation as long as possible, comprise about 16% of a population. These people are the most local in their outlook of all adopter categories. They tend to be suspicious of innovations. Their traditional orientation slows the innovation decision process to a crawl, with adoption lagging far behind awareness of a new idea. This resistance is entirely rational from their viewpoint.

This theory is important because it shows the impossibility of having all members of a population adopt an innovation at the same time. Change agents should anticipate different responses to their innovations and develop plans for addressing the concerns of all groups from innovators to laggards. Before deciding about your diffusion process, consider rating areas or people within your organization (see Table 17-3).

One Practical Example

To select hospital sites that had a higher potential for success of an information system implementation, Vanderbilt University Medical Center used Rogers' Diffusion theory coupled with past research in organizational change to create what became known as the Success Factor Profile©.[9] This profile was developed to assess each potential pilot site through a combination of structured interviews, visits/observations, and data from past experiences with each unit. Key questions included:

- *Success likelihood*—What is the unit's probability of successful development and implementation of new processes?

TABLE 17-3. Identification of areas or people by their projected acceptance of change

Areas or People	A	B	C	D	E	Currently Doing?	Need to Begin Doing as Soon as Possible	Strategies to Involve?

- **Innovation history**—Has the unit had success piloting programs in the past?
- **Unit champions**—Does the unit have nurse and physician champions?
- **Ability to generalize**—Will there be gains for the rest of the hospital from the processes developed within this unit?
- **Learning opportunities**—Will the unit provide quality feedback for development and implementation teams to improve processes?

The two units that rated the highest in this profile were selected for the implementation. In turn, both sites had successful implementations. Table 17-4 presents a checklist for the change agent.

TABLE 17-4. Success factor profile© for innovation (see reference[9])

	Success Likelihood	Innovation History	Ability to Generalize	Innovation Personality	Learning Opportunity	Pilot Rating
	Probability of prosperous implementation*	History of leadership and pilot success*	Relevant gains for rest of the hospital*	Enthusiasm for implementation, strength of leadership team*	Quality feedback for development and project teams to improve processes and products*	Quasi-scientific result based on Survey Team Assessment*
Unit A						
Unit B						
Unit C						
Unit D						
Unit E						
Unit F						
Unit G						
Unit H						

* Scale of 1 (low) to 8 (high).

Key Organizational Issues

Experience tells us that motivated, involved people can make bad systems work. After all, they have done it for years. In the same way, unmotivated— or even worse, negatively motivated—people can bring the best system to its knees. Which situation will we have? How well we perform the steps outlined above will often answer that question. Profound change initiatives come in many shapes and sizes. They can be as simple as a series of meetings on a crucial business objective or as complex as a corporate-wide "transformation."

The need for making major changes starts at the conceptual level. When we view majestic buildings, companies with outstanding profits, or a program so excellent it makes us envious, we need to step back and realize that these outcomes normally did not occur overnight. They started at the conceptual level. Then there was commitment and an understanding of what needed to occur to make that outcome happen. With a new building, someone first needed to decide that a building was needed for a specific purpose. Then the issues of where, when, how, etc., needed to be considered. The time and effort spent well before the groundbreaking occurs largely determine the ultimate value of all the activities performed from the groundbreaking to the completion of the building.

Creating a Vision for Change

Vision—what is it and where do you get it? Do you concentrate on not making buggy whips and become obsessive about that? Do you listen to the rosy promises that vendors whisper in your ear? How do you decide? Where do you begin?

In a personal conversation years ago, Russell Ackoff, one of the great minds in decision making and operations research, observed that we can envision the future; we simply cannot plan for it in great detail. He went on to say that everything an organization needs to determine future direction is known today (although we may not know it, of course, if we hide our heads in the sand like a threatened ostrich). We all know that listening to four gurus may produce at least five opinions. In the end, we all have to make our own judgments as to which part of the known information— to use Ackoff's concept—will be most relevant to our case.

The keys to successful creation of a vision are:

- Visionary leadership possessing a "can do" attitude
- Knowledge and understanding of the needs of the major stakeholders
- Knowledge and understanding of the organizational milieu, including both the opportunities and the constraints

These three keys provide the foundation that enables the creation of a meaningful vision. Once the vision is created, this foundation will also allow the vision statement to be translated strategically into statements of the "we want to be capable of" type. Creating a "capable of" statement is the step that translates the vision into a workable and understandable action-oriented goal. Many people might read the vision statement and say, "That sounds great." Unfortunately, they then return to their regular work, and the vision gathers dust on the shelf. In many ways, a vision is so big that it is somewhat like an elephant. First, the elephant is so big that even people with normal sight can examine it and draw very different conclusions. Second, it is difficult to decide how to "eat" that elephant. Often, there is endless debate about the process; then everyone agrees that it is indeed a beautiful creature but simply too big to eat. The "capable of" statement is action-oriented and helps people dissect an elephant, making the vision more manageable.

As an example of the concepts described above, a *vision statement* might be, "The organization will have a fully integrated information system." One of the many supporting *capable-of statements* might be, "The system will be capable of electronically accessing selected full-text library journal resources from the patient floor." This example clearly shows how "capable of" statements got their name.

The more contemporary approach to managing the complexity of the healthcare situation is to be somewhere in the center or to the right of center of the model. However, if the information systems person is functioning in an environment where the decisions are made on the far left side, then the information system planning needs to first acknowledge this environment and then needs to gather vision ideas from those who are on the right side of the model.

With this analysis completed, it is then necessary to approach the key power brokers within the organization, share the vision (perhaps in draft form) with them, and encourage each person to become involved and make inputs, and build ownership in the vision.

If the "capable of" statements seem to be "fuzzy," then it is critical for the person creating the vision statements to remove as much of this fuzziness as possible. When the concept of integrated information (IAIMS) was first presented at the University of Cincinnati Medical Center, it was clear that a few people understood and agreed with what was being said, but there were many "glassy" stares. At that point, the IAIMS leader created a scenario about an imaginary patient, Mary Smith, who became ill at 2 a.m.[1] Each clinical department was then asked what types of information and communication items they would need to effectively treat Mary Smith's problems. Poor Mary had many varied problems, of course, depending on the group being addressed. If it was the Department of Psychiatry, Mary had major psychiatric problems, and the issues of confidentiality received considerable attention. If Mary was a postoperative surgical patient, the Department of Surgery would express her complications in a very clear and distinct manner. If the physicians were from Internal Medicine, Mary had many problems that would pertain to the various specialties within Internal Medicine.

Key Change Leader Concerns

Change leaders who have to function at the "bleeding edge" are not always successful. To be successful, the informatics change leader must understand and constantly monitor four key concerns:

- Point-person role
- Knowledge and commitment
- Formal and informal power
- Rapid shifts in focus

In the following discussion, notice that some of these key concerns may involve issues that need to be resolved before the change leader assumes the role. If these issues cannot be resolved to the change leader's satisfaction, assuming the responsibilities is probably a big mistake.

Point-person Role

The change leader is the "point" person for the change that happens, and may well become a "symbol" of this change to those unhappy with it. This is a variation on the old "shoot the messenger" phenomenon. Stresses within the organization or the environment that do not directly involve the particular change will still often have an impact on the change leader. Suppose an organization is moving from the "big iron" mainframe-type information systems approach to a more decentralized approach. If the information system (IS) staff members feel that they may not have the skills for this new direction and perhaps feel that their future or even their jobs are threatened, they will probably resist the change vigorously. In one organization with more than 100 people in the IS department, volunteers were sought to assist in exploring the new direction for that institution. One person chose to go with the new group. As early small successes started to occur, many of the people within that IS department clearly realized that they did not have the appropriate skills for the future. Rather than upgrading their skills, they spent considerable time and energy resisting the new system and the efforts of the change leader in order to try and stop the system. Eventually the transition was made, but unfortunately the negativity toward the change leader "who had caused all the problems" lingered on.

Knowledge and Commitment

The change leader must be both knowledgeable and committed. Knowledgeable means an understanding of not only the organizational issues but also of the technology and the concept of systems. The person must be respected for his or her particular knowledge and must be firmly committed to the project. Any significant project will inevitably have its moments of euphoria and its moments of despair. A deep commitment—coupled with competence and confidence—is essential for weathering these lows.

Formal and Informal Power

The change leader must have the necessary formal and informal power within the organization to lead the change. The person could have formal organizational power, such as being the CIO, but without personal respect within the organization he or she will not be successful. However, someone may have high informal power within the organization but without formal power be blocked by a minority of the organization that does not accept that informal power. The change leader must be the authorized or legitimate organizational leader. It is critical that the organization sanction only one person to lead the effort and support that person through the highs and lows of the change process. If "competing" formal leaders are created by the organization, massive resources that could be dedicated to the change process will be wasted in "turf" battles.

Rapid Shifts in Focus

The role of change leader typically requires good skills in the technical, human, and conceptual areas, as discussed earlier. More important, the change leader has to be able to constantly and rapidly shift between these skill areas on any given day. This kind of mental flexibility is critical. Whereas successful change leaders must certainly have the ability to plan and organize well, they must also have the mental flexibility to deal with interruptions, changes in plans, and changes in the area and level of focus.

Organizational Leadership Commitment

The organizational leadership—CEO, president, vice presidents, deans, department chairs, etc.—must be *committed* to supporting the change process, not merely involved. They must ensure that there is broad and constant support for the process and the resulting projects. They must also "stay" with the change process in the sense of ensuring that all their decisions and actions are consistent with the values of the change process. The way for top leadership to kill a change process is for them to establish a vision, send some person or group off to implement that vision, and then proceed to make decisions not in accord with that vision.

It is critical that top management continuously integrates information planning into the overall organizational planning process rather than treating information issues as occasional problems to be solved on a crisis basis. Because healthcare organizations are so complex and constantly changing, the top organizational leaders are typically involved in the decision to implement major new technology systems. They then normally charge the person managing this effort with completing the implementation. At this point, top management gallops off to deal with other problems, feeling that this particular area has been handled. The information systems people then proceed to build the system that was approved for the organization. Unfortunately, major systems are not implemented overnight. By the time of actual implementation, the system that was envisioned as needed 1 or 2 years ago may not be the system that is needed today.

End-user Needs

The end users are key stakeholders in the implementation of any health informatics system. There are five key areas of concern involving these customers for the information system:

1. The end users must know and comprehend what the system will be realistically capable of doing. In the Mary Smith scenario mentioned earlier, the end users helped create the scenario for the information needs that they had with regard to Mary Smith. The role of the information managers and leaders is to effectively manage the end-user expectations because the expectations will always be greater than the capabilities of the technology, the software, and the people who can deliver the end products.

2. The end users must be included in the communications and information regarding changes that are being considered and/or developed.

3. The end users must believe that key people are committed to the success of the system. In one organization, the department head decides that he would develop a "tiger team" made up of several people from his group plus several people from the information systems group. The team met over a 2-month period and, using a very iterative process, developed a system that was accepted immediately. The system worked because the hand-picked user representatives brought high content knowledge to the project *and* constantly discussed progress and needs with their other colleagues. That system is still in use today and continues to be enhanced.

4. The gatekeepers and opinion leaders must support the system and push or pull through various times of success or failure. The gatekeepers and opinion leaders need not be the formal organizational leadership.

5. End users must "see and know" the results of their inputs as rapidly as possible. This is true whether it is helping the residency recruitment program, creating a discharge summary statement, clearly identifying all the drugs that a patient is taking, or identifying past medical problems. It is important that changes be seen immediately and not in 3 to 5 years after end-user participation in the process.

Summary

In early 1993, a managed care organization installed a new computer system in one of its pharmacies. The decisions regarding the system selection and installation followed the "usual and customary" processes. Namely, the decision was reached by a few people and then "sold" to the many who would be the ultimate users of the system. Complaints and anger were so strong that, rather than "force" the use of the system, the new person responsible for the clinical-based system decided to remove the expensive system from the pharmacy.

Normally, when an expensive system is "pulled," it goes to a "system sanctuary," also known as long-term storage. This time the system only had a short rest in the "sanctuary."

Having been selected as the person responsible for clinical-based systems and inheriting a disaster in the making, the new leader thought there must be a better way. He attended the International Medical Informatics Association Working Conference on the Organizational Impact of Medical Informatics and decided to rapidly put into practice many of the concepts he heard expressed. In a pharmacy in another location within the same managed care organization, the leader used involvement strategies for the people who would be the most affected by the system selected. The involved people spent many hours outlining their specific needs, desired processes, and so forth. In reviewing the possible systems that would meet their specific needs, it turned out that the system that was pulled from the first location would be an ideal match. The system was retrieved from the "sanctuary" and was installed. After more than a year in operation, the system was working very successfully for the people in the second location. They still feel strongly that "it" is their system and they made the decision to use this system.

Did something miraculous happen to the system when it was in the sanctuary or did the new involvement process make the difference?

Questions

1. You have just been selected to implement a major change. What are the first three agenda items that would create for you? The Information Systems Department? The broader organization?
2. What other physician resistance areas can you identify?
3. List what you would consider as the most successful strategies to gain clinician adoption of a new information system.
4. How much time do you really think needs to be spent on the type of topics discussed in this chapter? In reality, how much time do you think is spent on the type of topics mentioned here? Why? Why not?

5. If people say—all "this" sounds like common sense or generalities. If they are such common sense, why do you think most people do not follow these principles? Do you think not following principles such as outlined here leads to the almost 50% failure rate of information systems? Why? Why not?

References

1. Lorenzi NM, Riley RT. Managing Technological Change: Organizational Aspects of Health Informatics. New York: Springer-Verlag; 2004.
2. Edelson J. Physician use of information technology in ambulatory medicine. J Ambul Care Manage 1995;18(3):9–19.
3. Teach RL, Shortliffe EH. An analysis of physician attitudes regarding computer-based clinical consultation systems. Comput Biomed Res 1981;14(6):542–558.
4. Rogers EM. Diffusion of Innovations. 4th ed. New York: The Free Press; 1995.
5. Dixon DR, Dixon BJ. Adoption of information technology enabled innovations by primary care physicians: model and questionnaire development. In: Safran C, ed. Proceedings of the Seventeenth Symposium on Computer SCAMC Proceedings. New York: McGraw-Hill; 1994:631–635.
6. Hebert M, Benbasat I. Adopting information technology in hospitals: the relationship between attitudes/expectations and behavior. Hosp Health Serv Adm 1994;39:369–383.
7. Lomas J. Diffusion, dissemination and implementation: who should do what? Ann NY Acad Sci 1994;701:226–237.
8. Gundry L. Computer technology and organizational culture. Special Issue: Social Impact of Computers. Comput Soc Sci 1985;1:163–166.
9. Lorenzi NM, Smith JB, Conner SR, Campion TR. The Success Factor Profile for Clinical Computer Innovation. In: Fieschi M, ed. Medinfo 2004. Amsterdam: IOS Press; 2004:1077–1080.

Section 4
Going Forward

18
Evaluation of Electronic Health Record Systems

PAUL N. GORMAN

Evaluate: "To judge or determine the significance, worth, or quality of"[1]

The aim of this chapter is to provide an overview of issues and approaches relevant to the evaluation of electronic health records (EHRs), in the context of the evaluation of healthcare information technology (IT) in general. This chapter does not offer detailed guidance or specific "how-to" information on the design and conduct of evaluation studies—the field of health informatics is far too broad and its approaches too diverse to do so in a single book, much less a single chapter. Rather, this chapter discusses evaluation of healthcare information systems in terms of a collection of frameworks, which, it is hoped, can assist those who design and conduct evaluations of EHR systems (EHR-Ss) and those who use the information these evaluations provide.

The Necessity of Evaluating IT in Health Care

As new technologies are developed for health care, there is an ongoing tension between the need to introduce and disseminate them as rapidly as possible, so that patients and society may enjoy their benefits, and the need to evaluate them as rigorously as possible, to ensure that the benefits are real and outweigh the risks and costs. As a rule, developers and proponents of interventions, whether medical treatments, surgical procedures, or information technologies, are able to offer persuasive arguments about benefits based on early data and current understanding of the functioning of natural systems (whether biological systems or social and organizational systems). Often, these early data are supported by subsequent experience and the intervention stands the test of time and practice. Often, however, it does not, because of unforeseen harms and costs, because of inadequate understanding of the natural system in question, or because of inadequate evaluation.

Turning to medical practice, there is no shortage of examples of interventions initially, sometimes fervently, believed to be beneficial, which later proved to be harmful. A compelling example is routine administration of pure oxygen to healthy neonates in the late 1940s. It seemed obvious at the time that oxygen would benefit newborns, and many opposed conducting controlled trials on the basis that it would be unethical to deny newborns an obviously beneficial treatment. The practice was quickly abandoned after 1954, however, when a relatively new (to medicine) study methodology, the randomized controlled trial, demonstrated that oxygen was responsible for retrolental fibroplasia, a then increasingly common cause of blindness in infants.[2] Similarly, there was little doubt well into the 1980s that drug treatment was indicated to suppress cardiac rhythm disturbances. Physicians everywhere (including this author) routinely used an array of antiarrhythmic drugs for this purpose, believing this to be best for their patients. This practice, too, was quickly abandoned when the Cardiac Arrhythmia Suppression Trial demonstrated that these treatments were actually associated with an increase, in mortality, not a decrease.[3]

We expect, then, that some information technologies that we currently believe will be beneficial may turn out to cause unintended harm. For instance, software for administering treatments has been reported to have a role in treatment errors and even deaths from radiation therapy[4] and intravenous analgesic medications.[5] Even implementations of EHR-S components that are not directly involved in treatment administration have been reported to result in unforeseen problems, as with computerized order entry[6-8] and computerized physician documentation.[9,10]

One also finds in medical practice examples of the opposite: Interventions that proved to be beneficial despite a lack of predicted benefits based on then-current understanding of biological systems. Goodwin refers to this phenomenon as the "tomato effect": Rejection of effective treatment because of inadequate understanding of underlying mechanims.[11] Gold therapy for rheumatoid arthritis (RA), for example, was initially proposed when this disease was believed to be an infection—and heavy metals such as gold were being used to treat infections! Later, when this theory about the cause of RA was discarded, the treatment also was discarded—it did not make sense that it would work—only later to be resumed because, without knowing why or how, it became clear that it actually does help patients.[11] Similarly, for years it was universally understood that beta-blocking drugs must be harmful to patients with congestive heart failure: Use of these medications in such patients was contraindicated and considered a marker for poor quality care. Only recently have we discovered that beta-blocker medications actually reduce mortality in patients with heart failure, resulting in a complete reversal of practice recommendations,[12] so that *not* using them is now a marker of poor quality care.

An example connected to EHR-Ss is that of diagnostic expert systems. They have not been used in practice, although research has shown them to be more accurate than typical physicians.

Two recent editorials reflect this tension between the need to implement new technologies or practices ("we know what works, let's just do it")[13] and the need for rigorous evaluation ("sound evidence is needed before widespread adoption of interventions").[14] This debate is likely to continue unresolved, for both sides represent valid points of view. Like the patients and clinicians we hope will benefit from the EHR-S, we must often make decisions and take action based on imperfect evidence. It is important at the same time to remain aware of the strength of the evidence that is available, and where it is limited, to support rigorous evaluations, especially for expensive or risky interventions.

The Challenges of Evaluating IT in Health Care

Aside from this tension between deploying technology versus waiting for its evaluation, and aside from the usual difficulties evaluators face in designing rigorous evaluations within real-world constraints, IT in health care presents special challenges somewhat unique to the field.

Health informatics is an integrative discipline concerned essentially with two key questions, "How to build the right systems?" and "How to build the systems right?" (J. Moehr, personal communication). To explore these questions requires expertise and methodology drawn from a diverse array of fields in the natural and social sciences, from computer science to organizational behavior, from mathematics to medicine. Jochen Moehr has represented this diversity of fields in a space defined by two axes, from the theoretical ("pure") to the practical ("applied") and from the natural (physical) sciences to the social sciences (see Figure 18-1).

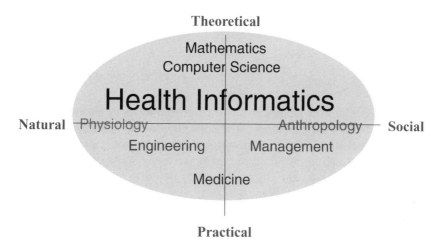

FIGURE 18-1. Informatics as an integrative discipline, with diverse paradigms and methods. (*Source:* Adapted from Jochen Moehr, University of Victoria.)

Real progress in health informatics, whether answering the first question or the second, requires multidisciplinary collaboration calling upon diverse theory and methods. This diversity of approaches required to make progress in health informatics research and development is equally important to conducting evaluations, sometimes bringing together different or even conflicting philosophical and epistemological points of view. The result can at times be disagreement about the kinds of evaluations that are needed and the interpretation of their results. On the one hand, adapting methods from other fields can lead to significant new insights, such as the application of receiver operating characteristic analysis in radiology and diagnostic testing,[15] or bringing the methods of anthropology to informatics.[16] On the other hand, rigid adherence to familiar methods ("when all you've got is a hammer, every problem needs a pounding . . .") can lead us to "ask inappropriate questions, apply unsuitable methods, and incorrectly interpret results."[17] As McManus has asked,

Can we imagine how randomised controlled trials would ensure the quality and safety of modern air travel . . .? Whenever aeroplane manufacturers wanted to change a design feature . . . they would make a new batch of planes, half with the feature and half without, taking care not to let the pilot know which features were present.[18]

To make progress in the field, it is important to move beyond disagreements about the relative merits of different research and evaluation methods, which have been most evident in debates over the validity and usefulness of qualitative versus quantitative techniques.[19] Sackett and Wennberg[20] call for an end to these debates about methods and emphasize the need to focus instead on the question:

The question being asked determines the appropriate research architecture, strategy, and tactics to be used—not tradition, authority, experts, paradigms, or schools of thought.[20]

Frameworks for Evaluating Information Systems

Therefore, evaluation studies in health informatics may involve a broad spectrum of methods, depending on the question being addressed. To guide the design, conduct, and interpretation of informatics evaluations, it is useful to consider the purpose, the perspective, the stage of development, the level of evaluation, and the quality of evidence.

Purpose of Evaluation

The first issue to consider as designer or consumer of an evaluation of an EHR is the purpose for which the evaluation is performed. Ideally, it would be more convenient and efficient if a single evaluation could serve multiple purposes, but in practice, it can be difficult or impossible to accomplish this. Chelimsky et al.[21] described three main purposes for which evaluations are performed: 1) Evaluation for Development, in which the intent is to provide data for immediate use in improving a program or project; 2) Evaluation for Knowledge, where the aim is to generate new understandings or discoveries, usually about the natural world or our interactions with it; and 3) Evaluation for Accountability, performed for the purpose of measuring the results, costs, and value of a program or intervention (see Table 18-1).[21] To be done well, each of these evaluation purposes requires different approaches, especially with respect to the relationship between the evaluator and the object of study. As indicated in Table 18-1, evaluations performed as part of the development process benefit from close interaction between developer and evaluator. These would be difficult or impossible without such relationship. In contrast, independence and objectivity are paramount with evaluations conducted to produce new knowledge or to assess program value and costs. Even with methods that are unimpeachable, such evaluations are subject to criticism when independence cannot be assured, as in a recent systematic review of computerized decision support systems, which noted a tendency for positive effects to be reported when evaluations are conducted by the developers themselves, implying a need for corroborating, *independent* evaluation to validate the findings.[22]

Perspective of Evaluation

The second issue that requires consideration, although it may seem an obvious one, is the perspective to be taken in the study. Again, although ideally a single evaluation might serve the needs of multiple clients or audiences, in practice this too is difficult to achieve. As Gremy and DeGoulet[23] note, "The people concerned by health informatics applications constitute a complex network of actors which is nearly impossible to model" (see Figure 1, from their article) (Figure 18-2).

Given the complexity of these systems and the technologies embedded in them, it is inevitable that the perspectives and goals of participants and stakeholders will at times conflict. As a consequence, it is also inevitable that evaluation performed from the perspective of one stakeholder group may not reflect or serve those of another. Consistent with Grudin's law,[24] an EHR component that produces benefits for a class of users at little cost will be adopted more rapidly by those users than one that increases effort with little benefit. Physicians may quickly adopt the laboratory results or PACS (picture archiving and communication systems) into routine use, but be slower to accept computerized progress notes or order entry. Nurses may readily recognize the value of physician order entry or computerized physician notes, but be less receptive to nursing documentation systems. More generally, EHR components that deliver benefits to IT managers (reduced

TABLE 18-1. The three perspectives and their respective positions along nine dimensions

Dimensions	Accountability Perspective	Knowledge Perspective	Developmental Perspective
Purpose	To measure results or value for funds expended; to determine costs; to assess efficiency	To generate insights about public problems, policies, programs, and processes; to develop new methods and to critique old ones	To strengthen institutions; to build agency or organizational capability in some evaluative area
Need for use to fulfill purpose	No	No	Yes
Typical uses	Policy use; debate and negotiation; enlightenment; governmental/agency reform; public use	Enlightenment use; policy; research and replication; education; knowledge base construction	Institutional or agency use as part of the evaluative process; public and policy use
Evaluator role regarding client	Distant	Distant or close, depending on evaluation design and methods	Close: The evaluator is a "critical friend" or may be part of a team
Independence	A prerequisite	Critical	Little need
Advocacy	Unacceptable	Unacceptable, but now being debated	Often inevitable, but correctable through independent, outside review
Acceptability to clients or users	Often difficult but may be helped by negotiation	Clients may ignore or shelve findings they do not like	Easy: No threat is posed
Objectivity	High	High (when advocacy is not present)	Uncertain (based on independence and control)
Position under policy debate	Can be strong (depending on leadership)	Can be strong (if consolidated and dissemination channels exist)	Uncertain (based on independence and control)

Source: Chelimsky and Shadish.[21]

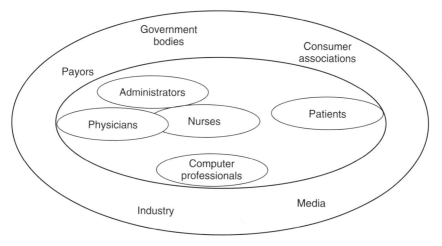

FIGURE 18-2. Participants and stakeholders in health IT. (*Source:* Gremy and DeGoulet.[23])

installation and maintenance costs, for example) or health system managers (improved documentation to meet regulatory requirements or access to data for management decision making) may not be acceptable to others who use the systems and actually enter the data. Tradeoffs among conflicting perspectives are unavoidable and must be confronted in making decisions about EHR development and implementation. To support these decisions, evaluations are needed that explicitly consider the perspective to be taken.

Stage of Development

The third major issue in designing, conducting, or making use of evaluations of EHR-Ss and their components is the stage of development of the technology. Stead et al.[25] provided a useful framework for this purpose, reproduced in Figure 18-3. As indicated in this figure, any substantial healthcare information system can be expected to pass through a series of stages, from initial concept, through the development and integration of components, through full implementation and real-world use.

Three key points follow from this conceptualization: First, the methods and metrics chosen to evaluate the system must be appropriate for the stage of development of that system or component. At the specification and early component development stages, techniques such as cognitive work analysis, task analysis, and verification and validation methods from software engineering are most appropriate. At the component development and integration stages, component-specific evaluation methods are needed, such as recall and precision studies of the information retrieval components, or

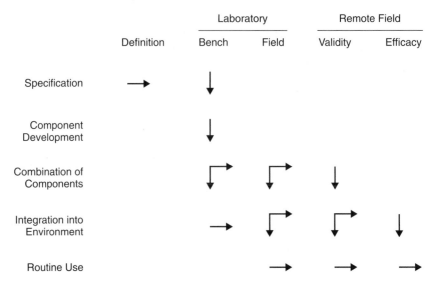

FIGURE 18-3. Relationship of System Development Stage to Level of Evaluation. (*Source:* Adapted from Stead et al.[25])

discount usability engineering techniques to evaluate and improve the user interface. At the implementation and routine use stages, methods and metrics are required that assess performance of real tasks by real users in real environments, as well as the broader organizational and economic impacts of the technology.

The second key point that follows from this conceptualization is that the evaluation is necessarily sequential—it makes no sense to conduct laboratory testing of component performance if the conceptual model upon which the design is based has not been validated. Similarly, it is premature to conduct comparative studies of outcomes or task performance by users with completed systems when the underlying components, including the user interface, have not yet been properly evaluated and improved.

The third key point, emphasized by Gremy and DeGoulet,[23] is that the farther one moves along this hierarchy the more complex the evaluation task becomes. To evaluate a system at one level, one must be sure that the subsystems each function effectively. Effective performance of these subsystems is necessary but not sufficient—a clinical system combining properly functioning subsystems in the laboratory may still not perform properly when integrated in real-world settings with real-world users. Ideally, the evaluation process must be sequential and also carried to completion in real-world settings.

For EHR-Ss, the old hospital information system modules (laboratory, pharmacy) have been evaluated primarily through practice. New compo-

TABLE 18-2. NASA technology readiness levels

Basic research	1. Basic principles observed and reported
Feasibility	2. Technology concept or application formulated
Technology development	3. Analytical and experimental function and/or characteristic proof-of-concept
	4. Component and/or breadboard validation in laboratory environment
Technology demonstration	5. Component and/or breadboard validation in relevant environment
	6. System/subsystem model or prototype demonstration in relevant environment (ground or space)
System development	7. System prototype demonstration in space environment
System test and operations	8. Actual system completed and "flight qualified" through test and demonstration
	9. Actual system "flight-proven" through successful mission operations

Source: Adapted from Mankins.[26]

nents—notes (CDA Architecture; see Chapter 12), automated coding (see Chapter 15)—remain to be evaluated as components, whereas others, such as computerized provider order entry (see Chapter 7) require evaluation at the level of Integration into the Environment, beyond the academic centers where they have had their initial evaluation.

This notion of tailoring the evaluation to the stage of development of the technology is of course not new or unique to healthcare information systems. A useful comparison is the Technology Readiness Levels (TRL) framework used by the United States National Aeronautics and Space Administration.[26] As indicated in Table 18-2, the TRL framework is similar to that described above in that it is sequential and hierarchical, proceeding through stages of concept development, proof-of-concept demonstrations, component development and validation, and combined system performance in the intended environment.

Level of Evaluation

After consideration of the stage of development, it is important to consider also the level at which system evaluation is to be or has been performed. Littenberg's general framework of technology assessment in health care (Table 18-3, from reference[27]) can be applied to IT in health care. This framework, similar to those above, is hierarchical, following the conceptual progression from the understanding of the underlying natural system through the demonstration of intended changes in that system, through to the demonstration of changes in important individual and social outcomes.

As an example, in the second column of Table 18-3, the technology for dissolving clots formed in the arteries of the heart that cause myocardial infarction began with the question of scientific plausibility—"Could throm-

TABLE 18-3. Healthcare technology assessment framework

Level	Clinical Example: Clot-dissolving Technology for Heart Attacks	IT for Healthcare System
Scientific plausibility	Could thrombolysis help patients with myocardial infarction?	Does the system design make sense?
Technical feasibility	Can thrombolysis be done safely?	Can the system be implemented?
Surrogate outcomes	Does thrombolysis open coronary arteries?	Does system improve patient care process?
Patient outcomes	Does thrombolysis improve survival?	Do patients benefit from system?
Social outcomes	Is TPA cost effective compared with SK?	Can we afford the system? (CEA, ROI)

Source: Adapted from Littenberg.[27]
TPA: tissue plasminogen activator; SK: streptokinase; CEA: cost-effectiveness analysis; ROI: return on investment [analysis].

bolysis help patients by dissolving coronary thromboses?" The question required investigation of the underlying natural system, to confirm that clots do, in fact, have a role in causing heart attacks, which was still being debated into the 1970s.[28] Next, the question of feasibility had to be addressed: "Can thrombolysis be done safely?" This amounts to a proof-of-concept study, a necessary prerequisite to further evaluation. Third, the question of outcomes must be addressed—initially demonstrating a change in some intermediate outcome, believed to be related to the underlying process, often something that is readily measured. In the early 1980s, studies demonstrated that after the use of clot-dissolving drugs, the arteries of the heart remained open for some time, an important intermediate outcome. But the fact that the arteries remain open does not necessarily imply that patients are better off, with fewer symptoms, better function, or longer lives, and so this technology remained "unproven" until 1986 when the first study demonstrating lower mortality was published,[29] soon to be followed by others confirming this finding. Finally, there is the question of societal benefit: Once the benefit has been demonstrated for individuals, the question remains, "Can we afford this?". In the case of clot-dissolving treatments, this question arose when an improved agent, tissue plasminogen activator, was introduced, requiring that additional studies be conducted to determine whether the additional benefits to patients were worth its much higher costs to administer.

An analogous approach can be used in evaluating information technologies, as seen in the rightmost column of Table 18-3. Initially, questions must be answered about the underlying system, process, or behavior to be addressed, to answer the question, "Does the system design make sense?" in terms of our current (albeit sometimes fallible) understanding of the natural process. Next, it is necessary to examine the feasibility of the system through proof-of-concept demonstrations that answer the question, "Can the system be implemented?" Third, using the Littenberg framework, it is necessary to answer the question, "Are intermediate outcomes improved?" usually by examining some process measure such as numbers of diagnostic tests performed or treatments ordered. Next, it is essential to answer the question, "Do patients benefit?" by examining patient health outcomes such as functional status, symptom relief, or mortality. Finally, it is important to consider the costs to society of realizing whatever benefits the system produces. Studies at this level, such as cost-effectiveness analysis, potentially provide the ability to compare IT interventions with other healthcare interventions, so that the value of the investments in the technologies can be compared.

Of course, it can be exceptionally difficult to conduct evaluations at this level, for a great many reasons. As Friedman and Wyatt[30] point out,

The relationship between an information resource and patient outcome is usually quite remote when compared to more standard medical interventions, such as drugs. In addition, the actual function of an information resource and its impact may depend critically upon feedback from patients and or healthcare workers. It is thus unrealistic to expect, and evaluate for, quantifiable changes in patient outcome following the introduction of many information resources, and wiser to look for changes in the structure or processes of healthcare delivery[30]

In part, this is attributed to the complexity of the system and the remoteness of the information system supporting health care and the actual patient outcome. In part, it may be attributed to the fact that, although better patient and social outcomes are always desirable, information systems in health care are often implemented for other more proximate goals. In this case, tailoring the evaluation framework to the type of system and intended user may be more appropriate. In his address at the (1991) Symposium on Computer Applications in Medical Care (whose theme was "Assessing the Value of Medical Informatics"), David Eddy outlined a hierarchy for information system validation that progresses through intended changes in user knowledge and behavior, using the example of a decision support system

TABLE 18-4. Eddy information system validation framework

	Question	Validation
First-order validation	Does the system work?	Computer doesn't crash
Second-order validation	Are the results correct?	System produces correct advice in response to submitted case scenarios
Third-order validation	Does knowledge change?	Clinician users learn about current management
Fourth-order validation	Do actions change?	Clinician users order tests or treatments in accordance with recommended guidelines
Fifth-order validation	Do outcomes change?	Patients have fewer strokes, heart attacks, etc.

Source: David Eddy, personal communication, 1991.

for hypertension (Table 18-4). This approach is analogous to the technology assessment framework of Littenberg in Table 18-3, but it explicitly lends itself to examination of intermediate outcomes of the sort intended by information systems, for example changes in user actions such as ordering of tests or treatments. It can be adapted to a wide variety of EHR components, from nursing documentation, to pharmacy decision support, to physician diagnosis and treatment planning. A recent review by Roderer[31] illustrates the spectrum of such outcomes that has been examined in information system evaluations.

Quality of Evidence

The final issue to be considered by designers or consumers of EHR evaluations is the quality of the evidence being examined. As the Evidence Based Medicine movement has taught us, healthcare interventions ought to be based on the most valid scientific evidence available. Why should health informatics interventions, which also are costly and have the potential for harm as well as benefit, be any different? The EBM movement has also taught us that not all scientific evidence is equally valid or valuable. The importance of controls cannot be overemphasized. To quote Sackett's early observation, "studies with enthusiasm generally lack controls, while studies with controls generally lack enthusiasm."[32] This forms part of the basis for the now-familiar hierarchy of study designs in clinical epidemiology, seen in Table 18-5. The hierarchy is based on the notions that controlled studies, properly conducted, are more likely to offer valid results than studies without controls; that collections of studies that lead to the same or concordant conclusions provide greater confidence than individual studies, and that actual demonstration of benefit in a given individual (or setting) is more likely to be valid than application of results from other individuals (or settings).

TABLE 18-5. A hierarchy of strength of evidence for treatment decisions

N of 1 randomized trial
Systematic reviews of randomized trials
Individual randomized trials
Systematic reviews of observational studies
Individual observational studies
Physiologic studies
Unsystematic observations

Source: Guyatt, et al.[33]
A much more complete listing is available at the Oxford Centre for Evidence Based Medicine: http://www.cebm.net/levels_of_evidence.asp.

After controls, a second key element for valid scientific evidence is hypothesis testing. Although there continues to be scientific discussion about the relative standing of conclusions based on accommodating or explaining existing data,[34] it remains true that we justifiably place greater credence in those studies that successfully predict what will occur in the future or withstand rigorous hypothesis-testing experiments.[35]

Of course, randomized controlled trials are not suitable for all interventions[36]; not all evaluations of EHRs will fit into this clinical-epidemiology paradigm, as the previous sections have discussed. Still, in an approach similar to that of the United States Preventive Services Task Force,[37] it is possible to weigh the evidence by asking four key questions: First, is the design of individual studies suitable for the question being addressed? Second, given those study designs, were the studies conducted with sufficient rigor to rely on their findings? Third, do available studies provide an internally consistent body of evidence? Fourth, what is the magnitude of the beneficial effect, relative to costs and potential harms? This approach can be applied whether the evaluation is a discount usability engineering study to improve the design of a user interface, or a return on investment analysis to determine whether a specific EHR investment makes sense for an individual organization at a particular time.

Conclusions

It can be seen that evaluation of the EHR is a difficult and complex subject, for the reasons outlined. Many approaches and frameworks have been proposed.[23,38–40] It requires a step-by-step approach, each step being necessary but not sufficient, each more complex than the last as higher-order systems depend on proper function of multiple lower-order systems. Each level requires a wider and wider repertoire of methods and measurement of relevant variables, as evaluation moves from conceptual model or design, to testing the laboratory, testing in the field, and finally testing in routine use. It is hoped that this bricolage* of frameworks drawn from within informatics and without will provide EHR evaluators with a useful starting point for the design and conduct of their studies. Equally important, it should provide those who make decisions about EHR development, purchase, and deployment with a set of useful questions to ask when choosing evaluation studies on which to base their decisions.

---

* The late Claudio Ciborra, of the London School of Economics, suggested the use of this term in the context of health IT.

References

1. Random House (firm). Webster's Encyclopedic Unabridged Dictionary of the English Language. Revised Edition ed. New York: Gramercy; 1996.
2. Silverman WA. Human experimentation: a guided step into the unknown. Oxford [Oxfordshire]; New York: Oxford University Press; 1985.
3. Echt DS, Liebson PR, Mitchell LB, et al. Mortality and morbidity in patients receiving encainide, flecainide, or placebo. The Cardiac Arrhythmia Suppression Trial. N Engl J Med 1991;324(12):781–788.
4. Leveson NG, Turner CS. An Investigation of the Therac-25 Accidents. IEEE Computer 1993;26(7):18–41.
5. Vicente KJ, Kada-Bekhaled K, Hillel G, Cassano A, Orser BA. Programming errors contribute to death from patient-controlled analgesia: case report and estimate of probability. Can J Anaesth 2003;50(4):328–332.
6. Borden S. Computer Entry a Leading Cause of Medication Errors in U.S. Health Systems. United States Phramacopeia News Release 2004 20 December.
7. Berger RG, Kichak JP. Computerized physician order entry: helpful or harmful? J Am Med Inform Assoc 2004;11(2):100–103.
8. Koppel R, Metlay JP, Cohen A, et al. Role of computerized physician order entry systems in facilitating medication errors. Jama 2005;293(10):1197–1203.
9. Embi PJ, Yackel TR, Logan JR, Bowen JL, Cooney TG, Gorman PN. Impacts of computerized physician documentation in a teaching hospital: perceptions of faculty and resident physicians. J Am Med Inform Assoc 2004;11(4):300–309.
10. Hammond KW, Helbig ST, Benson CC, Brathwaite-Sketoe BM. Are electronic medical records trustworthy? Observations on copying, pasting and duplication. AMIA Annu Symp Proc 2003:269–273.
11. Goodwin JS, Goodwin JM. The tomato effect. Rejection of highly efficacious therapies. Jama 1984;251(18):2387–2390.
12. Shibata MC, Flather MD, Wang D. Systematic review of the impact of beta blockers on mortality and hospital admissions in heart failure. Eur J Heart Fail 2001;3(3):351–357.
13. Leape LL, Berwick DM, Bates DW. What practices will most improve safety? Evidence-based medicine meets patient safety. Jama 2002;288(4):501–507.
14. Shojania KG, Duncan BW, McDonald KM, Wachter RM. Safe but sound: patient safety meets evidence-based medicine. Jama 2002;288(4):508–513.
15. Lusted LB. Signal detectability and medical decision-making. Science 1971;171(977):1217–1219.
16. Forsythe D, Hess DJ. Studying those who study us: an anthropologist in the world of artificial intelligence. Stanford, Calif.: Stanford University Press; 2001.
17. Heathfield H, Pitty D, Hanka R. Evaluating information technology in health care: barriers and challenges. Bmj 1998;316(7149):1959–1961.
18. McManus IC. Engineering Quality in Health Care [editorial]. Quality in Health Care 1996;5:127.
19. Poses RM, Isen AM. Qualitative research in medicine and health care: questions and controversy. J Gen Intern Med 1998;13(1):32–38.
20. Sackett DL, Wennberg JE. Choosing the best research design for each question [editorial]. Bmj 1997;315(7123):1636.
21. Chelimsky E, Shadish WR, editors. Evaluation for the 21st Century. Thousand Oaks, CA: Sage; 1997.

22. Garg AX, Adhikari NK, McDonald H, et al. Effects of computerized clinical decision support systems on practitioner performance and patient outcomes: a systematic review. Jama 2005;293(10):1223–1238.

23. Gremy F, DeGoulet P. Assessment of health information technology: which questions for which systems? Proposal for a taxonomy. Medical Informatics 1993;18(3):185–193.

24. Norman DA. Things that make us smart: defending human attributes in the age of the machine. Reading, Mass.: Addison-Wesley Pub. Co.; 1993.

25. Stead WW, Haynes RB, Fuller S, et al. Designing medical informatics research and library–resource projects to increase what is learned. Journal of the American Medical Informatics Association 1994;1(1):28–33.

26. Mankins JC. Technology Readiness Levels. A White Paper: Advanced Concepts Office, Office of Space Access and Technology, NASA; 1995 April 6.

27. Littenberg B. Technology assessment in medicine. Academic Medicine 1992;67(7):424–428.

28. Robbins SL. Pathologic basis of disease. Philadelphia,: Saunders; 1974.

29. Effectiveness of intravenous thrombolytic treatment in acute myocardial infarction. Gruppo Italiano per lo Studio della Streptochinasi nell'Infarto Miocardico (GISSI). Lancet 1986;1(8478):397–402.

30. Friedman CP, Wyatt J. Evaluation methods in medical informatics. XIX. New York: Springer; 1997.

31. Roderer NK. Outcome measures in clinical information systems evaluation. Medinfo 2004;11(Pt 2):1096–1100.

32. Anonymous. How to read clinical journals: I. why to read them and how to start reading them critically. Cmaj 1981;124(5):555–558.

33. Guyatt GH, Sinclair J, Cook DJ, Glasziou P. Users' guides to the medical literature: XVI. How to use a treatment recommendation. Evidence-Based Medicine Working Group and the Cochrane Applicability Methods Working Group. JAMA 1999;281(19):1836–1843.

34. Stanger-Hall K, Allchin D, Aviv A, et al. Accomodation or Prediction? [letters]. Science 2005;308(5727):1409c–1412.

35. Lipton P. Testing Hypotheses: Prediction and Prejudice. Science 2005;307(5707): 219–221.

36. Rees J. The Problem with Academic Medicine: Engineering Our Way into and out of the Mess. Public Library of Science: Medicine 2005;2(4):e111.

37. Harris RP, Helfand M, Woolf SH, et al. Current methods of the US Preventive Services Task Force: a review of the process. Am J Prev Med 2001;20(3 Suppl): 21–35.

38. Stoop AP, Berg M. Integrating quantitative and qualitative methods in patient care information system evaluation: guidance for the organizational decision maker. Methods Inf Med 2003;42(4):458–462.

39. Van Der Meijden MJ, Tange HJ, Troost J, Hasman A. Determinants of success of inpatient clinical information systems: a literature review. J Am Med Inform Assoc 2003;10(3):235–243.

40. Kaplan B, Shaw NT. Future directions in evaluation research: people, organizational, and social issues. Methods Inf Med 2004;43(3):215–231.

19
Grand Challenges of Information Technology in Medicine

ELAINE REMMLINGER, GERARD M. NUSSBAUM, JASON OLIVEIRA, and
STACY MELVIN

The release in late 1999 of the Institute of Medicine report "To Err Is
Human" focused public interest on improving patient safety and quality of
care.[1] Subsequent Institute of Medicine reports touted the potential positive impact of advanced clinical information technology (IT) in reducing
errors, improving care coordination, enhancing efficiency, reducing duplication, and increasing the amount of time dedicated to direct patient care.
Although progress has been made in the adoption of many of these IT tools,
there remains significant opportunity for further advances; with recent
efforts increasing optimism that progress will accelerate.

Implementation rates, in the inpatient setting, for advanced functionality
such as computerized physician order entry (CPOE), clinical decision
support systems, and multidisciplinary documentation remain at less than
10%.[2] The Leapfrog Group, an organization composed of employers and
other purchasers of health care focused on patient safety and quality, indicates that only 4% of hospitals have fully implemented CPOE.[3] CPOE is
seen by many as a key element in improving patient safety and quality of
care and thus has been a substantial target for many in the industry. For
successful CPOE, a partial electronic health record system (EHRS) is a key
foundational element.

Greater progress has been made in the ambulatory care environment.
Electronic medical record (EMR)[4] implementation in ambulatory settings
is nearing 40%, according to some studies.[5] However, it is unclear how these
investments translate into direct utilization of advanced functionality by
caregivers, or the extent to which the EMR acts as a replacement of paper-
based medical records with electronic charts.

A major challenge to the more widespread adoption of EHRs has been
the immaturity of many of the products provided by healthcare information system vendors. Healthcare providers and their vendors have been on
a decade-long exploration of how to create a system that is useful, efficient,*

---

* Efficiency is a key requirement. Any "solution" that takes more time to use than
the old-fashioned paper and pencil, or dictating orders to a nurse, will meet with
stiff physician resistance.

and able to be integrated into the care process. Although progress is being made, failure to overcome these challenges may make achievement of the government's stated goal of widespread adoption of fully interoperable EHRs in 10 years[6] virtually unachievable. The good news is that significant interest in EHR technology and significant momentum exist within the industry, which has the potential to translate into real improvements if the existing barriers to adoption can be surmounted.

This chapter considers some of the larger challenges to achieve the EHR vision. We highlight changes necessary to avoid cementing challenges into barriers. Ultimately, overcoming these grand challenges requires effort on multiple fronts, and above all, willingness to change fundamental approaches and practices over several years.

Industry Factors Impacting the Deployment and Use of EHRs

Basic industry factors that prevent deployment and use of EHRs include financial factors, immature products combined with long lead times, and unmet research needs.

Funding Constraints Hamper the Adoption of EHRs

Although the implementation of clinical IT is clearly on the minds of the majority of provider organizations, the financial investment required to successfully implement and support these systems represents one of the most significant inhibitors to the widespread deployment of the EHR. The 2004 HIMSS Leadership Survey indicates that, once again, the lack of financial support is the most significant barrier to implementing IT.[7] Given the financial state of the healthcare industry, the funding of major projects is a fiercely competitive process that often favors projects that more readily demonstrate a clear return on investment.

To date, there has been little evidence demonstrating significant financial improvement for provider organizations as a result of investments in clinical information systems, including EHRs. By and large, those that most directly benefit from use of clinical information systems are the payers, employers, patients, and malpractice underwriters. Although the financial results from fewer medical errors, reduced duplication, and improved quality of care benefit those responsible for paying for our system of health care, the providers are faced with funding these initiatives. Furthermore, many physicians in private practice are concerned with the potential negative impact that the use of an EHRs may have on productivity and, as a result, their income. Some organizations are forced to delay EHRs funding until the initiative proves more economically beneficial to the organization overall and to the clinicians directly.

There has been discussion regarding rewarding providers for use of and offsetting some of the costs of EHR-Ss. Incentives might be in the form of direct increases to health insurance and/or Medicare and Medicaid reimbursement for providers that demonstrate use of technologies such as an EHR-S, allowing providers to share in the financial benefits that accrue to the payers.

Indirect incentives may be provided to healthcare organizations that can demonstrate delivery of the highest quality of care or achievement of other performance benchmarks, which would result in bonus payments. In this scenario, not only will the achievement of these benchmarks be facilitated by the implementation of the appropriate systems, but IT will support easy collection, analysis, and reporting of required data. The federal government is considering both Medicare reimbursement for use of an EHR-S and Medicare "pay-for-performance" programs that will reward clinicians for delivering the highest quality care instead of the highest volume of services.[8]

The United States (US) government has acknowledged that provider organizations need financial assistance to support these initiatives to offset significant upfront costs. In October 2004, $139 million was approved through HHS' Agency for Healthcare Research and Quality (AHRQ) to be used for grants and contracts to provider organizations.[9] However, the level of funding allocated, to date, is substantially below the funding estimates necessary for the automation of the entire US healthcare industry. In addition, the government is evaluating the possibility of encouraging the banking industry to provide low-rate loans for technology adoption. It appears unlikely that government funding or related efforts alone will provide sufficient monies to achieve the levels of automation envisioned for EHRs adoption. Provider, and state and federal budgetary constraints seem to stand in the way. Beyond simply footing the bill, government funding will be critical in establishing the communications and standards infrastructure prerequisite for a nationwide EHR.

As a result, provider organizations are seeking more creative ways to fund the upfront and ongoing costs of an EHRs. For example, the payment model for acquiring an EHRs may shift from large upfront capital investments by providers, with accompanying heavy annual maintenance costs, to a usage-based charge. It may be feasible for software vendors, and other industry players, to bundle IT and clinical transformation into a usage-based charge, which may be billed to the patient, or their insurance carrier. Some vendors are already providing their solutions on a subscription basis to assist customers in smoothing cash flow and eliminating large up-front costs.

David Brailer, National Health Information Technology Coordinator, has called for vendors to deliver an EHR solution for $100 per month to assure the ability of small and medium physician practices to utilize EHR solutions.[10] To realize the full potential for a national interoperable EHR, the participation of individual physician practices is essential.[10] Whether the industry is able to rise to this challenge is an open question.

Greater use of standards may also help to lower the costs of EHRs. More widespread adoption of EHRs can spread the fixed costs of development and maintenance, thus reducing the per provider costs. The key to success of a nationwide EHR is participation, as widespread adoption will also serve as a basis for lower per user costs.

Immature Products Combined with Long Lead Times Will Delay Full EHR Implementation

The technology available to the healthcare industry today is vastly improved; however, vendor products remain challenged to meet the needs and expectations of a sophisticated and demanding user base. These users are being asked to replace their comfortable and reliable paper-based system, however inefficient, with one that appears infinitely more complicated. Users expect applications to be intuitive, user-friendly, fast, and easily accessible. To achieve the necessary level of acceptance, the EHRs must support fast access to necessary information, and not be viewed as a hindrance to clinical care.

Furthermore, providers expect clinical applications to provide functionality that is not available with the current paper-based system, such as easy exchange of information, robust clinical decision support, embedded access to knowledge sources, niche capabilities to support subspecialty needs (e.g., cardiology, oncology, critical care), and data entry mechanisms that balance ease of use for physicians and other caregivers. To be successful, an EHRs must also support the capture of data in a codified manner for research and reporting purposes. To the dismay of many, current offerings remain challenged to meet these requirements for the multitude of potential users.

Given the need for more sophisticated functionality to provide minimally capable systems and the total cycle time to develop any new solution, it is likely that vendor offerings will remain relatively immature for some time. Generally, the major software vendors require as long as 3 to 5 years to develop initial versions of next-generation capabilities. Given the current EHRs capabilities available in the marketplace, healthcare organizations may be required to acquire and implement one to two more generations of technology solutions before the full spectrum of desired EHRs functionality is available in the marketplace. Thus, absent a major shift, it will likely be a minimum of 5 to 10 years before EHRs functionality reaches the levels necessary for the broad adoption throughout the industry to achieve EHR success.

Continued mergers and acquisitions in the healthcare information technology (HCIT) vendor marketplace could lead to further delays in the

development of new EHRs technology. Newly merged vendor organizations often devote their primary efforts to consolidating disparate products,
to the detriment of developing new functionality that is a prerequisite for
full EHRs adoption. The fallout from HCIT mergers causes disruption
for healthcare provider organizations because installed products often
lose support and lack ongoing development, which requires provider
organizations to take costly detours to replace unsupported EHRs
products.

Exacerbating development and implementation delays is the reality that
the majority of vendors are publicly traded companies that must answer to
Wall Street demands. An emphasis on positive quarterly earnings performance results in premature product introductions and the attendant failures that slow innovation and reduce the "believability" of the EHR as a
viable solution.

Furthermore, a shift from the large capital-sale model of selling EHR
applications to a usage-based model may be ruled out by the need to "meet
the numbers" for Wall Street.

Even if the healthcare IT industry is able to overcome existing obstacles
to develop mature EHRs applications, it takes as long as 5 to 8 years before
a major new clinical system, including an EHRs, is fully implemented in a
provider setting. The process leading to the system acquisition decision and
obtaining the necessary funding may take up to 2 to 3 years. Once the decision is made, it takes an average healthcare provider organization 3 to 5
years for selection, negotiation, and full implementation of the new system.
If one factors in the EHR development and implementation timelines, estimated above, the healthcare industry may not see full adoption of the full
EHR until the 2015–2025 timeframe (see Figure 19-1).

Research Needs Are Not Met by Current EHR-Ss; Future Developments Must Address This Deficiency

Existing EHRs offerings focus on supporting direct clinical care, and generally are unable to meet the more sophisticated demands of clinical trials,
public health epidemiology, and clinical and translational research. As a
result, many academic medical centers and research centers have turned to
in-house development of wrap-around technologies, as well as creation of
complete, EHRs solutions to support their research needs. This approach is
fraught with risk as the provider strays from the core business of health
care and becomes software developer. It also further silos the data and
limits the ability to share EHR data for clinical purposes across institutional
boundaries.

As longitudinal repositories and business intelligence tools are developed, and data elements standardized, the research value of the data cap-

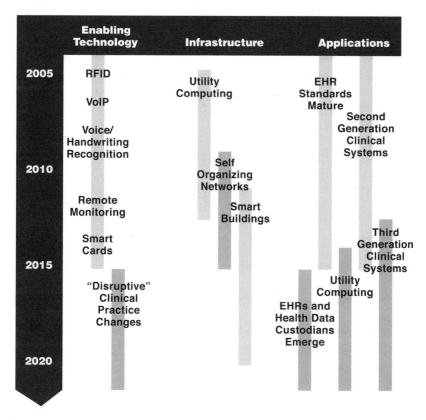

FIGURE 19-1. Future deployment of healthcare information technologies. (*Source:* By permission of Kurt Salmon Associates.)

tured in EHRs will grow exponentially. To demonstrate value and return on investment of their products, commercial software vendors need to address the needs of clinical and translational research, particularly in academic medical centers, cancer centers, and other research environments. If complementary uses of the EHR are viable, research and other private industry funding may help defray some of the costs of a comprehensive EHRs.

Both researchers and treating clinicians must sit at the EHR design and acquisition table to balance the needs of clinicians and researchers. However, failure to provide for the needs of treating clinicians will negatively impact the EHR implementation and leave researchers with no data and the EHR effort will lose crucial backing.

Technical Architecture Factors Affecting the Deployment, Interoperability, and Use of the EHR

The envisioned next-generation EHR-Ss remain theoretical discussions until they become technical architectures where information is captured, managed, processed, and delivered to recipients. The industry is faced with two strategic approaches to designing and building architectures: The EHR solution as a hand-crafted, custom-made work that stands alone or as an agreed upon common architectural standard.

Greater use of standards may help to lower the costs of the development, implementation, and maintenance of EHRSs, and therefore promote adoption. Also, to be successful both within and across healthcare institutions, an EHR-S must support the capture of data in a codified and sharable manner to enable functionality of clinical decision support, research, and knowledge management processes.

Unlike countries with a universal health IT architecture (see Chapter 10), the American challenge is to enable a highly fragmented infrastructure, application, and data environment to communicate and share appropriately. The choice of the strategic approach may seem obvious. However, as the industry and vendors face long development cycles, whether to wait for architecture standard setting processes to unfold before designing and building interoperable EHR architectures, or to forge ahead with proprietary solutions is a difficult choice. Given the various pressures on vendors to bring solutions to market quickly, the choice is often to forge ahead with proprietary architectures even though this will hamper standards adoption and keep the cost of development and maintenance high. Notwithstanding these market pressures, there is a wealth of experience, existing standards, resources, and processes upon which the industry and vendors can begin building the next-generation EHR architectures.

EHR Data Architecture Standards to Enable Interoperability

The basis for achieving the US government's goal of widespread adoption of fully interoperable EHRs by 2010[11] rests on a foundation of EHR data architectural elements being standardized, adopted, and incorporated in the next-generation solutions for provider organizations (see Table 19-1). These architecture standards to date including the following.

A Universal Health Data Model

At either end of any health information exchange are the applications and health data stores that comprise the EHR. Interoperable EHRs across the nation require a universal data model, a shared language, which stan-

TABLE 19-1. Data architecture standards

Data Architecture Component	Purpose	Prevailing Standard
Universal Health Data Model	Industry standard data model of health and medicine subject-area definitions	Health Level-7 Version 3 Reference Information Model
Controlled Medical Vocabulary	Within the Universal Health Data Model, a standard lexicon of terms and values	College of American Pathologists SNOMED-CT
Standard Identifiers	Standard identification of providers, payers, sites of care, and patients across all healthcare participants	The identifier standards mandated by HIPAA of 1996
Metathesaurus	In the short term, there remain numerous domain-specific versions of data models and lexicons. A metathesaurus serves as a translator between these models	Unified Medical Language System of the National Library of Medicine
Medical Knowledge Representation Model	A cognitive automation model to know, update, perceive, and understand the content and structure of medical science and its application	None

dardizes how we describe and communicate health and medicine subject matters. This is an essential step to enable the efficient exchange of electronic healthcare data and alleviate the need for proprietary point-to-point data interchanges and translations between disparate data models. The benefit of adopting a unified data model is that once applications and information networks can freely understand each other's conceptual view of the healthcare world, the effort required to design and maintain the interconnections is greatly reduced.

Controlled Medical Vocabulary

Creating the syntax of a language to enable data interchange between EHRs is only one element of interoperability. There is also the need to create an agreed upon vocabulary, within the linguistic syntax, so the EHRSs understand what is being said regarding key concepts of medical science and its practice. The medical record largely remains a collection of free-form natural language text and images. It is only through controlled, structured, electronically legible and understood terms that the value of clinical decision support, alerts, clinical rules, and clinical research is realized. Key terms that should be described by a controlled medical vocabulary include organisms, substances, symptoms, diagnoses, procedures, and diseases.

Standard Identifiers

Standard identifiers for people, places, and roles are an essential prerequisite to sharing healthcare data across caregivers, care processes, and societal functions. Identifiers, at a minimum, are required for providers, payers, sites of care, and more controversially, patients. The current identifier systems, created largely for state and federal reimbursement purposes,** have a number of strengths, but, because of their inherent proprietary weaknesses, must be overhauled to fully meet the needs of a universal EHR.

Metathesaurus

Ubiquitous adoption of a universal health data model and a controlled medical vocabulary will take many years. In the interim, there will be numerous domain-specific versions of data models and coded-value libraries. In addition, it is not practical to think, at least short-term, that there will be universal adoption and translation of terms and terminologies in the thousands of legacy systems and data stores throughout the US. Therefore, there is a need for a meta-model, integrating domain-specific models, and a thesaurus to translate terms from one system into another and back again—a metathesaurus.

Medical Knowledge Representation

As the sheer mass of medical information generated grows exponentially, gleaning relevant information from the wealth of available data is increasingly difficult and so time consuming that it becomes impossible for the clinician. The ability to leverage IT to search and integrate volumes of medical knowledge and bring it to the point of patient care requires a system to know, update, perceive, and understand the content and structure of medical science and its application. This cognitive model is the basis for multiple capabilities essential to deriving benefits from an EHR, including intelligent clinical alerts, evidence-based medicine, and diagnostic expert systems.

Although there remain significant architectural components that need further definition and development, there are significant experience and existing standards upon which the interoperable EHRSs of the future can start being built today.

** Universal Provider Identification Number (UPIN), DEA provider numbers, and numerous state-based Medicaid provider numbering systems are examples of the duplication and fragmentation of provider identification systems.

The Federal Government Will Provide Momentum, but Adoption of EHR Data Architecture Standards Will Continue to Move Slowly

What has historically been lacking in EHR standards adoption is a unifying force to bring the whole industry to the same conclusion. The role of the U. S. government is indispensable in promoting, coordinating, and serving as the custodian for a public domain standards framework. Despite the absence of a federal legislative mandate for an interoperable EHR standards framework, the U.S. Government is creating a de facto national standard through its Consolidated Health Informatics (CHI) effort.[12]

The goal of the CHI effort is to bring together and coordinate the infrastructure of 23 federal agencies including Health and Human Services, Department of Defense, Centers for Disease Control, Veterans Administration, and other agencies under a Federal Health Architecture (FHA). The CHI effort establishes health information interoperability standards as the basis for electronic health data transfer in all activities and projects among all federal agencies. As these federal agencies, combined, represent a significant amount of the health care financed and delivered in the U.S., the effort could stimulate adoption of the standards architecture throughout the industry.[13] The expectation is that the FHA would be coordinated and interoperable with the private-sector equivalent through shared adherence to standards.

Some have advocated that the government should extend its role even further and support the certification of vendors to compliance of standards.[14] Other voices argue strongly that certification of vendors should be undertaken via private efforts.*** It is most likely that the future guidance and direction of the CHI and FHA effort will be governed under the newly appointed Office of National Coordinator of Health Information Technology (ONCHIT); as well as the recently formed American Health Information Community (AHIC).

HHS and ONCHIT, under the leadership of Secretary Michael Leavitt and Dr. David Brailer respectively, have sponsored several initiatives. Four contracts have been awarded by HHS to streamline standards development; develop criteria to certify and evaluate health IT products; develop solutions to address variations in business policies and state laws that affect privacy and security practices; and the development of Regional Health Information Organizations (RHIO) architectures towards a Nationwide Health Information Network (NHIN). As part of the contracts, these partnerships will deliver reports to the American Health Information Commu-

---

*** The Certification Commission for Healthcare Information Technology, A Voluntary, Private-Sector Initiative to Certify HIT Products, has already been created to bring together the major stakeholders. More information may be found at CCHIT.ORG.

nity (the Community), a new federal advisory committee that is chaired by Secretary Leavitt and charged with providing recommendations to HHS on how to make health records digital and interoperable.

While leadership is helpful, the government must be careful that its process does not stifle innovation and unnecessarily prevent consideration of alternatives. The response of the private sector, working cooperatively with governmental bodies has shown great promise and will be a critical element of EHR success.

Health IT Vendors Have a Key Role in Speeding Adoption of EHR Data Architecture Standards

Whereas the health information systems used within federal agencies such as Tri-Care and VistA are mostly self-developed, the majority of the clinical information systems, including EHRSs used by providers, are vendor supplied. Today's industry portfolio of applications has been developed over many years, by many commercial vendors as well as internal development groups, and have been implemented in various ways. It is a safe generalization to say that these application solutions were not designed or deployed with interprovider operability as a design requirement.

As discussed above, the federal government will have a significant role as arbiter and "tipping point" for full adoption and deployment of standards, both within the Federal Health Architecture, and working collaboratively with the commercial marketplace. The federal government is already incorporating its selected architecture standards in all requests for information and requests for proposals issued to contractors as required by the Office of Management and Budget.[15] The government will also incorporate the standards, as appropriate, in federally funded grant requests.

Commercial health IT vendors faced with this double pressure to incorporate standard EHR interoperability components into their solutions from both their nonfederal and federal client base will start to do so—or risk failure in the marketplace.

The good news for vendors is that many of the internal federal standards already are, or will be, made available in a variety of ways:

- Public domain such as the Unified Medical Language System[16]
- Copyrighted such as Regenstrief Institute's laboratory controlled medical vocabulary LOINC[17]
- Commercially available licensing such as the SNOMED-CT (systemized nomenclature of medicine–clinical terms) controlled medical vocabulary currently available at no cost through the National Library of Medicine.[18]

Therefore, there is little reason for commercial vendors to delay incorporating these architectural standards into next-generation EHR solutions brought to market.

Clinician Adoption and Use of EHR-Ss Will Be Influenced by the Development of Several Technical Infrastructure Components

Ability to leverage technology will enhance the availability of the EHR-S at the point of care. Point of care includes the bedside, examination room, the patient's home, and wherever the medical professional is located when trying to diagnose, evaluate, and treat the patient. Access from fixed locations, such as a physician's office, is usually not an issue; rather, it is mobility that is crucial to point-of-care EHR access (see Table 19-2).

Wireless

A key element in mobile EHR access is the widespread implementation of wireless networks. Most institutions think of EHR access from the perspective of their own facilities. Virtually all new healthcare facilities include provisions for wireless computing within the buildings. More forward-thinking institutions extend wireless access throughout their campus. However, to achieve unfettered EHR access, the four walls of the institution cannot serve as the boundary. Public wireless networks are part of the EHR-access solution.

Wireless networks for EHR access require pervasive access to the underlying information systems, the use of devices associated with them, and the ability to access and update information unbounded by location or device. The primary challenges to the connectivity aspect of pervasive access are

TABLE 19-2. Technical infrastructure components that enable clinician adoption

Technical Infrastructure Component	Clinician Adoption Challenge	Technical Infrastructure Solution
Wireless	Provisioning of access to information and decision support anywhere and anytime in as pervasive a mode as the telephone	Campus and community wireless networks that provide pervasive connectivity
Mobile devices	Mobility is a key to delivering access to clinicians at point of care and elsewhere	In most patient-care settings, the device of choice will be a tablet-style computer that weighs 1–3 pounds and has the dimensions of a clipboard stuffed with papers. In other settings, it will be a PDA or multifunction cellular telephone.
Human machine interface (HMI)	Clinicians will resist using the computer-based patient record if it remains more time consuming and less intuitive than the paper chart and verbal orders	Appropriate application of voice recognition, natural language processing, and handwriting recognition

cost and security. Whether on an internal wireless network or over the public cellular data network, security must assure confidentiality of the data, as well as the availability of the wireless network and ability to reach the appropriate servers, while blocking unauthorized use of the wireless network.

Handheld/Tablet/Mobile Devices

In most patient-care settings, the preferred device is a tablet-style computer that weighs 1–3 pounds in the dimensions of a clipboard stuffed with papers. For any mobile device of this nature, the challenges for use include loss rate, security, functionality, and form factor.

Although portability, size, and weight are critical to the device's usability, these attributes also make the device subject to theft, damage, or loss. The replacement cycle for mobile devices is much shorter than for desktop workstations. A desktop workstation is replaced every 3 to 4 years, whereas the mobile device may have a life of only 1 to 2 years because of damage and other causes of loss. Replacement costs can represent a significant ongoing budget item.

Form and functionality are intertwined. Mobile technology must accommodate human capabilities that influence decisions on screen and keypad size and resolution. Alternative input modalities, such as voice and handwriting recognition, and greater use of preformed response (via drop-down lists and check boxes) may address input modality issues. However, the user must be able to view the screen and it must be large enough to display relevant information without excessive scrolling. Furthermore, design requires consideration of the human–machine interface (HMI), discussed below.

As EHR access is extended outside the four walls, a different type of EHRs access device may be required for portability. A personal digital assistant (PDA) or multifunction cellular telephone that uses the public wireless networks and a Web browser to securely access the EHRs may be a good option. Because a user carries cell phone, pager, electronic date book, and PDA, these "consumer" devices will continue to converge into a single portable device that can serve multiple voice and data functions.

The Human–Machine Interface

Advances in the human machine interface (HMI) are critical to clinician adoption and use of EHRSs. A bad interface will result in an EHRs access solution that does not contribute to effective and efficient patient care. Clinicians will resist using the EHR if it remains more time consuming than the paper chart and verbal orders.

Including human factors research in the design of EHR products will help validate the benefits of speech recognition, natural language processing, and handwriting recognition in particular circumstances and environments. The challenge is selecting the right technology for the environment. For example, in a direct patient care setting, use of speech recognition may be inappropriate for privacy reasons, as well as to shield the patient from the direct communication necessary for clear records; in a radiology reading room, speech recognition and control may be an appropriate mode to access and update the EHR.

Handwriting recognition, especially when used in conjunction with tablet computers, most closely mimics current approaches of writing and therefore makes the user feel comfortable. However, continued advances in handwriting recognition technology quality and speed will be required to be as efficient as pen and paper. Further redesign of EHRSs, to use drop-down lists and check boxes, will accelerate the potential for this approach.

Organizational, Legal, and Regulatory Issues Will Complicate the Adoption of EHR-Ss

Although technical aspects pose some of the major challenges to nation-wide adoption of EHRs, the social challenges—including legal and regulatory issues, as well as the new combinations of skills and knowledge required to support and implement the EHR—may be an even greater hurdle.

Data Ownership and Constraints on Sharing Health Information Must Be Resolved Before Community-wide EHR Capabilities Are Feasible

Having the technical capabilities to accumulate and share health information is just the beginning. Ownership of medical data is unclear and may present an obstruction to sharing health records. Laws regarding ownership of medical data can be changed if all interest groups, through the political process, can agree.

Under the laws of most states, providers currently "own" the medical record. Although individuals have a right to access their medical record, providers may refuse to provide access to the entire record, especially in the case of psychiatric notes. As a matter of professional courtesy, providers usually make available *portions* of the patient record to another treating provider. This, however, does not change the physician's perspective that the record and its contents are the physician's property.

If each individual provider owns his records, they may be less likely to contribute them in their full detail to a common repository, or permit them to be linked into a shared EHR. The provider's control of the patient information, an aspect of ownership, serves a competitive advantage because it helps bind the patient to a particular physician or health system.

The Health Insurance Portability and Accountability Act (HIPAA) reinforces the right of a patient to have access to her/his medical record, but does not alter the provider's basic ownership rights of the medical record. The HIPAA privacy rule imposes barriers to the seamless sharing of clinical data by restricting the access to the patient record, to the minimum necessary portion of the record. Controlling access to the minimum necessary portion of the patient's record presents significant challenges in the creation and maintenance of a community health information system.

Changes in the law, at both state and federal levels, and clarification of rules promulgated under HIPAA, are required to address ownership rights in the record and to overcome barriers to appropriate information sharing. The best outcome is a requirement that providers contribute to the community-wide EHR at the request of the patient, all medical data, while preserving the providers' ownership in their own records.

A Central Repository to Compile and Maintain a Comprehensive Longitudinal Patient Health Record Will Be Crucial

One aspect of the medical error rate is a set of related failures: Failure to have access to information, failure to have consistent information, and failure to use information. "Information about the patient, medications, and other therapies should be available at the point of patient care" because "providers who don't have all of the necessary information about patients are more likely to misdiagnose or mistreat."[19] Clearly, any discussion regarding the availability of accurate information for patient care must stress the need for electronic databases and interfaces to allow them to be fully integrated. The development of integrated computer-based databases and knowledge servers is necessary to accomplish this goal.

To meet this need, a new player, the health data custodian (HDC), is required. The HDC acts on the consumer's behalf to both house an individual's entire clinical record and broker access to this information as directed by the consumer.[20] The existence of a comprehensive health record maintained by the health data custodian will lead to more effective treatment and reduction in duplicative testing, which can potentially reduce costs.[20] HDCs are envisioned as private corporate entities that exist in a fiduciary relationship to the individual.[20] The HDC is the trusted intermediary for management of data and control over access (see Figure 19-2).

The HDC assures capture of all relevant clinical data at the point of its creation. Significant quality and cost benefits can be achieved if clinically specific data are captured once at the point of care. Then all other legitimate data needs are derived from those data.[21] To be of maximum value, the HDC will contain information from all of the providers who care for the individual.

The data maintained by the HDC have a variety of potential uses. Included among them are:

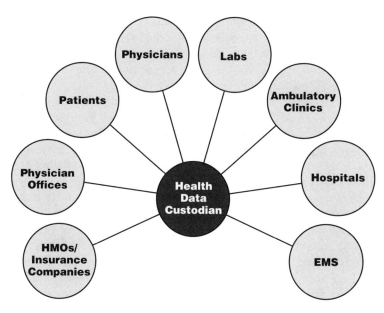

FIGURE 19-2. HDC's relationship to other stakeholders. (*Source:* By permission of Kurt Salmon Associates.)

1. Providing for anticipated and emergency care of the individual[22]
2. Reimbursement and eligibility transactions relating to past, present, or future care[23]
3. Use in public health alerts and improvements[24]
4. Use in the creation of research databases[25]
5. Creation of an income stream for the patient from the selective release of information in exchange for remuneration, i.e., selling access to the patient or the data[26]
6. Support achievement of the JCAHO goal to accurately and completely reconcile medications across the continuum of care.[27]

These differing scenarios argue for a more nuanced approach to disclosure of the volumes of data that would be in an individual's EHR. Any system that would provide access to protected health information would need to comply with the HIPAA Privacy Rule.[28] The model of role-based access, when combined with the minimum necessary[29] perspective, provides an implicit suggestion that some form of controlled granular access system would be appropriate.[30]

One approach to providing this granular access approach would be for the patient and their primary healthcare coordinator to distribute their health information into buckets representing varying levels of confidentiality.[31] Each bucket would be labeled to indicate the degree of protection or confidentiality assigned to the information in the bucket. To be useful, the data and the buckets would need to adhere to a standard scheme, uniformly adhered to across the nation and, potentially, the world.[32] Although this setup may initially be time consuming, the overall benefit to preserving patient confidentiality would be well served over a simple all or nothing approach for access to the patient data.

Although the HDC may initially be loaded with summary data, once real-time links between the HDC and the electronic health information systems internal to the various providers are established, automation and standards can be leveraged to assure the relevant and current data are transferred from the internal EHR to the HDC. This approach to leveraging a central repository may be more beneficial than merely establishing pointers to disparate data stores and will also enhance the degree of security that could be applied to assure confidentiality.

As part of the security model, to assure confidentiality of the data and appropriate patient consent, the HDC would rely on patient biometric data, as well as clinician biometric data to assure proper match and authorization for data access. Through the use of a variety of biometric**** identifiers, such as hand geometry, fingerprints, footprints, and retinal patterns, the system could provide access in the event of emergencies when formal patient consent was unavailable.

A key advantage of the HDC, over merely linking to the many disparate repositories of patient information, is the potential that, especially for smaller entities such as individual physician offices and small clinics, the HDC could easily become the primary EHR. This would lead to cost savings and enable even smaller entities to leverage the economies of scale of the HDC.

The HIPAA Security Rule "provides that covered entities that maintain or transmit health information are required to maintain reasonable and appropriate administrative, physical, and technical safeguards to ensure the integrity and confidentiality of the information and to protect against any reasonably anticipated threats or hazards to the security or integrity of the information and unauthorized use or disclosure of the information."[33] This onus would be on the HDC to assure compliance for information it maintains as well as compliance during the delivery of the protected health information.

There are, however, numerous challenges to the creation of HDCs. Among these are: The complex nature of clinical data,[34] lack of complete and comprehensive standards,[35] costs of implementing the needed information systems, and the need to identify funding sources.[36] Nontechnical barriers to the creation and operation of HDCs include the need for enormous cultural and behavioral shifts in the provision of medical care,[37] confused ownership of the medical records (with hospitals, clinicians, and patients all asserting a right of ownership),[38] and the need to address privacy and security issues.[39]

**** Biometric is the use of physical attribute to identify and authenticate a person.

Changes in the approach to sharing information, both legal and clinical, are required before HDCs become a reality. However, HDCs offer a locus and model to make patient health information stored in the EHR available.

As Information Systems Become More Closely Intertwined with the Direct Delivery of Clinical Care, the Potential for Increased Regulation of Software and Equipment Increases

Whereas medical devices[40] and certain computer systems, such as prenatal risk evaluation software,[41] blood bank,[42] and picture archiving and communications systems (PACS)[43] are subject to Food and Drug Administration (FDA) regulation, information systems and the networking infrastructure are not. For general computer systems, the FDA has adopted an approach that the systems are not subject to regulation unless directly intended to diagnose or treat a patient.[44]

As medical devices become more intertwined with information systems, the FDA may assert its authority to regulate the computer systems themselves as devices intended for use in the diagnosis or treatment of patients[45] or as a component subject to regulation as part of a recognized medical device.[46]

Specific areas in which regulatory interest may be seen include:

- Patient-connected monitoring equipment including embedded software that triggers changes in the treatment via a closed feedback loop. Thus, a monitoring system that measures blood levels and has the capability to alter, according to a treatment protocol, the rate of infusion of an intravenous fluid might be considered a medical device. If the treatment protocol were downloaded from the clinical information system, the clinical information system itself might also be subject to additional regulation.
- Use of clinical alerts—especially the composition and nature of alerts and methods used to document alert overrides.
- Use of embedded clinical pathways and treatment protocols that are used to guide or define the course of treatment of specific patients.

Some of these areas may impact EHRSs if they are seen directly as a device or function of a medical device. Furthermore, if EHRSs are seen as having a measurable impact on health and safety, the FDA may consider it within its scope to regulate, or, in reaction to safety concerns, Congress can expand the FDA's regulatory scope to include EHRSs.

Complying with regulatory requirements adds substantial costs to product development and maintenance. The process of obtaining regulatory approval, both upfront and ongoing, can take substantial time, which delays innovation in the marketplace. If the FDA does become involved, recently introduced user fees for device-related regulatory filings[47] may curb the development of EHR-related software.

Continuation of the current approach of limited regulatory oversight of software systems would remove a potential obstacle to the further development of EHRSs. To assure this limitation continues, the shapers and influencers of policy will need to understand the distinctions and argue persuasively for less regulatory oversight.

Legal Restrictions on the Practice of Medicine May Act as a Barrier to the Best Care

Today, technology has the potential to support care across geographic boundaries, but legal restrictions on the practice of medicine within a given state may act as a barrier to obtaining the best care.

The practice of medicine is regulated by each state individually. To legally practice medicine within a state, the physician must be licensed by that state. A physician who wants to practice in every state must be licensed in all 50 states.[48]

These licensure barriers have survived despite the lengthy experience with telemedicine, such that out-of-state physicians who treat an in-state patient via telemedicine must be licensed within the state where the patient is located.[49]

Location-independent clinical technologies, including telemedicine consults and office visits, remote intensive care unit monitoring, remote radiologic reading, and remote laboratory services, are limited because all require the clinician to be licensed in the state where the patient is located. This means that the specialist who may be an expert in the given condition may be prevented from providing the treatment.

The current work-around is that the remote expert consults and advises the doctor at the patient's location who then provides the treatment. However, even this approach will fail as the technology permits remote procedures based on technologies used in microsurgery and robot-assisted procedures where the physician works by wire, not by physical contact.

All of these remote knowledge activities are based on the EHR. Even a patient-initiated review of the data in the EHR, especially those augmented by images, video, and other multimedia modalities, may be considered illegal practice of medicine if performed by a physician who is not licensed in the state where the patient is located.

The experience with telemedicine has not been encouraging. For the location-less access aspects of the EHR to have full utility, a means to support the review and treatment of a patient that is blind to the geographic location of the parties must be defined. This will require changes in licensure approaches, perhaps moving to some level of federal licensure or reciprocity among all 50 states. Achieving these changes will require overcoming powerful economic interests who have a strong voice at the state level. Issues of liability in the event of alleged malpractice will also need to be addressed to surmount licensure challenges.

As the Demarcation Between IT and Clinical Technology Further Blurs, the Responsibilities and Qualifications of Those Who Manage the Technology Becomes Muddled

As IT becomes more involved in and a critical part of the direct clinical care process, the delineation of the roles and accountability for managing, maintaining, troubleshooting, and repairing clinical technology becomes unclear. The current model within most healthcare providers is to place the majority of the responsibility for the operation and management of enterprise-wide clinical information system on the IT function, the IT Department.

However, departmental systems that maintain segments of the patient record, e.g., PACS, radiology information systems, laboratory systems, and cardiac catheterization systems, are often maintained by clinical technicians within each department. Systems that have direct patient contact—medical devices such as infusion pumps and monitors—are often maintained by bio-medical engineering.

At the point of care, the use of closed-loop decision models enables the use of algorithms to continuously adjust treatment. Within this environment, clinicians may wish to set parameters and alert levels for specialty-specific treatment approaches and those suitable for their personal needs. The clinician is responsible for "coding" their personal settings, even if this "coding" relies on information stored in the EHR. Therefore, no single entity is responsible. Given the disparities in roles, knowledge, and skills, today's model does not readily permit any one department to take broader responsibility and accountability.

To address this challenge, healthcare providers must broaden the capabilities of central information management departments (IMDs). IMDs will need to possess skills and capabilities in medical decision making and bio-medical engineering, as well as core IT and health information management, to be able to manage the widely varying range of interconnected and interdependent systems (See Figure 19-3).

To bring together all segments of the patient record, the IMD must also have primary responsibility for underlying systems and storage; and thus must have greater clinical knowledge to support specialized departmental needs. This will provide focus to address the challenge of having key elements of the current patient record scattered across the enterprise in individual system silos. In addition to enhancing the ability to achieve a comprehensive EHR, unifying control of data will enhance security and business continuity operations.

One challenge is that information system design has often separated roles that require clinical knowledge and technology skills. For example, image management in a PACS system is part database administration, an IT skill, and part study management, a clinical role tied to the operation of the

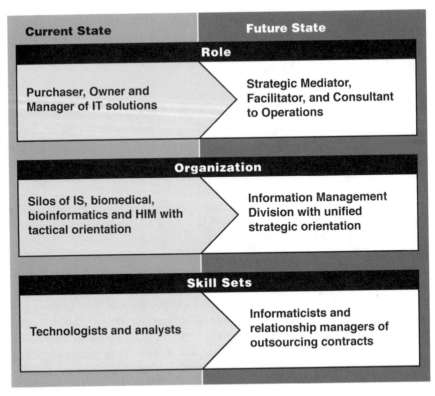

FIGURE 19-3. Anticipated shifts in roles, organizations, and skill sets. (*Source:* By permission of Kurt Salmon Associates.)

department. Archiving and restoration is one part storage modality management, a central IT role, and one part radiology administration to assure that relevant data from both current and prior studies are accessible.

To address the design, maintenance, and remediation roles today often requires significant cross-departmental effort among multiple support organizations, which often have different agendas, conflicting priorities, and individual missions, plus vastly differing skill sets. To meet the challenges of an integrated environment with the EHR as the centerpiece of a state-of-the-art treatment process will require significant cross training of personnel and a unified organizational approach.

This challenge is primarily organizational, not technical, although technical aspects of system design are also implicated. The formation of information management departments with broader scope and skill sets, including extensive cross-training, will be pivotal in meeting this challenge. Part of an EHRs selection approach must include the operational aspects of managing the system, including the organizational structure and skills appropriate to that management.

Conclusion

Significant progress has been made toward the overall goal of a universal EHR. However, many challenges remain. As health care entered the 21st century, EHR adoption rates were less than 10%. However, progress continues and interest in EHRs remains high. Significant IT-related challenges remain, although the high level of industry and governmental focus will support resolving these issues.

Funding constraints are a significant barrier to the achievement of the government's goals for fully interoperable EHRs by 2010. However, even if all of the necessary funding were made available, lengthy system development and implementation life cycles would slow full achievement of this goal. No amount of money can overcome these process-based delays within a short time frame, although the funding is critical to expediting overall progress.

Also critical to fully interoperable EHRs are the creation and adoption of uniform standards for data models, controlled medical vocabularies, medical knowledge representations, and metathesauri. Although these efforts have moved slowly in the past, recent federal government interest and nascent efforts to facilitate the creation of the necessary standards has been critical in bringing together the necessary parties and encouraging the health IT vendors to incorporate the standards into their products.

Governmental leadership is necessary to remove legal barriers to the creation of EHRs. Clarification of HIPAA privacy rules will support the ability to aggregate and share protected health information and lead to the formation of health data custodians. Resolution of issues embedded in state law, including data ownership and licensure will be necessary to be able to gain full benefits from EHRs. These legal challenges are not insurmountable, but will require coordinated state and federal governmental action.

Technology developments in handheld computing and pervasive computing infrastructures are mature. Further attention to HMIs will be needed as part of the EHR development effort. EHRs rely on integrating clinical and information technology. As EHR and other clinical IT applications become more prevalent, the skills and locus of control needed for integration and resolution of problems must change. Merging of IT, clinician, and biomedical expertise into a single organizational unit will be indispensable to building and maintaining the EHR. Leading organizations are already making these organizational shifts and will lead the way for others.

Although much progress has been made, because of the large challenges discussed above, it seems unlikely that full implementation of the EHR will occur before 2015. Although this may be considered by many a large-scale miss on the 2010 goal, it will mean that health care has made more progress in 10 years than it made toward achieving EHR success in the last 25. This is a cause for hope and renewed effort—as well as encouragement when it seems that the challenges may be insurmountable.

References

1. Institute of Medicine. To Err Is Human: Building a Safer Health System. Washington, DC: National Academy Press; 1999.
2. KLAS Enterprises. CPOE Digest. Orem, Utah. February 2003:5.
3. Leapfrog Group Survey, Press Release November 16, 2004. Available at: http://www.leapfroggroup.org/media/file/Leapfrog-Survey_Release-11-16-04.pdf. Accessed December 20.
4. The electronic medical record (EMR) is one component of the overall electronic health record (EHR) that is situated within the care institution and focuses mainly on clinical data.
5. HIMSS Ambulatory Technology Survey. February 9, 2004:1, 5. Available at: http://www.himss.org/content/files/ambulatory_tech_survey_0209.pdf. Accessed November 16, 2004.
6. President George W. Bush. Technology Agenda. April 26, 2004. Accessed January 6, 2005.
7. The 2004 HIMSS Leadership Survey. Available at: http://www.himss.org/2004survey/ASP/healthcarecio_final.asp. Accessed November 16.
8. Thompson TG, Brailer DJ. The Decade of Health Information Technology: Delivering Consumer-centric and Information-rich Health Care Framework for Strategic Action. U.S. Department of Health and Human Services. July 21, 2004. Available at: http://www.hhs.gov/news/press/2004pres/20040721.html. Accessed January 5, 2005.
9. United States Department of Health and Human Services. HHS Awards $139 Million to Drive Adoption of Health Information Technology. October 13, 2004. Available at: www.hhs.gov/news/press/2004pres/20041013.html. Accessed November 16, 2004.
10. BRAILER 1104. Healthcare IT News. November 2004. Available at: www.healthcareitnews.com/NewsArticleView.aspx?ContentID=1876&Con-tentTypeID=3&IssueID=12. Accessed December 31, 2005.
11. Thompson TG, Brailer DJ. The Decade of Health Information Technology: Delivering Consumer-centric and Information-rich Health Care Framework for Strategic Action. U.S. Department of Health and Human Services. July 21, 2004.
12. Consolidated Health Informatics, www.whitehouse.gov/omb/egov/gtob/health_informatics.htm. Accessed January 5, 2005.
13. H.R. Committee on Energy and Commerce Subcommittee on Health, Tommy G. Thompson Secretary Department of Health and Human Services (22 July 2004) (Administration's efforts to increase the use of information technology throughout the health care industry).
14. W. Edward Hammond, III, *Electronic Medical Records—Getting It Right And Going To Scale* (Commonwealth Fund January 2004).
15. 69 Fed. Reg. 65599.
16. Unified Medical Languages System. U.S. National Library of Medicine. Available at: http://www.nlm.nih.gov/research/umls/. Accessed 5 January 2005.
17. Logical Observation Identifiers Names and Codes. The Regensteif Institute, http://www.regenstrief.org/loinc. Accessed January 5, 2005.
18. SNOMED Clinical Terms®. http://www.snomed.org. Accessed January 5, 2005.
19. Davis JB. Road to Recovery, 89 ABA J. 50. 2003. Quoting Alan S. Goldberg of Gouldston & Storrs. Washington, DC.

20. Wietecha M, et al. A View of the U.S. Health Care System and Implications for Provider Year 2020. New York: Kurt Salmon Associates; 2004.

21. National Committee on Vital and Health Statistics, Report to the Secretary of the U.S. Department of Health and Human Services on Uniform Data Standards for Patient Medical Record Information, 7, 6 July 2000.

22. Schoenberg R, Safran C. Internet based repository of medical records that retains patient confidentiality. BMJ 2000;321:1199.

23. Schoenberg R, Safran C. Internet based repository of medical records that retains patient confidentiality. BMJ 2000;321:1199, 1200.

24. Shaping a Health Statistics Vision for the 21st Century. Executive Summary, x. National Committee on Vital Statistics, Department of Health and Human Services, Final Report, November 2002. (Identifying the overarching mission of the health statistics enterprise "to efficiently provide timely, accurate, and relevant information that can be used to improve the population's health.")

25. Tang PC. Key Capabilities of an Electronic Health Record: Committee on Data Standards for Patient Safety, Institute of Medicine, Letter Report, 2. The National Academies Press, 31 July 2003. (Citing the critical need for a more advanced health information infrastructure as "crucial for . . . various forms of biomedical and health systems research.")

26. Kostyack P. The Emergence of the Healthcare Information Trust, 12 Health Matrix 393. Summer 2002. (Discussing the creation of data warehouses, the Health Information Trust, of secondary information that would be managed for the advantage of the beneficiary by accepting assignment of the patient's property interest in their medical information). Given the discussion above, see Part III, and the explicit acknowledgment in the Privacy Rule that individuals did not have property interests in their medical record, see note 86 supra, this may be difficult to achieve.

27. 2005 Hospitals' National Patient Safety Goals, Joint Commission on Accreditation of Healthcare Organizations. Available at http://www.jcaho.org/accredited+organizations/patient+safety/05+npsg/05 npsg hap.htm. Accessed December 15, 2005.

28. 45 CFR 160. et seq.

29. 45 C.F.R.§164.514(d)(1).

30. Schoenberg R, Safran C. Internet based repository of medical records that retains patient confidentiality. BMJ 2000;321:1199.

31. Schoenberg R, Safran C. Internet based repository of medical records that retains patient confidentiality. BMJ 2000;321:1199.

32. National Committee on Vital and Health Statistics, Report to the Secretary of the U.S. Department of Health and Human Services on Uniform Data Standards for Patient Medical Record Information, 6–13, 6 July 2000.

33. 68 Fed. Reg. 8334.

34. National Committee on Vital and Health Statistics, Report to the Secretary of the U.S. Department of Health and Human Services on Uniform Data Standards for Patient Medical Record Information, 13, 26 July 2000.

35. National Committee on Vital and Health Statistics, Report to the Secretary of the U.S. Department of Health and Human Services on Uniform Data Standards for Patient Medical Record Information, 14, 26 July 2000.

36. National Committee on Vital and Health Statistics, Report to the Secretary of the U.S. Department of Health and Human Services on Uniform Data Standards for Patient Medical Record Information, 13, 26 July 2000.

37. National Committee on Vital and Health Statistics, Report to the Secretary of the U.S. Department of Health and Human Services on Uniform Data Standards for Patient Medical Record Information, 13, 6 July 2000.

38. Schoenberg R, Safran C. Internet based repository of medical records that retains patient confidentiality. BMJ 2000;321:1199.

39. Privacy and Security were two prongs underlying the passages of the Health Insurance Portability and Accountability Act of 1996 ("HIPAA") [Pub. L. No. 104–191, 110 Stat. 1936 (1996)] as discussed in Standards for Privacy of Individually Identifiable Health Information, "In enacting HIPAA, Congress recognized the fact that administrative simplification cannot succeed if we do not also protect the privacy and confidentiality of personal health information. The provision of high-quality health care requires the exchange of personal, often-sensitive information between an individual and a skilled practitioner. Vital to that interaction is the patient's ability to trust that the information shared will be protected and kept confidential." 65 Fed. Reg 82462, 82463. December 28, 2000.

40. 21 U.S.C. 360c. The FDA classifies devices into one of three categories; most active devices are either Class II, such as infusion pumps, or Class III, such as implanted pacemakers.

41. Class III device.

42. 21 C.F.R. 864.9175 (Blood Bank systems are Class II).

43. 21 C.F.R. 892.2050 [Picture Archiving and Communications Systems (PACS) Class II Devices].

44. FDA Policy for the Regulation of Computer Products, 1. November 13, 1989 DRAFT. Available at: http://www.fda.gov/cdrh/ode/351.pdf. Accessed December 24, 2004.

45. 21 U.S.C. 321(h) (device includes instrument, apparatus, implement, machine, implant, including any component, part, or accessory, which is intended for use in the diagnosis of disease or other conditions, or in the cure, mitigation, treatment, or prevention of disease, in man or other animals).

46. FDA Policy for the Regulation of Computer Products, 1–2.

47. Medical Device User Fee and Modernization Act of 2002, Pub. L. No. 107–250§738(a)(1)(A)(2002). The fee for 2004 was $206,811 (Guidance for Industry and FDA: User Fees and Refunds for Premarket Approval Applications, 2, U.S. Department of Health and Human Services, Food and Drug Administration, Center for Devices and Radiological Health. Available at: http://www.fda.gov/cdrh/mdufma/guidance/1224.pdf. Accessed November 24, 2003.

48. Lugn N. Medical Licensure and Telemedicine: Necessity or Barrier? Suffolk Transnatl Law Rev 2001;165:186. (In the United States, medical licensure regulations vary; some regulations prohibit the importation of medical information from other states or countries. To practice within a state, a physician must hold that state's license. A physician wanting to practice medicine in all states must apply for and obtain 50 different licenses.)

49. Silverman RD. The changing face of law and medicine in the new millennium. Am J Law Med 2000;255:268.

20
Grand Challenges of Medicine and Health for Information Technology

Yves A. Lussier and Edward H. Shortliffe

Both medicine and information technology (IT) are fields characterized by rapid change and remarkable contributions to new knowledge. In this chapter, we consider the relationships between the fields, acknowledging the evolving trends in IT and discussing implications for the practice of medicine and associated decision-making processes. We have identified challenges in medicine and health related to IT, with an emphasis on how the computer-based patient record (CPR) is influencing them and, at the same time, being influenced by changes in these two arenas.[1]

This chapter is divided into four sections, beginning with this introduction outlining key trends in medicine. In the second section, we address the importance of improving the decision making of health professionals in the era of exploding data, information, and knowledge. The third section discusses the evolving roles of stakeholders in the healthcare environment and their impact on IT. The concluding section provides a perspective on the relationship between IT and the financing of medicine.

CPRs are the core technology on which almost all IT-related innovations in health care are built. The patient record (PR) is a keystone to patient–provider encounters, recording decisions of pivotal moments that determine significant allocations of health resources. The number of computer-based components of PRs is rapidly increasing. From an early base in the automated management of data from clinical laboratories, increasing amounts of data are now managed by computer in industrialized countries after being derived or abstracted from PRs. These include administration and billing records, clinical research records, data reported to the World Health Organization, public health records, disease registries, and the like. Furthermore, the "computerized" components of some PRs have insidiously become invisible, as was predicted by Donald Norman.[2] The "invisible CPRs" range from pervasive communication devices, such as two-way pagers that exchange clinical information among providers, to IT-enabled medical devices (e.g., a blood glucometer that is capable of sending objective data to a repository) and IT-enabled prostheses (e.g., implantable cardioverter defibrillators that record arrhythmias for remote monitoring[3]).

Arguably, storage-enabled medical devices and their remote monitors together form a modest CPR system as they contain specialized patient data that are reusable via admittedly unconventional storage and retrieval mechanisms. However, the written clinical interactions among providers over devices, such as two-way pagers, challenge the very definition of the type of interactions that should be recorded in the PR and may altogether extend or even partially disintermediate CPR repositories. As medicine and its devices evolve, "invisible CPRs" face unique integration challenges. A successful outcome may lead to the timely reuse of crucial and valuable observations for enhanced decision making, amid risks for segregated, inaccessible, or untapped patient data.

In the last decade, several novel trends in healthcare processes have achieved wide acceptance. To keep up with demands for patient empowerment, clinicians have developed new strategies to address the continuum between being healthy and being disabled. As a result, many healthcare services are focused on "healthcare consumers" instead of making an arbitrary distinction between healthy individuals and patients. In addition, as the aging population becomes increasingly educated and computer literate, opportunities are arising to engage them successfully in communications with their providers via e-mail. Patient–physician e-mail has been used to such an extent that professional societies have developed guidelines for their members, especially in light of requirements for confidentiality and data privacy.[4] E-mails in clinical care have thus become a new component of the clinical record.

On a related note, the notion of individualized medicine is appealing and heavily promoted by pharmacogenomics companies. However, the term implies much more than merely tailored medications. Because individual cognitive factors affect compliance with optimal treatment, individualized education based on CPRs has been developed to provide a continuum of materials across a combination of finely tailored "states," calculated from cognitive variables and clinical data as described by Cimino and colleagues.[5] Support for tailored decision making from CPRs and other decision-support tools have been developed for more than four decades. Nevertheless, such tools generally are incapable of integrating the myriad personal variables that are pertinent when providing individualized care.

In parallel to the emerging needs of individualized medicine, genomic medicine has been anticipated for more than two decades and is just now emerging as an area of intense interest.[6] Recent clinical publications have established the significance of analyzing components of an individual's genome when attempting to optimize therapy.[7] Additionally, genomic medicine is likely to be as knowledge-intensive as evidence-based and error-free medicine. A recent publication in the *New England Journal of Medicine* confirms that genomic approaches to the discovery of biomarkers in clinical trials are scientifically, medically, and economically valid. Indeed, Liu and Karuturi[8] demonstrate that the development of accurate markers derived from microarray data may require 10 times fewer patients (116 to 285 patients) when compared with the development of a valid single molecular marker (400 to 1000 patients). However, the interpretation of the results of a genome-based biomarker comprising thousands of relevant genes requires computational assistance and cannot be memorized easily, as the behavior of individual genes is less informative than that of their clusters. Because genomic medicine is data- and knowledge-intensive, redefining diseases with their molecular etiology, it is likely to challenge our model of medical practice and consequently its decision-making processes.

Genomic medicine is one of many changes in medicine that has significantly affected decision making. Not long ago, during medical training, health professionals carried pearls of knowledge recorded on paper or printed in small booklets that would fit in the pockets of their white coats. Today, personal digital assistants are gaining in popularity among clinical trainees; they present distinct advantages over paper in terms of volume of knowledge stored, and have been shown to be particularly useful for assessing drug interactions while writing prescriptions. Accordingly, it seems that we are beginning to exceed the capacity of a trainee's white coat to carry the required amount of printed knowledge for reliable decision making. Indeed, the quantity of knowledge required for optimal decision making has increased exponentially. Evidence-based medicine (EBM) was advocated more than three decades ago by Archie Cochrane[9] and has since become a recognized criterion for determining the quality of care. EBM is knowledge intensive by definition; one should be able to categorize each decision according to whether it is based on "scientific evidence," a "consensus-based guideline," or "best practices." The application of EBM principles has been shown to reduce medical errors and has become increasingly recognized with two recent publications of the Institute of Medicine in 2000 and 2001.[10,11] However, as with the other challenges, very few implemented CPRs formally incorporate EBM-enhanced decision-support features.

Challenges of Optimal Decision Making in Medicine and Education

The pace of innovation experienced by clinicians continues to accelerate rapidly. In response to these changes, clinicians have successfully divided their discipline into specialties over the last 30 years. The emergence of subspecialties within the scope of these existing specialties further reveals the tremendous societal pressure to balance competencies and continuing education. IT offers the opportunity to seamlessly integrate decision making and education into the processes of health care. Medicine is faced with the challenge of supporting the competencies of its professionals beyond the scope of traditional venues, such as professional meetings and journal articles, seeking to provide clinical updates via nontraditional forms, such as decision support tools and other derivatives from journal articles, such as distilled excerpts and summaries. In some sectors of medicine, clinicians are progressively favoring evidence-based databases over the traditional primary medical literature.[12,13] Pushing the paradigm shift further, MedBiquitous, a nonprofit knowledge-management organization, creates technology standards to connect the leading entities in professional medicine and enables them to make medical education more effective, accessible, and traceable.[14] Furthermore, Greene proposes the Sharable Content Object Reference Model (SCORM), a successfully validated theoretical and technological framework, to directly link EBM to safety and quality.

While these trends in medicine and IT illustrate strategies for decision making, they also incrementally improve the CPR. Medicine accordingly has to promote fundamental IT research, which may yield powerful new data structures and decision-support mechanisms for the CPR. For example, very few CPRs use the semantics of ontologies for database queries. Additionally, organizational theory and cognitive ethnography should be used to model healthcare processes further in order to design more effective clinical information systems.[15] CPRs incorporating clinical decision-support systems (CDSSs) and computerized physician order entry (CPOE) have been shown to increase quality and reduce errors.[2,10] However, optimal decision making in patient care remains challenging, because it involves assessments based on incomplete facts about best diagnoses and therapies for a specific patient. Likewise, optimal decision making in allocating healthcare resources within a society is based on gathering the right facts. Public health databases must derive increasingly accurate datasets from primary CPRs because, in the context of limited overall societal resources, enhanced decision making in public health remains one of the salient challenges of the new century.

Shifting Roles of Stakeholders in the Healthcare Environment

As discussed earlier, health care in the future will be subjected to a profound metamorphosis if it is to become economically viable and efficient in the context of an increasingly aged population and constantly enhanced offerings of healthcare products and services.[16]

Blurred Roles Between Clinicians and Healthcare Administrators

The Hippocratic Oath emphasizes patient advocacy. Arguably, every model of clinical practice distorts, in distinct ways, patient-centered medicine as advocated in the Hippocratic Oath. Indeed, fee-for-service (FFS) promotes expenditure by rewarding superfluous procedures. FFS incentives and disincentives have progressively been replaced or transformed by those of "Managed Care" (MC). In this model of practice, physicians' traditional role as caregivers conflicts with their "additional" role as explicit rationers. Furthermore, MC administrators and insurers are not held to behavioral standards that would be consistent with the legal obligations of clinicians or a stated standard of care.[17] In the midst of shifting roles of clinicians and models of practice, decisions to acquire or update a CPR are also being deferred.

Additionally, although those who pay for health care and the primary users of CPRs generally have different needs, several new trends in health care have mandated enhancements to CPRs that meet the needs of both clinicians and healthcare administrators: 1) The Health Insurance Portability and Accountability Act (HIPAA)-mandated security, focused on protecting data integrity, confidentiality, and availability, and 2) the Institute of Medicine reports that assert the valuable role of CPOE systems and CDSSs in reducing errors and enhancing safety and quality.[10,11] As CPOE systems and CDSSs are integrated with an underlying CPR, there is increasing pressure for organizations, administrators, and clinicians to invest in such advanced CPR systems. However, in the context of declining margins of profit caused by reduced reimbursements, and escalating costs of competing healthcare technologies, such as medical devices and medications, the case for investing in advanced CPRs is far from compelling, either to practitioners or to provider organizations. Indeed, the needs of patient-driven demand plus the high visibility of powerful pharmaceutical companies/products and of clinical subspecialty procedures, combined with decreasing budgetary allocations, tend to drive investments toward products in which fees can be charged to an individual patient (and reimbursed accordingly) rather than toward integrative technology. In addition, fully functional CPRs are typically acquired by large groups that often favor cost-effective systems for their organizations over ones that would be optimal for clinicians, creating a gap in acceptance criteria between the purchaser and the clinical user. Therefore, there is a dilemma in medicine: While physicians and healthcare administrators are increasingly exposed to a complexity of motivations (e.g., the patient's versus the insurer's perspective of "optimal" care), their respective roles are reshaped and possibly distorted by healthcare financing models. Furthermore, whereas product innovations in health care as well as managed care may have the secondary effect of discouraging healthcare organizations or physicians to support investment in CPRs, studies that confirm the cost-reducing potential of CPRs coupled with documentation of valued trends such as data integrity, data confidentiality, quality, and safety may be the key determinants of their increased usage.

Patient Empowerment in Diagnostic and Therapeutic Decision Making

Benefits of patient self-management in chronic diseases have been well established in clinical studies for conditions such as asthma or diabetes.[18] As a result, specialized and well-funded clinics nationwide have been focusing on promoting, educating, and reinforcing patient self-management for these conditions. With increasing patient empowerment and access to diagnostic tests and over-the-counter drugs, there is a resurgence of the apothecary model: Patients as purchasers and decision makers regarding drug choices and biomedical devices. The explosion in direct-to-consumer advertising is further evidence of this trend. Although self-management education is not yet available or agreed on for a large number of chronic illnesses, its development is likely to complement current practices in health care.[19] In contrast, although patient empowerment in diagnostics is fundamentally different from the patient's role in therapeutic decision-making, because it distintermediates and challenges the traditional roles of medical centers and clinicians, it benefits direct marketing of generally available therapeutic products, especially if they do not require a clinician's prescription.

IT has been demonstrated as one important mechanism for patient empowerment. Indeed, patients use the World Wide Web to locate knowledge about their disease and to engage in asynchronous or synchronous communications with peer communities about specific health issues. In recent years, patients have been offered increasing numbers of alternatives from which to choose when submitting samples for laboratory testing. Some laboratories even provide Web sites for direct access by patients. One challenge faced by clinicians has been the impact of increased knowledge of one's symptoms or illness by patients who come to their clinical appointments prepared with printouts of their clinical data or with information about their conditions (or *possible* conditions). Clinicians have accordingly had to transform their assumptions and working habits to cope with changes in the patient–physician relationship brought about by ubiquitous IT innovations such as the Web and e-mail. For example, accounts of patient communications with physicians, traditionally recorded by clinicians in the medical record, are now occurring via e-mail, are considered a legitimate practice,[20] and must be suitably documented and archived. E-mails in clinical practice can be handled by specialized software in a HIPAA-compliant manner and integrated directly with the CPR, but such approaches require additional investments in technology by the clinician when compared with the simple practice of printing out standard e-mail and inserting it into a paper chart. Web-based IT has also been used to provide patients with custom-tailored information,[5] to manage patients' expectations in the context of increasing direct-to-consumer marketing of pharmaceuticals,[21] and will in time be used to facilitate patients' decision making regarding diagnosis and treatment.

One challenge of medicine will be dealing with innovations in devices that increasingly incorporate intelligence and thereby empower patients for self-care. Initially, incremental improvements to prevalent medical devices such as digital glucometers or sphygmomanometers may provide advice on the right medication dosage according to patient-specific information including the individual's recorded history of response to the same or similar agents. Eventually, novel adaptations of common nonmedical devices for new healthcare purposes are foreseeable. For example, automated teller machines are deployed worldwide and could be used as a model interface for decision-making software and delivery of prescriptions or nonprescription medication, disintermediating clinicians and drugstores altogether. Finally, worldwide medicine also faces a challenge with the digital divide, which may be the source of a worrisome "medical divide." As innovations increase the mediating role of IT in patient-centered decision making and care delivery through medical devices, access to IT may be regarded as a health-related right that becomes an intrinsic part of the care system for individuals.

The Evolution of Health Demographics and Healthcare Financing

Table 20-1 provides an international perspective on varying models of health care, with healthcare indicators, age demographic measurements, and financing information on five countries including the United States (US), deliberately chosen for their different approaches to healthcare financing and excellence in medical practice. Whereas each selected country other than ours invests about 6% of their gross domestic product (GDP) in *public* health care, the US invests two to five times as much GDP in *private* health care. In addition, countries other than the US and Canada are already

TABLE 20-1. Healthcare indicators

	US	Canada	Japan	Norway	UK
Public health expenditure (% of GDP, 2001)	6.2	6.8	6.2	6.9	6.2
Private health expenditure (% of GDP, 2001)	7.7	2.8	1.8	1.2	1.4
Population age 65 and above (2002, % total)	12	13	18	15	16
Population age 65 and above (2015, % total)	14	16	26	18	18
Physician/100,000 people (2003)	279	187	202	367	164
Maternal mortality ratio adjusted per 100,000 live births (2000)	17	6	10	16	13
Under-five mortality rate in 2002 per 1000 live births (<5 years)	8	7	5	4	7
Life expectancy in 2002 (years)	71.5	73.2	73.3	74.4	72

Source: Adapted from the World Health Organization.

encountering the burden of an aging population equivalent to that which the US will face 10 years from now. Age-adjusted GDP expenditures for the the US are significantly higher than those of other countries. The population homogeneity of Japan and Norway may partially account for better health indicators than those in the US, because this homogeneity likely facilitates public health policies. However, Canada has achieved excellent health indicators despite a population heterogeneity that is not dissimilar to our own. Thus, lessons can be learned for improving financing of health care or medical practice in the US by studying countries that have contained the escalating costs of medicine despite an inverse age pyramid more pronounced than in the US. For example, most of these countries, most notably the United Kingdom (UK) and Japan, have influential public health policies and infrastructures, which reuse healthcare data generated in CPRs. Indeed, the UK's National Health Service, in particular, has developed socially acceptable and sustainable methods by which to code clinical data in primary care and reuse them for public health purposes.[22,23] In addition, Japan has instigated successful large-scale preventive medicine programs generating clinical repositories, such as the "human dry dock" examinations and the automatic multiphasic health testing system (AMHTS).[24-26]

Impact of Financing and Innovation: CPRs and Implied Challenges

Four scenarios are illustrated in the quadrants of Figure 20-1. Our conjecture is that the differential growth of the two axes of medicine (*Financing* and *Practices*) will determine the growth and impact of CPRs. Ultimately, the prevailing scenario (which may vary by country and even by region or system within countries) will determine how CPRs are perceived in the future. There are contemporary CPRs and sectors of health care in all four quadrants; these can help to illustrate their future counterparts and are provided as examples.

Scenario 1: *Current CPRs. Conventional healthcare practices and increased expenditures for CPRs.* This is a future in which incremental changes occur in the practice of medicine and the use of centralized CPRs, however, the current paper-based component of the practice of medicine disappears progressively, leading to the emergence of a paperless office. With increased expenditures, additional streams of data are integrated in traditional ways and standards for interoperability progress and compete without a ubiquitous dominant one—a status quo. Contemporary examples are large-scale institutions with multifaceted CPRs integrating patients as well as clinician portals for data entry and reuse.[27,28]

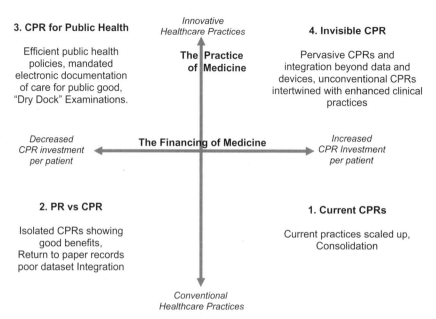

FIGURE 20-1. Scenarios of the future of CPRs according to two axes: Financing of Medicine and Healthcare Practices.

Scenario 2: *PR versus CPR. Conventional healthcare practices and decreased expenditures for CPRs.* This scenario delineates a somber future in which there is a reversal or stagnation of the computerization of patient records. In a majority of medical centers, contemporary patient records are generally hybrid, partially paper and electronic. This picture does not provide much insight except for emphasizing that reduced investments in CPRs are unlikely to foster innovation or investment in other types of clinical information system. For example, over the last decade, small private practices have seen their market share and profit margins reduced in the US because of the reorganization in healthcare financing favoring managed care. Thus, CPR companies targeting small private sectors have generally found very weak markets for their product and have accordingly transformed their offering for other sectors, such as medical centers or HMOs.

Scenario 3: *CPR for Public Health. Innovative healthcare practices and decreased expenditures for CPRs.* In this scenario, decreased investments in CPRs are associated with optimal yield using innovative healthcare practices. It is likely that in an environment conducive to creative new practices, despite its paradoxical financing constraint, the most practical approach to sustaining innovation is dependent on a judicious use of resources favored by influential public health policies and infrastructures. In addition, to be viable, such a system would necessarily entail fundamental transformations to control further unreasonable legal practices or unwarranted healthcare consumerism. For example, the efficacy of individual health-risk appraisal and nationwide preventive medicine in Japan is based on longitudinal analyses of an AMHTS and "human dry dock examination" databases.[24-26]

Scenario 4: *The Invisible CPR. Innovative healthcare practices and increased expenditures for CPRs.* We could forecast that the trend observed in cost-intensive specialties of medicine that harbor pervasive CPRs (e.g., remote monitoring of implantable cardioverter defibrillators, Schoenfeld et al., 2003) accelerate. Standards for interoperability, sharing data and knowledge are achieved. Intelligent devices provide advice on diagnosis and treatment directly to customers. The CPR emerges as a set of coordinated processes, mediated in a variety of ways, rather than as an object or a uniform centralized or distributed dataset.

Summary

Healthcare financing and practices are driving forces that influence research and development regarding CPRs. For example, healthcare financing in medical devices related to cardiology and neurosurgery means that CPRs in these disciplines are likely to remain differentially emphasized when compared with the investment in CPRs for other sectors. This differential financing of CPRs will continue to foster the development of innovative subspecialty-centric CPRs tightly interoperating with their related medical devices and therapeutic interventions. In addition, novel business models arising with the deployment of CPRs that interoperate with processors embedded in medical devices may accelerate further the implementation of interoperability standards for CPRs throughout health care. Healthcare decision makers, educators, researchers, and developers must leverage those valuable CPRs solutions for the broad benefit of our healthcare delivery system.

References

1. Patel VL, Kushniruk AW, Yang S, Yale JF. Impact of a computer-based patient record system on data collection, knowledge organization, and reasoning. J Am Med Inform Assoc 2000;7(6):569–585.
2. Norman DA. The Invisible Computer: Why Good Products Can Fail, the Personal Computer Is So Complex, and Information Appliances Are the Solution. Cambridge, MA: MIT Press; 1999.
3. Schoenfeld MH, Compton SJ, Mead RH, et al. Remote monitoring of implantable cardioverter defibrillators: a prospective analysis. Pacing Clin Electrophysiol 2004;27(6 pt 1):757–763.
4. Kane B, Sands DZ. Guidelines for the clinical use of electronic mail with patients. The AMIA Internet Working Group, Task Force on Guidelines for the

Use of Clinic-Patient Electronic Mail. J Am Med Inform Assoc 1998;5(1): 104–111.

5. Kukafka R, Lussier YA, Patel VL, Cimino JJ. Developing tailored theory-based educational content for WEB applications: illustrations from the MI-HEART project. Medinfo 2001;10(pt 2):1474–1478.

6. Sikorski R, Peters R. Genomic medicine. Internet resources for medical genetics. JAMA 1997;278(15):1212–1213.

7. Bullinger L, Döhner K, Bair E, et al. Use of gene-expression profiling to identify prognostic subclasses in adult acute myeloid leukemia. N Engl J Med 2004;350:1605–1616.

8. Liu ET, Karuturi KR. Perspective: microarrays and clinical investigations. N Engl J Med 2004;350:1595–1597.

9. Cochrane AL. Effectiveness and Efficiency: Random Reflections on Health Services. Nuffield Provincial Hospitals Trust; 1972.

10. Kohn LT, Corrigan J, Donaldson MS. To Err Is Human: Building a Safer Health System (2000). 1st ed. Institute of Medicine, ed. National Academies Press; April 15, 2000, 287 p.

11. Institute of Medicine, ed. Crossing the Quality Chasm: A New Health System for the 21st Century. National Academies Press; June 1, 2001, 364 p.

12. Peterson MW, Rowat J, Kreiter C, Mandel J. Medical students' use of information resources: is the digital age dawning? Acad Med 2004;79(1): 89–95.

13. Koonce TY, Giuse NB, Todd P. Evidence-based databases versus primary medical literature: an in-house investigation on their optimal use. J Med Libr Assoc 2004;92(4):407–411.

14. Greene PS, Smothers V. Collaborating Across Healthcare to Improve Education: Online Learning Using SCORM and MedBiquitous Standards. Public Health Information Network (PHIN) Conference, Atlanta, May 25, 2004. Available at: http://www.cdc.gov/phin/04conference/05-25-04/.

15. Staccini P, Joubert M, Quaranta JF, Fieschi D, Fieschi M. Modelling health care processes for eliciting user requirements: a way to link a quality paradigm and clinical information system design. Int J Med Inform 2001;64(2–3):129–142.

16. Sprinkle RH. A moral economy of American medicine in the managed-care era. Theor Med Bioeth 2001;22(3):247–268.

17. Peppin JF. Book review of medicine and the marketplace: the moral dimensions of managed care. J Med Ethics 2000;26:293.

18. Warsi A, Wang PS, LaValley MP, Avorn J, Solomon DH. Self-management education programs in chronic disease: a systematic review and methodological critique of the literature. Arch Intern Med 2004;164(15):1641–1649.

19. Bodenheimer T, Lorig K, Holman H, Grumbach K. Patient self-management of chronic disease in primary care. JAMA 2002;288(19):2469–2475.

20. Brailer D. Interview with National Health Information Technology Coordinator David Brailer, MD, PhD. BMJ 2004;329(7471):E328–329.

21. Mansfield PR, Mintzes B, Richards D, Toop L. Direct to consumer advertising. BMJ 2005;330(7481):5–6.

22. Gray J, Orr D, Majeed A. Use of Read codes in diabetes management in a south London primary care group: implications for establishing disease registers. BMJ 2003;326:1130.

23. Brown PJB, Warmington V, Laurence M, Prevost AT. Randomised crossover trial comparing the performance of Clinical Terms Version 3 and Read Codes 5 byte set coding schemes in general practice. BMJ 2003;326:1127.
24. Aoshima T, Tanaka Y, Shibata S, et al.; Committee of Health Evaluation Support System Council of Japan AMHTS Institutions. Development of a health guidance support system for lifestyle improvement. Methods Inf Med 2002; 41(3):209–212.
25. Sasamori N. A health condition survey of Japanese people in the prime of life, based on national MHTS and human dry dock statistics. Methods Inf Med 1998; 37(2):134–139.
26. Tamura M. Elimination of inter-institutional discrepancies in health check-up results: standardization of diagnostic decision level and uniformity of examination data. Methods Inf Med 1998;37(2):140–142.
27. Wald JS, Bates DW, Middleton B. A patient-controlled journal for an electronic medical record: issues and challenges. Medinfo 2004;2004:1166–1172.
28. Starren J, Hripcsak G, Sengupta S, et al. Columbia University's Informatics for Diabetes Education and Telemedicine (IDEATel) project: technical implementation. J Am Med Inform Assoc 2002;9(1):25–36.

Appendix: Acronyms

AAFP	American Academy of Family Physicians
AAP	American Academy of Pediatrics
ACID	atomicity, consistency, isolation, durability
ACIP	Advisory Committee for Immunization Practice
ACR	American College of Radiology
AHIC	Australian Health Information Council
AHIMA	American Health Information Management Association
AHMAC	Australian Health Ministers' Advisory Council
AHRQ	Agency for HealthCare Research and Quality (US)
AMA	American Medical Association
AMIA	American Medical Informatics Association
ANSI	American National Standards Institute
ASTM	American Society for Testing and Materials
BICS	Brigham Integrated Computing System
caBIG	Cancer Biomedical Informatics Grid
CAP	College of American Pathology
CAT	computer-assisted tomography
CBD	computer-based documentation
CDA	Clinical Document Architecture
CDC	Centers for Disease Control and Prevention (US)
CDEs	common data elements
CDISC	Clinical Data Interchange Standards Consortium
CDR	clinical data repository
CDS	clinical decision support
CDT	Current Dental Terminology
CEN	European Committee for Standardization
CEO	chief executive officer
CfH	Connecting for Health
CHCSII	Composite Health Care System II (DoD)
CHI	Consolidated Health Informatics
CIA	confidentiality, integrity, availability
CIAS	Clinical Image Access Service

CL	computational linguistics
CLIA	Clinical Laboratory Improvements Amendments
CMS	Center for Medicaid and Medicare Services
COAS	Clinical Observation Access Service
CORBA	Common Object Request Broker Architecture
COSTAR	Computer Stored Ambulatory Record System
COTS	commercial off-the-shelf
CPI	Consumer Price Index (US)
CPOE	computerized provider order entry
CPR	computer-based patient record
CPT-4	Current Procedural Terminology
CTMS	Clinical Trials Management System
DCOM	Distributed Component Object Model
DEC	Digital Equipment Company
DHHS	Department of Health and Human Services (US)
DICOM	Digital Imaging and Communications in Medicine
DoD	Department of Defense (US)
DoH	Department of Health (US)
DRG	Diagnostic Related Groups
DSM	Diagnosis Codes for Mental Disorders
DSTU	Draft Standard for Trial Use
DTD	document type definition
EAV	entity, attribute, value
EBM	evidence-based medicine
ECDL	European Computing Driving License
EDSF	Emergency Data Sets Framework
EHR	electronic health record
EHRi	electronic health record infostructure
EHR-S	electronic health record system
EMR	electronic medical record
E-PHI	electronic protected health information
EPR	electronic patient record
ER	entity-relationship
ETP	electronic transmission of prescriptions
EU	European Union
FDA	Federal Drug Administration
FHA	Federal Health Architecture
FIPP	Fair Information Practice Principles
FIPS	Federal Information Processing Standards
GDP	gross domestic product
GE	General Electric
GEM	Guideline Elements Model
GP	general practitioner
GLIF	Guideline Interchange Format
GUI	graphical user interface

HCHP	Harvard Community Health Plan
HCIT	health care information technology
HCR	health concept representation
HCP	healthcare professional
HCPCS	Healthcare Common Procedure Coding System
HDC	health data custodian
HDTF	Health Domain Task Force
HEDIS	Health Plan Employer Data and Information Set
HELP	Health Evaluation through Logical Processing
HHS	(Department of) Health and Human Services (US)
HIAL	Health Information Access Layer
HIBCC	Health Industry Business Communications Council
HIMSS	Health Information Management Systems Society
HIPAA	Health Insurance Portability and Accountability Act
HIS	hospital information system
HISA	Health Informatics Service Architecture
HIT	health information technology
HL7	Health Level-7
HRG	Healthcare Resource Group
HTML	hypertext markup language
IAIMS	Integrated Academic Information Management System
ICD-9-CM	International Classification of Diseases–Clinical Modification
ICF	International Classification of Functioning, Disability & Health
ICU	intensive care unit
IDS	integrated delivery system
IEEE	Institute of Electrical and Electronic Engineers
IETF	Internet Engineering Task Force
IHE	Integrating the Healthcare Enterprise
IM/IT	information management/information technology
IMD	information management department
IOM	Institute of Medicine
IP	Internet Protocol
IRB	institutional review board
ISAM	Indexed Sequential Access Method
ISO	International Organization for Standardization
IT	information technology
ITMRA	Information Technology Management Reform Act of 1996 (Clinger–Cohen Act)
ITU	International Telecommunication Union
JCAHO	Joint Commission on Accreditation of Health Care Organizations
JDBC	Java Database Connectivity
JPEG	Joint Photographic Experts Group

KR	knowledge representation
LCS	Laboratory of Computer Sciences
LINC	Laboratory Instrument Computer
LOINC	Logical Observation Identifiers Names and Codes
LQS	Lexicon Query Service
LSP	local service provider
MAGE-ML	MicroArray and Gene Expression Markup Language
MathML	Mathematical Markup Language
MHS	Military Health Systems
MLS	multi-level security
MRI	magnetic resonance imaging
MTFs	military treatment facilities
MUMPS	MGH Utility Multi-Programming System
N3SP	N3 Service Provider
NAHIT	National Alliance for Health Information Technology
NASP	National Application Service Provider
NCHS	National Center for Health Statistics
NCI	National Cancer Institute
NCICB	NCI Center for Bioinformatics
NCQA	National Committee for Quality Assurance
NCRS	National Care Record Service
NCVHS	National Committee on Vital and Health Statistics
NDC	National Drug Codes
NCPDP	National Council on Prescription Drug Programs
NEHTA	National e-Health Transition Authority
NEMA	National Electrical Manufacturers Association
NCG	National Guideline Clearinghouse
NHIG	National Health Information Group
NHII	National Health Information Infrastructure
NHIN	National Health Information Network
NHIS	National Health Interview Survey
NHS	National Health Service (UK)
NIST	National Institute of Standards and Technology (US)
NPfIT	National Program for Information Technology (UK)
NTP	Network Time Protocol
ODBC	Open Data Base Connectivity
OLTP	online transaction processing
OMB	Office of Management and Budget (US)
OMG	Object Management Group
OSI	Open System Interconnection
PACS	picture archiving and communication systems
PAR	participatory action research
PBS	Pharmaceutical Benefits Scheme
PCASSO	Patient-Centered Access to Secure Systems Online
PGP	Pretty Good Privacy

PHI	protected health information
PHR	personal health record
PHWG	Connecting for Health Personal Health Working Group
PIDS	Patient Identification Services
PIN	personal identification number
PMRI	patient medical record information
PPA	prescription pricing authority
PROMIS	Problem Oriented Medical Information System
RAD	Resource Access Decision
RAM	random access memory
RBRVS	Resource Based Relative Value Scale
RCRIM	Regulated Clinical Research Information Model
RDP	requirements development process
RDR	research data repository
RFI	request for information
RFP	request for proposals
RIM	Reference Information Model
RIS	radiology information system
RMI	Remote Method Invocation
RM/ODP	Reference Model for Open Distributed Processing
ROC	receiver operating characteristic
ROI	return on investment
RPC	Remote Procedure Calls
RSNA	Radiological Society of North America
SAM	Sequential Access Method
SAML	Security Assertion Markup Language
SARS	severe acute respiratory syndrome
SAVS	SmartAccess Vocabulary Server
SCP	Service Class Provider
SCU	Service Class User
SDLC	system development life cycle
SDOs	Standards Development Organizations
SHA	Strategic Health Authority
SNOMED	Systemized Nomenclature of Medicine
SNOP	Systematized Nomenclature of Pathology
SOA	Service-Oriented Architecture
SOAP	Simple Object Access Protocol
SQL	Structured Query Language
SSN	Social Security Number
TC	Technical Committee
TCP	Transmission Control Protocol
TF	technology framework
TMIS	Technicon Medical Information System
TMR	The Medical Record
TOL	TRICARE Online

TPN	total parenteral nutrition
TRL	technology readiness levels
UCSD	University of California at San Diego
UPI	unique patient identifier
UPN	unique patient number
URL	uniform resource locator
VA	Veterans Administration
VHA	Veterans Health Administration (US)
VISTA	Veterans Integrated Service and Technology Architecture
VPN	Virtual Private Networks
VSAM	Virtual Storage Access Method
VUMC	Vanderbilt University Medical Center
WADO	Web Access to DICOM-persistent Objects
WHO	World Health Organization
WWW	World Wide Web
W3C	World Wide Web Consortium
XML	Extensible Markup Language

Index